Virtual Reality Technologies for Health and Clinical Applications

Series Editor

Paul Sharkey, University of Reading, Moulsford, UK

The series, edited by Paul Sharkey at the University of Reading, UK, comprises four volumes. The first two volumes discuss advances in the field in terms of Physical and Motor Rehabilitation (Vol. 1) and Psychological and Neurocognitive Interventions (Vol. 2). Volume 3 is devoted to Virtual Reality Games for Rehabilitation. Volume 4 underpins the content of Volumes 1 to 3 and is based on the underlying knowledge, expertise, or skills that enable such research and development. Titled Virtual Reality Technology in Health: Design, Technologies, Tools, Methodologies, and Analysis, this volume can be seen essentially as a tutorial guide to the underlying subject matter required to run successful projects. This volume will be highly referenced by the other three volumes and serve as a key technical reference for the interdisciplinary subject as a whole.

Eva Brooks • David J. Brown
Editors

Virtual Reality Games for Rehabilitation

Springer

Editors
Eva Brooks
Department of Culture and Learning
Aalborg University
Aalborg, Denmark

David J. Brown
Department of Computer Science
School of Science and Technology
Nottingham Trent University
Nottingham, UK

ISSN 2199-4684 ISSN 2199-4692 (electronic)
Virtual Reality Technologies for Health and Clinical Applications
ISBN 978-1-0716-3369-4 ISBN 978-1-0716-3371-7 (eBook)
https://doi.org/10.1007/978-1-0716-3371-7

This Springer imprint is published by the registered company Springer Science+Business Media, LLC, part of Springer Nature.
The registered company address is: 1 New York Plaza, New York, NY 10004, U.S.A.

Paper in this product is recyclable.

Introduction

Playing Virtual Reality (VR) games in rehabilitation activities has shown to be effective for improving different kinds of functions, such as motoric in relation to stroke, cerebral palsy, or fibromyalgia syndrome. Such game-based training is considered as motivational and engaging as well as feasible for use in rehabilitation among a diversity of target groups. This book approaches VR from a broad perspective by representing a set of computer-produced images and sounds representing a situation in which a person can take part (https://dictionary.cambridge.org/). Within this broad definition, a variety of games and technologies in rehabilitation settings are considered as VR and include, among others, tabletop games, VR simulations, sensor-based multimodal media technology, commercial games, and serious games systems. Recently, the use and development of both commercial and custom-made VR-based games has increased significantly. This development, together with improved technical performance and accessible prices, supports new attractive game-based solutions for rehabilitation practices (Gustavsson et al., 2021). The use of adaptive, augmented, and game-based environments, as well as multimodal and multimedia interaction tools, are examples of this in different rehabilitation contexts.

The emerging and expanding digital technology solutions are even accelerating at such pace that current technological hypes, such as VR games or Internet of Things, soon can become obsolete. Therefore, we see it as a challenge to explore potentials in new enabling technologies, which require involvement of various disciplines as well as stakeholders across existing disciplines and practices. A current challenge lies in fostering new ecosystems of innovation to harness holistic rehabilitation processes and a development of more inclusive societies.

Including a VR game environment in rehabilitation activities has potentials to create an immersed sense of being in another world separated from reality. Expressed differently, this feeling is often described as experiencing flow, where a person is immersed and focused on the task, forgetting everything else. Movements in VR-based games can also be perceived as more spontaneous and automatic compared to movements in real life, which can be experienced as a positive feeling of being capable in an activity (Csíkszentmihályi, 1996). This is to say that it is pivotal to seriously considering rehabilitation training methods that are motivating and enjoyable (Gustavsson et al., 2021). Motivation and joy are key matters of any training application. For example, direct feedback from a game itself can be important features that can motivate and spur participants to reach beyond the expected.

This book is first and foremost an introduction to a broader, social understanding of designing and using VR games in an era of digitalization. We present some interrelated frameworks that especially focus on the design of game-based applications and on games in use as well as on emerging practices in different rehabilitation fields. Hopefully, we can learn from these examples and get inspired to take even newer steps towards future, democratic, and inclusive solutions of rehabilitation environments including improved designs and uses of VR games.

Eva Brooks
David J. Brown

References

Cambridge Dictionaries Online. Cambridge University Press. Available from: https://dictionary.cambridge.org/

Csíkszentmihályi, M. (1996). *Creativity: Flow and the psychology of discovery and invention*. Harper Collins.

Gustavsson, M., Kjörk, E. K., Erhardsson, M., & Murphy, M. A. (2021). Virtual reality gaming in rehabilitation after stroke – User experiences and perceptions. *Disability and Rehabilitation, 44*, 6759. https://doi.org/10.1080/09638288.2021.1972351

Sutton-Smith, B. (2008). Play Theory: A Personal Journey and New Thoughts. *American Journal of Play*, 80–123.

Obituary: Penny Standen, Professor of Health Psychology and Learning Disabilities: 1949–2022

Posted by Deborah Kitson in News on Wednesday, 20 July 2022.

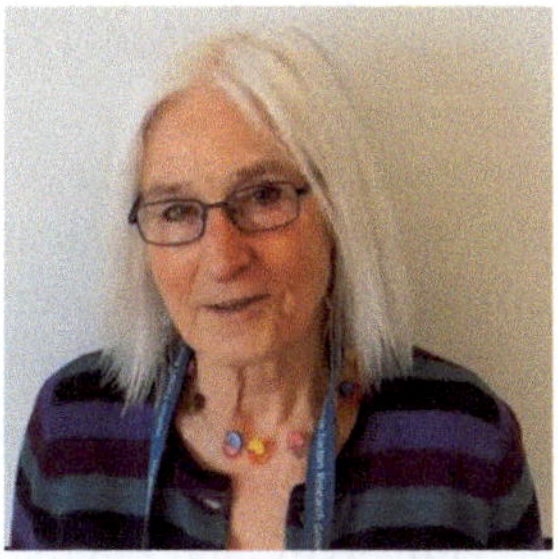

It is with great sadness that I have to share the news that Professor Penny Standen, Trustee of Ann Craft Trust, died on 8 July after a brave battle with cancer.

Penny was a supporter of the Ann Craft Trust since its inception in 1992, and she worked with Ann Craft on several research projects. She became a Trustee after her retirement in 2017, and despite her illness she continued in this role contributing and advising on the future direction of the charity until the very last.

Penny was Professor of Health Psychology and Learning Disabilities in the School of Medicine at the University of Nottingham. However, her academic career was nearly over before it began when her car was stolen with the only copy of her thesis on the back seat – in the days before computers. The car and its contents were never found, and Penny had to re-write her entire thesis.

After this unusual start, Penny forged a distinguished academic career, including serving as Head of School of Health Sciences. Throughout her career her main responsibilities were teaching medical students and trainee psychiatrists, supervising PhD students, and carrying out research to improve the quality of life of people with learning disabilities and those who care for them.

A key focus of her research was designing and evaluating information technology for people with learning disabilities and using approaches that involve them in the design process. In this she was helped by the Nottingham International Consortium on Educational Research, a group of people with learning disabilities who provide research consultancy and for whom Professor Standen acted as co-facilitator.

Penny was deeply committed to the lives of people who have a learning disability. She always sought to work *with* – rather than just *for* – people with learning disabilities. In addition to her academic work she was an active supporter of the leaver's group at Shepherd School, now Oakfield, sharing many memorable trips together at international conferences.

Beyond her work, Penny lived a full and varied life. For someone whose PhD was about the behavior of ducks, she imprinted herself on people far and wide. Before becoming an academic she held many different jobs: as a croupier, as a hand model – her hands featured in catalogues holding electrical components – and as a barmaid, where she once served the Kray twins! Penny also loved animals, competing in dressage competitions on her horse "Mrs O" and sharing her home with greyhounds rescued from a life of racing.

Since the sad news of her death, many colleagues within the university and beyond have shared memories of how Penny helped and supported them. Her years of work in medical education meant that during her cancer treatment she would often meet ex-students, many of whom have written on staff noticeboards about how influential she was in enabling them to successfully complete their qualifications.

Many academics across the University and beyond owe their career to Penny's supervision and early career support. The ACT team is grateful for her commitment and contribution to their work. Penny was a great and loyal friend and colleague to so many and will be sadly missed by all.

https://www.anncrafttrust.org/obituary-penny-standen-professor-of-health-psychology-and-learning-disabilities-1949-2022/ (accessed 10/11/2022).

Preface

> I believed that, when most of [the] scholars talked about play, they fundamentally presupposed it to be either a form of progress, an exercise in power, a reliance on fate, a claim for identity, a form of frivolity, an issue of the imagination, or a manifestation of personal experience. My argument held that play was ambiguous, and the evidence for that ambiguity lay in these quite different scholarly ways of viewing play. Further, over the years it became clear to me that much of play was by itself—in its very nature, we might say—intentionally ambiguous (as, for example, is teasing) regardless of [...] general cultural frames. (Sutton-Smith, 2008: 112)

So, what is it to play virtual reality games in rehabilitation activities, then? It is seriousness and frivolity, reality and make-believe, rules and freedom. Within these antinomies lies humans' experience of game play, where dichotomies are resolved through action. A main aim of this book lies in the vital role that practices of games play as drivers for inclusion and participation in everyday, training, and learning activities as well as for new innovations in virtual reality games for rehabilitation. The development and use of both commercial and custom-made games has increased significantly in recent years and have changed the ways we live our lives at an accelerating pace, which has created challenges for implementing them not only efficiently but also in meaningful ways. We can see increased societal interest in well-being, inclusive and equitable quality education, and lifelong learning opportunities for all. Recent years we have also seen a proliferation of concepts and research in game studies, such as serious games, pervasive games, alternate reality games, or playful game design elements for, among others, development of welfare and educational solutions.

This book discusses, and demonstrates, challenges and possibilities in relation to designing, developing, and using games in rehabilitation, both in terms of amplifying abilities and experiences and in terms of establishing inclusive and multimodal design approaches. This is done from diverse and multidisciplinary perspectives, which we mean can carry important potential for developing new knowledge, as well as forms of practice together with new ways of using virtual reality games in rehabilitation.

We would like to acknowledge all researchers that in different ways have assisted in shaping this book. We would also like to direct our sincere thanks to all authors that have contributed to this book. You are all in one way or another colleagues, research partners, and/or like-minded friends. We are grateful for your knowledge, insights, and trust. Last but not the least remains to thank the Springer support staff, especially Pinky Sathishkumar, whose patience and driving meant a lot for the finalization of this book.

Aalborg, Denmark — Eva Brooks
Nottingham, UK — David J. Brown
June 2022

Contents

Chapter 1
Games for Stroke Rehabilitation: An Overview

Pratik Vyas, Matthew C. Harris, David J. Brown, and Luke Shires

Introduction

Stroke is the most common disease in the UK with approximately 100,000 strokes every year (Stroke statistics, 2018). The chance of a stroke increases rapidly with age and gender (Patel et al., 2020). Lifestyle choices can also have a significant effect on the chance of stroke. High levels of alcohol intake, smoking, obesity and low levels of physical activity are all considered contributing factors (Rutten-Jacobs et al., 2018). Modern lifestyles are becoming increasingly sedentary, whilst obesity levels are on the rise, leading to increased stroke incidence at a younger age (Kissela et al., 2012).

Stroke is the leading cause of long-term disability (Adamson et al., 2004; Herpich & Rincon, 2020), with a higher disability impact compared to most other chronic diseases. There are estimated to be 1.3 million stroke survivors living in the UK (Stroke statistics, 2018). Stroke is estimated to cost over £45,000 per person in the first year and over £20,000 in subsequent years. The total cost for NHS and social care may be as high as £8.6 billion (Patel et al., 2020).

A stroke occurs when essential oxygen supply through blood to the brain is hindered either by formation of blood clots, causing ischaemic stroke, or by the less common rupture of blood vessel in the brain, called a haemorrhagic stroke (American Association of Neurological Surgeons (AANS), 2022). Blood flow needs to be resumed to normal levels within minutes in order to avoid permanent physiological damage to the brain and other parts of the body. Drugs may be used for the more common ischaemic stroke to quickly clear the clot and restore normal blood flow,

P. Vyas (✉) · M. C. Harris · D. J. Brown · L. Shires
Interactive Systems Research Group, Department of Computer Science, NTU, Nottingham, UK
e-mail: pratik.vyas@ntu.ac.uk; matthew.harris@ntu.ac.uk; david.brown@ntu.ac.uk, luke.shires2013@my.ntu.ac.uk

E. Brooks, D. J. Brown (eds.), *Virtual Reality Games for Rehabilitation*, Virtual Reality Technologies for Health and Clinical Applications,
https://doi.org/10.1007/978-1-0716-3371-7_1

whilst haemorrhagic strokes are far less common and are more difficult to treat, but surgery may be used to stem significant bleeds. Both types of strokes can result in long-term damage to the brain tissues and the effects can vary significantly between patients. Common symptoms may include altered or damaged sensory perception, reduced motor functions, altered emotional reasoning and damaged cognitive functioning.

Successful rehabilitation following stroke is key to helping stroke survivors regain independence in activities of daily living (ADL), increasing their quality of life. Successful rehabilitation can also allow some survivors to return to work, reducing the economic burden of stroke. Rehabilitation following stroke falls into three stages. The acute phase immediately follows the stroke, whilst the patient recovers in hospital. During the first few days, some brain tissue that was only partially damaged during the stroke may recover; this gives the patient a fast initial recovery rate. After this period, the longer-term impact of the stroke becomes more apparent. Patients are likely to be treated in a dedicated stroke unit and will begin the second phase (termed rehabilitation) as soon as they are physically and emotionally able. The rehabilitation phase is personalised for each symptom of the stroke (Krakauer, 2006). Common areas for rehabilitation include physical, occupational (focusing on daily living activities), speech and vision. Stroke rehabilitation is resource intensive and requires a great deal of one-on-one therapists' contact time. Guidelines recommend a minimum of 45 min therapy per area of treatment for 5 days a week (Intercollegiate Stroke Working Party, 2016). However, UK stroke patients are unlikely to receive more than 2 h of therapy a day during their hospital stay, with fewer therapist face-to-face contact hours compared to other European countries (Luengo-Fernandez et al., 2019).

The third phase is the recovery phase, and it follows hospital discharge where patients may receive therapy by a visiting therapist or outpatient facilities. Allowing the patient to recover at home can provide a more comfortable and relaxed rehabilitation setting. Therefore, early supported discharge (ESD) aims to quickly get patients from hospital back into their home setting. Being in the home may also help the patient focus on recovering the abilities they require the most for their day-to-day interaction with the environment. Evidence suggests that patients who undergo ESD have improved scores on the activities of daily living scale (Rodgers & Price, 2017). However, in the recovery stage, the daily contact time with a therapist is significantly reduced. To overcome the limitation of therapist contact time, patients will often be given a schedule of exercises and repetitions to perform independently every day. Undertaking a high number of exercise repetitions can be tedious and patients may not adhere to them over time. According to Alankus et al. (2010), "only 31% of patients perform the exercises recommended by their therapists". Furthermore, the only record of exercise dosage is that which the patient reports to the therapist.

The post-recovery phase begins when the patient has regained normal functionality, or their recovery rate has plateaued. Most survivors would be expected to reach this stage at around 3–6 months post-stroke. Survivors who have not regained full motor function may have to make lifestyle changes to accommodate their new reduced physical capabilities; many will be dependent on a carer for help with activities essential for daily living. Depression and low motivation is common in stroke survivors as the debilitating effects of the stroke are sudden and can often cause a significant change in a person's life (Fitzsimons et al., 2020). However, research suggests that long-term rehabilitation can be helpful to recovery, both physically and mentally (Luengo-Fernandez et al., 2019).

Whilst the long-term effects of a stroke differ between patients, motor deficits are extremely common and found in most stroke survivors. Motor impairments following stroke are mostly caused by the damage and loss of neural pathways in the brain that control specific joint movements, and the patient may re-learn the lost limb movements by building new neural pathways through repeated exercising (Galeoto et al., 2019). Rehabilitation exercises are designed to encourage a specific set of joint movements, usually the joints that have reduced motor control following the stroke. Because these joints are much more difficult to use, patients can often use compensatory movements, underusing or incorrectly moving their impaired joints to quickly regain functionality. This is generally bad in the long term, and by using compensatory movements, they will not recover and may lead to a non-functioning arm through learnt non-use. Compensatory movements can be unnatural and can lead to strain or injury. As stated by researchers (Wee et al., 2014), "Compensatory movement behaviours may improve upper extremity function in the short-term but be detrimental to long-term recovery". It is therefore important to recognise compensatory movements and provide feedback to the patient during rehabilitation.

Technological systems are used for stroke rehabilitation without the requirement of face-to-face therapist contact, increasing the total amount of available guided therapy time to the patient. Low invasive technologies are deployed in the home (Burke et al., 2009; Brusco et al., 2022), which reduce the requirements for travel to outpatient facilities and allow rehabilitation to continue in a relaxed setting that may be more comfortable to the patient. It allows a patient to continue rehabilitation independently, and by doing so, patients could enter ESD sooner. Further, gamification has shown to have become an important part of these technological solutions and provides a source of engagement and enjoyment. These technological solutions exist on a spectrum from fully mechanical orthoses, e.g. custom fabricated orthoses (Stuck et al., 2014), to fully virtual digital solutions (via an immersive head-mounted display). Mechanical devices are cheaper and can be custom built for any rehabilitation exercise through the use of weights, sensors, levers, etc. However, they require more physical space to store and need to be initially installed and regularly calibrated and provide set functions to the user with limited scope of diversification in exercise. On the other hand, virtual technologies for rehabilitation have evolved a lot in the last decade reducing the barriers to recovery (Galeoto et al., 2019).

Whilst both mechanical orthoses and virtual digital technologies provide a variety of benefits, this chapter focuses on the impact of virtual technologies on stroke rehabilitation. VR is a broad term used to describe a spectrum of systems from non-immersive to fully immersive technologies. Non-immersive virtual environments encompass technologies that usually comprise a 2D environment and provide for an experience of an outsider watching in (like watching television, computer screen, etc.) On the other hand, immersive virtual environments are systems where the users are fully integrated into the environment (often using a head-mounted display). Both kinds of system can allow the user to interact with the virtual environment through tracking the user's movement and by the use of embedded sensors. Such systems might track the user's rehabilitation exercises and use this to provide key feedback and even motivate and entertain them through gamification. In addition to this, further techniques in machine learning are evolving to create personalised gamification experiences during rehabilitation exercises. However, compared to specially built orthoses, commercial off-the-shelf (COTS) VR systems tend to be aimed at the gaming market, rather than at rehabilitation use cases. An exception to this is the GestureTek IREX (GestureTek Health, n.d.), which comes packaged with games that can be customised to the patient's needs. Therefore, this chapter explores the aspects of virtual technologies that can be of advantage to the process of stroke rehabilitation whilst recognising the present challenges and weaknesses present in these systems (Stuck et al., 2014; GestureTek Health, n.d.).

Independent Use

As previously stated, when performing exercises independently, patients may not always perform them correctly. This may happen through compensating for the lack of motion in one joint through moving another (Alankus, 2011). Current thinking in motor learning also suggests that frequent shorter therapy sessions with breaks may potentially be more beneficial to the patient as they promote memory recall (Dobkin, 2004). "Telerehabilitation" is a potential solution that allows rehabilitation to take place over the Internet, allowing the therapists to review the patients' exercises as they complete them at home. In such settings, the therapist can monitor multiple patients at the same time. However, this still requires therapist time and does not guarantee that patients will not compensate during practise outside of these sessions.

Mitigating compensatory movements is currently an open problem but could be solved as technology to track patients' movements becomes more sophisticated. For example, Sarsfield et al. (2019) have developed and evaluated an algorithm capable of segmenting exercise repetitions in real time, enabling responsive feedback for the user. This was possible using a single consumer-level depth sensor and could be used as part of a larger system to give feedback to the patient on their exercises. Further, VR-based therapy has shown promise in having a positive effect on patient recovery with Laver et al. (2017) reporting that VR therapy had shown to be as effective as conventional therapy for improving upper limb function within their study criteria. Artificial intelligence and augmented reality-based solutions are now aiding the creation of virtual technological systems that provide similar services as a therapist. Such digital virtual therapists can help patients and overcome the problem of compensatory movement in stroke patients in non-supervised settings. Thus, virtual technological systems have great potential for independent use, helping patients to achieve the high volumes of repetitive exercises needed for recovery, reducing costly therapist time.

Lewis et al. (2011) present a study attempting to analyse results from patients' perspectives rather than purely clinical statistical methods. Patient feedback identified one particularly interesting suggestion for future directions. The suggestion from the patients was that the virtual technological systems should continue to be developed for use in homes and not just the clinical settings likc labs. This is because the patients wanted to continue with community-driven social interaction that they received in clinical settings. This suggests that if virtual technologies are to be used in home settings, social aspects are just as important as the games themselves. Player interaction in commercial games, where Internet-based social gaming has long been established, could form a key area for investigation when applying virtual technologies for stroke rehabilitation. The patient may live alone and can benefit from online community participation. Thus, independent use of a virtual technological system is also important when considering its suitability for use in a home setting (Alankus, 2011; Sarsfield et al., 2019; Lewis et al., 2011).

Home Deployment

Many virtual technological systems use varying novel motion capturing technologies that can have certain environmental constraints, limiting the types of settings and locations that they can be successfully deployed in Laver et al. (2017), and Dobkin (2004). This is particularly important if the goal is to create a home-based recovery system as a clinical setting may allow tighter control over the environment. The following is a list of the key environmental variables that should be evaluated when considering a system's suitability for home use.

- Space requirements for any hardware: A contained system may require its own display device, peripherals and a desk or workspace to set up the equipment. It may not be physically or technically feasible for the end user to set up and take down the system for every use, so the system would take up a permanent space in the environment.
- Space required for usage: Commercial off-the-shelf (COTS) systems, such as game consoles, that take up relatively little hardware space but require a larger area when in use. How much space is required to safely use the device when it is in operation remains dependent on the app being used. Similarly, issues of safety that can result from a user being immersed in the environment remain a concern.
- Required lighting conditions: A variety of tracking methods have been demonstrated to have potential in this application of stroke rehabilitation. Lighting level and colour may affect recognition software and intensity of sunlight could also interfere with the infrared tracking devices that are associated with systems that utilise tracking.

- Cost of the hardware: Beyond the initial development cost, widespread use of the device will have an associated unit cost. The system may also require additional displays, speakers, etc. Integration with displays that may already be present in the home, such as a television, should be considered.

As some studies have already considered the application of COTS video gaming systems for applications in stroke therapy, these systems should set a benchmark for home use as they are designed specifically with this scenario in mind. Whilst what was historically thought of as a COTS game is of little interest for rehabilitation use, there has been a trend towards motion-controlled gaming. These same systems can be used to support remote rehabilitation solutions. The systems that are proposed for stroke rehabilitation should follow the principles of usability. For example, the system must be easy and intuitive to start up and use, especially by non-technically aware patients. It must be completely usable by those with poor limb coordination and motor control, which is challenging due to diversity of ability that different stroke patients present with. Similarly, using the system for rehabilitation, the user must be able to effectively start and stop the system when required and be able to navigate and use all system menus. COTS have a potential downfall in this regard as commercial game consoles can have relatively complex start-up menus before a game can be started. Patients would have to learn to use and navigate these. For bespoke built systems, this is less of an issue, as menu systems can be streamlined based on user feedback and adapted as required. However, no study has yet been found that investigates patient proficiency in starting and using the menu systems of VR rehabilitation systems, as well as focusing on the effectiveness of the rehabilitation aspects.

Marker-less vision systems are of interest as they don't require the user to physically interact with devices. This feature has some advantages as patients with different levels of manual dexterity may not be able to pick up or manipulate all controller peripheral devices. Investigation with the Microsoft Kinect also provides individual hand tracking that does potentially allow for more complex interactions and clinical tracking of the patient's recovery. Sensor-based systems require the user to pick up and manipulate an object that contains one or more sensors that can be tracked. Research using COTS such as the Nintendo Wii fall into this category as the patient interacts with the game by using the Wii Remote. Studies investigating the rehabilitation potential of this system have shown that holding and manipulating the sensor device can be difficult at times for patients (Alankus et al., 2010). The Wii Remote is a relatively complex device, with buttons on both sides that can be hidden from view or accidentally pressed when used. Also the patient is required to keep a closed hand to avoid dropping the device; therefore patients with low hand and arm strength may struggle to do this for an extended period of time. A system where the user is required to pick up a basket with an attached sensor has been presented (Ma et al., 2007). The system is only able to detect arm movement, but it still requires grab and hold movements from the patient so this kind of sensor-based recovery may have advantages in promoting exercises beyond gross arm movement.

Engagement

One of the main justifications of using games for stroke rehabilitation is the potential for games to aid in many encouraging ways (Alankus et al., 2010). The fun aspect and engaging environment that games create is likely to encourage the patient to continue their rehabilitation, even if the activities are perceived as repetitive exercises. However, this is a huge generalisation of the very broad field of games. Some virtual games can promote high levels of engagement and encourage players to use them for hours on end. Additionally, the sheer variety of virtual games developed in the last decade means there is a greater choice of available virtual games to treat each patient's mobility and rehabilitation needs. Some new emerging social games make use of time-based strategies encouraging players to periodically revisit the game. Therefore, there is a need to explore the key concepts in game design and how these can help in the context of stroke rehabilitation.

In a seminal analysis, Csikszentmihalyi (1978) describes some important features for intrinsically motivating activities:

1. The activity should be structured so that the actor can increase or decrease the level of challenges he is facing, in order to match exactly his skills with the requirements for action.
2. It should be easy to isolate the activity, at least at the perceptual level, from other stimuli, external or internal, which might interfere with involvement in it.
3. There should be clear criteria for performance; one should be able to evaluate how well or how poorly one is doing at any time.
4. The activity should provide concrete feedback to the actor, so that he can tell how well he is meeting the criteria of performance.
5. The activity ought to have a broad range of challenges, and possibly several qualitatively different ranges of challenge, so that the actor may obtain increasingly complex information about different aspects of himself.

An alternative framework has been produced, with each section explained in detail (Malone, 1981) (Fig. 1.1).

Researchers Burke et al. (2009) have identified two principles of game design that they believe to be relevant to rehabilitation games, the main points of which have been condensed below:

Meaningful play:

- The player should be able to perceive how their actions affect the game.
- Use of feedback to show how their actions have affected the game. Feedback can be conveyed orally, visually and/or haptically and be in the form of achievements, graphs, scores, etc. as well as in-game incentives, such as new skills or game elements. These incentives can increase motivation and provide a desire to complete tasks.
- It is mentioned that in COTS games, players exhibiting poor gameplay are expected to be penalised in some form to encourage them to learn from their

I. **Challenge**
  A. Goal
    1. Personally meaningful goals
    2. Obvious or easily generated goals
    3. Performance feedback
  B. Uncertain Outcomes
    1. Variable difficulty level
      a. Determined automatically
      b. Chosen by learner
      c. Determined by opponent's skill
    2. Multiple level goals
      a. Score-keeping
      b. Speeded response
    3. Hidden information
    4. Randomness
  C. Toys vs. Tools
  D. Self-esteem

II. **Fantasy**
  A. Intrinsic and extrinsic fantasies
  B. Cognitive aspects of fantasies
  C. Emotional aspects of fantasies

III. **Curiosity**

Optimal level of informational complexity

  A. Sensory curiosity
  Audio and visual effects
  B. Cognitive curiosity
    1. "Good form" in knowledge structures
      a. Complete
      b. Consistent
      c. Parsimonious
    2. Informative feedback
      a. Surprising
      b. constructive

Fig. 1.1 Framework for a theory of intrinsically motivating instruction. (Adopted from Malone, 1981)

mistakes; by not including incentives for successful gameplay, the player is less likely to engage effectively with the game. However, in the case of rehabilitation games, it is recommended to handle failure more conservatively, with the initial goal to be engagement and thus reward all engagement with success; the difficulty should be paced so failures do not catastrophically affect the flow of the game and handled in a positive manner to keep the patient engaged and motivated.
- Providing a virtual representation of the patient has been positively received by stroke patients as it allows instant and continuous visual feedback. Any interactions with game elements should be clearly presented, such as highlighting the item, playing a sound, etc.
- It is common to use scoring mechanisms as a means to observe improvement over a period; it may be beneficial to reward the player for range of movement or time engaged in play, etc.

Challenge:

- A new player generally desires a low level of challenge to meet their low level of ability/familiarity with the game.
- Many games use levels to structure difficulty requiring the player to reach the necessary skill to advance to the next level, which may build upon skills learnt in previous levels or require the acquisition of new skills to complete.
- Another approach to maintaining a level of challenge is to dynamically adjust the difficulty based on the performance of the player.
- An approach taken by a physiotherapist to maintain challenge is also described: "A physiotherapist will usually begin by conducting a series of assessments (e.g. Action Research Arm Test, Motricity Index, Line Cancellation Test) to ascertain both the person's physical and cognitive abilities – these will provide data on, inter alia, the person's grip and pinch strength and gross movement in the affected limbs. Informed by this data, the physiotherapist will then devise a set of tasks for the person to practise. The physiotherapist typically works closely with the person with stroke, monitoring engagement and progress. As the rehabilitation continues over a period of weeks, the physiotherapist can increase the difficulty of the tasks to ensure that an optimum challenge is presented to the user". This approach corresponds to the third bullet point of the challenge table as the difficulty of the tasks is adjusted based on the patient's performance.

However, there is a need to explore these key concepts further in the context of stroke rehabilitation. An activity is said to be intrinsically motivational if there is no obvious external reward associated with the activity (Malone, 1981). A game might be played because it is engaging, rather than because there is any reward for playing it. Conversely, an extrinsically motivated activity is one that leads to a reward such as money or food. In cases where a game is being designed for stroke rehabilitation, the activity could be both intrinsically and extrinsically motivating.

Engagement Using VR Vs Conventional Therapy

Unlike traditional regular physical therapy with simple physical equipment, a gamified approach (which could use virtual/augmented reality or motion control systems) has the potential to be more intrinsically motivating (if designed correctly). Simply using VR is unlikely to be more motivating than conventional therapy if the software deployed on the system does not conform to the features described by Csikszentmihalyi or Malone (above).

Further work on this subject (Westera, 2015) discusses both the extrinsic and potential intrinsic motivating factors in serious games. It is identified that extrinsic reward systems are associated with shallow learning rather than deep processing (Habgood & Ainsworth, 2011); this may mean that when serious games are used with stroke patients, compensatory movements may be used to "cheat" with regard to performing the exercises correctly to get to the reward faster. If extrinsic reward systems are used, they should be relevant to the tasks at hand. If these issues are carefully considered, serious games have the potential to be motivating for stroke patients. Motion-controlled interactive games (such as the Kinect or Wii) or headset-based AR/VR technologies have the potential to be used in conjunction with gamification approaches. These interactive technologies encourage the physical activity needed for rehabilitation whilst also having the potential to deliver the motivational benefits of gamification. In addition to this, they can provide environments with a high level of control of the parameters for each user (Johansson, 2011). Laver et al. (2017) and Domínguez-Téllez et al. (2020) conducted systematic reviews and found that VR interventions can be effective when used in conjunction with conventional therapies.

Feedback to Patients

Burke et al. (2009) discuss two principles of game design for creating what they refer to as "meaningful play" and "challenge". "Meaningful play" differentiates game-based rehabilitation from regular physical therapy in that game-based approaches should relate the user's actions to the system's outcome. Regular physical therapy may not provide the user with direct feedback on their progress developing their skills. Digital game-based feedback could be in the form of numerical scores, progress bars, etc. These elements can motivate users to continue playing. In addition to positive feedback, negative feedback and failure are often used in successful commercial games. Burke et al. (2009) argue that the goal of a game designed for rehabilitation should be to reward all engagement with success. Stroke survivors might not be familiar with games, so they may not engage with the game if the reward mechanism involves punitive measures.

Another factor to consider is the difficulty of the game and "Challenge" that users face: A stroke patient will get bored if they do not feel sufficiently challenged. If the challenge is too difficult, they will become frustrated. Stroke survivors may have more difficulty in interacting with the game if their symptoms are more severe. Rand et al. (2004) found that commercial motion-controlled games had potential for use with stroke survivors, although they found that many of the games were too fast paced for many of the participants. This has changed in recent years and many more options are now available (Laver et al., 2017). Therefore, the best approach may be games designed with stroke survivors in mind, with support for different levels of severity.

An approach to support stroke patients suffering symptoms of differing severity is to use dynamic difficulty adjustment (Hocine et al., 2015). This is where the game dynamically adjusts to the user's abilities and performance within the game.

Evaluating Engagement

There are several ways of evaluating a game design with regard to engagement and motivation. Brockmyer et al. (2009) developed a questionnaire and analysed the data with Classical Test Theory and the Rasch rating scale model (Snyder & Sheehan, 1992) to quantify a player's absorption, flow, presence and immersion to determine their level of engagement. A more recent study by Rogers et al. (2020) recorded brain activity using electroencephalography (EEG) to determine a player's engagement in real time whilst using a tabletop VR system. This was correlated with presence questionnaire scores. The suggestion that simply using games to encourage patient engagement needs careful evaluation. Whilst stroke is more common in the elderly, all age groups, genders and personality types can suffer a stroke. So, creating a single experience that promotes high levels of engagement in a wide range of patients would be challenging. Furthermore, maintaining engagement would be a challenge considering that game therapy must be started early on in the rehabilitation process and continue beyond the traditional 6-month recovery period. A major shortcoming evidenced in current literature regarding the application of games for stroke rehabilitation is that most studies tend to be relatively short term (Laver et al., 2017). This does not give a meaningful insight into how engagement and enjoyment changes over time. Usually, any evaluation takes the form of asking the participants to simply comment at the end of the study on whether they enjoyed the games or not.

The second issue evidenced in the current literature from this perspective is that most studies are focused, justifiably, on measuring the effectiveness or feasibility of using the technology surrounding games for rehabilitation. Studies of effectiveness are important to identify if game-based systems have any scope for rehabilitation; therefore it is natural that they would precede studies focused specifically on the design of games for stroke rehabilitation. Whilst the potential for different technologies to be used for rehabilitation is an important issue, if they are to be used to drive game-based experiences, more advanced game design principles will have to be employed and investigated. This currently seems to be the missing step required to move these systems away from technology-driven prototypes and into patient-focused systems for rehabilitation (Galeoto et al., 2019).

An important stage in determining the level of engagement is to compare stroke survivors' playing experiences to those of a non-impaired group. Measures of presence and enjoyment were recorded in three groups of players using two games built for the (now obsolete) COTS gaming system, the PlayStation EyeToy (Rand et al., 2004). These included a healthy young group who closely matched the system's target market, a group of healthy elderly players and a group of seven stroke survivors. The results raised two points of interest. Firstly, that the results for engagement, enjoyment and exertion are largely similar between the healthy young and elderly groups, all scoring highly. The player performance is identical for the Wishy-Washy game, whilst the younger group performed significantly better at the Kung-Foo game. Despite the better score in this latter game, it does not seem to have created any significant difference in enjoyment between the two groups. This suggests that the novel interface method and simple game design could allow greater accessibility for groups that would not traditionally be interested in video games.

The second point is that when looking at the stroke survivor group's levels of engagement and enjoyment, these are significantly higher than both healthy groups. The stroke survivors rated both games 5 out of 5 for enjoyment whilst giving a Scenario Feedback Questionnaire (SQF) score of 27 out of 30. This is even more fascinating when comparing the stroke survivors' scores to the other groups. Even though stroke survivors scored lower points in the game, they were still engaged with it. Clearly there are some unique attributes of the stroke survivor group that explains these high levels of engagement compared to the healthy groups. It is suggested that because the players understand the therapeutic value of the games, they are simply happy to engage in any activity that will help recovery, although at the time of the study it was unknown whether there would be any therapeutic benefits. This might indicate that patients were simply willing to engage hoping that they would benefit.

Designing games for people with a physical disability will also surely present some unique challenges. Making commercial games accessible for disabled users is an area that has been largely ignored in the past according to some researchers (Schrier & Gibson, 2011). In recent years there has been some drive to promote accessible design (Paiva et al., 2021). A previous study has provided an adaptive challenge level to keep the game within the limits of the patient's capability whilst maintaining interest (Burke et al., 2009). Unfortunately, this study only tests the player's engagement with the games developed specifically using these suggestions. This gives absolutely no basis for comparison to games that do not make use of these design ideas. Therefore, it is very hard to weigh up the merits of each suggestion. It should be mentioned that modern game design has already adopted all these ideas in current commercial games, highlighting the need to properly apply modern game design theory from the commercial sector in games for rehabilitation.

In summary, the review of the state of the art so far indicates the following emerging trends:

- Intrinsic motivation of games may not be the driving factor for stroke survivors who want to engage with them.

- Stroke survivors are a large and varied population. Therefore, a one-size-fits-all approach to game design might not be appropriate.
- Although there are some studies (Alankus et al., 2010; Tamayo-Serrano et al., 2018) that investigate what types of games would be of interest and engaging to stroke survivors, research in this area requires further analysis. Particular exploration of emerging markets such as Facebook games that are popular amongst the non-traditional gaming demographic should be investigated.
- Tracking recovery information to give meaningful feedback could be an important motivator for patients and may reinforce the actual reason they are engaging with the game.
- Social aspects present in recreational therapy (RT) provide important motivators for participation and may help fulfil patient needs beyond recovery.
- Borrowing social mechanics from commercial games should be investigated. Games that allow patients to socialise outside a clinical setting could provide more reasons to participate.

Control over the Parameters

In terms of physical interaction with devices, two categories emerge, each with its own advantages and disadvantages. Vision-based systems rely on camera devices and tracking algorithms to detect motion from the user and sensor-based devices, where the user must physically hold and manipulate a sensor device. A second category of marker-based vision systems has been identified in the past, although due to advancements in computer vision technology, these no longer have any significant advantages.

Both kinds of VR system provide the benefit (over mechanical systems) of allowing a practitioner to adjust the parameters in the game to patients' needs. Since the effects of stroke differ between patients, a patient might find an activity too difficult and become frustrated. In the same way, another patient might find an activity too easy and become bored (and also not see any improvement in their condition). A trained practitioner could adjust the types of exercises and repetitions to avoid this. This was an approach adopted in a previous study (Alankus, 2011); games focusing on arm movements were chosen based on a set of exercises that a therapist would have recommended as part of standard therapy. This resulted in the participant experiencing improvements in their ability to use her affected arm.

Control over parameters has developed in the domain of games for stroke rehabilitation. An early example has been the vision-based system applied in the PlayStation EyeToy. This consisted of a low-cost camera peripheral connected to a PlayStation 2 game console. The device was only able to sense motion by looking for changes in pixel values between frames. It also allowed for playing whilst seated, essential for many stroke patients with mobility problems. The EyeToy is now discontinued, and buying an EyeToy and PlayStation 2, as well as the accompanying games, proved to be very expensive with advent of better technologies. However, if we were to consider using the lessons learnt to build a similar bespoke device, a simple colour camera provides key advantages. Significant costs will likely come from what kind of computational device will be used to perform the games processing and if any display equipment is also required.

Following EyeToy, commercial technological devices like the Microsoft Kinect for Windows became available. This camera-based device with primary input consists of infrared light projected depth sensors that allowed the device to work regardless of ambient room lighting or even in complete darkness. The Kinect for Windows and official SDK provided the ability to develop bespoke applications and therefore overcome the disadvantages of COTS games for stroke rehabilitation. The Kinect consists of two raw visual streams of data. The first is an RGB image and the other is a depth image; this is similar to an RGB image, but instead of encoding the colour value at each pixel, a greyscale value based on the depth is stored. These data streams can be used to implement tracking algorithms to detect users, objects and actions. The depth stream has some advantages over conventional colour-based tracking as the difference in depth value makes background segmentation much more straightforward. Microsoft's SDK also has a built-in skeletal tracking algorithm that outputs a series of joint positions and orientations. However, following the commercial discontinuation of the product, development of the technology has slowed.

The technology of skeletal tracking used by Kinect remains appealing, providing joint positions and orientations in real time; the tracking as applied in Kinect did however have some disadvantages; specifically, the skeletal joint estimations are not always accurate and jitter can occur, especially when occlusion occurs between the camera and the joint. For the hand it currently only detects three locations, centre of hand, tip of hand and tip of thumb, but Microsoft has demonstrated a fully articulated hand-tracking algorithm (Microsoft Handpose, 2014) that may be released to the SDK in the future. Currently, unless bespoke hand-tracking algorithms are created, the default tracking is unable to track useful grabbing and fine motor control gestures. The Kinect SDK provided a seated tracking mode as well as standing (Fig. 1.2). This could be useful for tracking patients that are unable to stand unassisted and allows them to perform upper limb rehabilitation in a seated position.

To overcome the drawbacks of the commercial technologies at the time, Pareto et al. (2011) used a desktop-sized workbench environment that could be set up in a patient's home who required no more intervention. The workbench is connected to the Internet so a therapist can monitor the patient's performance from a distance. The desktop-sized workbench is relatively low in space footprint and requires no maintenance from the patient. The system uses a large amount of specialist hardware, with stereoscopic display used for a game display, a standard display for telecommunication with the therapist, a robotic haptic stick for 3D space tracking and force feedback and an electronic Grip-it device, used to measure the grip force of patients. As specification of each hardware item is unknown, a real price cannot be calculated, but the cost is certainly significantly higher than COTS and low-tech systems.

The Nintendo Wii was another commercial gaming system that was designed with motion input as the primary form of interaction rather than a secondary add-on

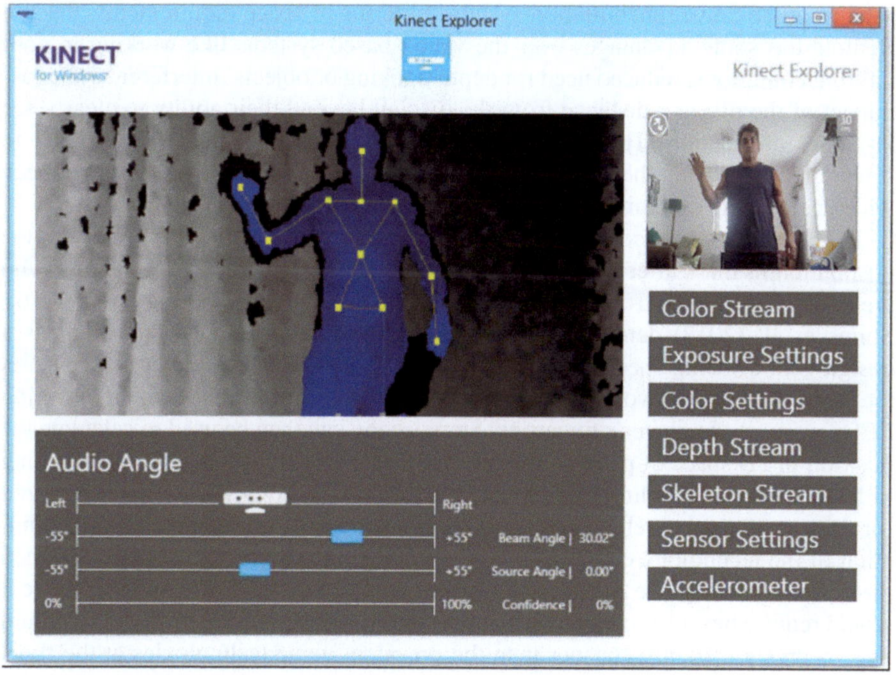

Fig. 1.2 Kinect for windows tracking

with a peripheral. This had the effect of widening the console gaming market far beyond the traditional gaming audience by offering a seemingly intuitive and far less intimidating method of interacting with the system. Unlike the hands-free system of the EyeToy, the Wii requires the player to interact using a motion controller. This device has several buttons like a traditional gaming peripheral but also contains a set of accelerometers to track the motion of the controller and an infrared camera that tracks a sensor bar mounted around the display device, allowing the player to point at the screen. Even though the Nintendo Wii has been discontinued, studies are still being conducted using this technology because of the high usability and intuitive user interface. This includes studies on the add-on devices, such as the "balance board" that provide use for rehabilitation (Carregosa et al., 2018). Though games such as Wii sports have shown benefits for physical therapy (Silva et al., 2020; Unibaso-Markaida & Iraurgi, 2021), there remains a need for customisation and prescription for stroke rehabilitation. Whilst most of the games tested teach the player to perform the real-world equivalent of the action that they are trying to achieve in the game, e.g. swing their arm to throw a bowling ball, it seems that most activities can be done in a much smaller range of motion. Also, as the Wii Remote is tracked (rather than the player), there is no distinguishing between standing and sitting whilst playing, which as mentioned before is a key factor for stroke rehabilitation. Furthermore, the Wii Remote is incapable of detecting compensatory movements and therefore would require another device to perform this task if it is to be used as an effective rehabilitation system. In terms of space requirements, the Wii Remote has some advantages over the vision-based systems like working in poor lighting conditions, reduced need for depth tracking or objects' interference and less impact of the player's distance from the display beyond their ability to clearly see in-game information. Though the EyeToy, Kinect and Wii have contributed to research investigating the role of games for stroke rehabilitation, there has not been wide-scale stable implementation.

High platform costs could make large-scale deployment difficult especially at the post 6 months mark after stroke when resources tend to be allocated to patients who are in early stages of stroke recovery (Intercollegiate Stroke Working Party, 2016). Shires et al. (2013) demonstrate their prototype home-based system that has a design goal of being specifically low cost and uses a bespoke system that reverses the Wii technology. Two Wii Remotes are used and an infrared camera detecting LEDs worn on the player's fingertips. Stereoscopy can then be used to calculate the position in 3D space of patients' fingertips. This allows for more complex tracking of hand gestures including rotation and pinch/grab. The two Wii Remotes required for the system used to retail at around £40 for the pair at the time but the discontinuation of the technology could make acquiring them difficult. The custom-designed electronics for the glove consist of a simple battery pack and LED; however since it would require bespoke manufacturing, it is hard to estimate costs involved but could have been significantly cheaper than the prevalent game technologies at the time. The studies identified using these technologies evaluated the device based on its effectiveness as a method of rehabilitation rather than assessing the practicalities of using it outside of a conventional therapeutic context. This has contributed to these technologies becoming those of the past and not technologies of the present.

Within the last decade, high fidelity consumer-grade VR systems first became widely available (Samsung Mobile Press, 2014). These systems are able to simulate a virtual environment through use of a "6 degrees of freedom" (6DoF) head-mounted display and controllers. 6DoF systems track the user's orientation and position in 3D space, allowing them to explore the virtual environment by walking around. They support much higher display resolution of realistic environments compared to their predecessors. Examples of systems released around this time include the original HTC Vive and Oculus Rift. However, these systems are required to be connected to a high-performance PC, which both increases the overall cost and adds to set-up complexity. They require "base stations", which assist in tracking the headset and controllers' movement in space, further increasing set-up complexity. Such equipment requires space and setting them up requires time and effort. Mobile phone-based VR systems were introduced as a response to these issues and often involve the user inserting their phone into a headset, which they use to drive the VR experience. The now discontinued Google Cardboard (Google Cardboard – Google VR, n.d.) and Samsung Gear VR (Samsung Gear VR with Controller, n.d.) are examples of this kind of technology. These work well for simple 360 experiences such as viewing 360 videos; however, these systems are only capable of tracking the orientation (not position) of the headset. This is known as 3DoF tracking and limits the user's immersion somewhat. A study exploring how geographically separated users could interact in social VR, Moustafa and Steed (2018) distributed Samsung Gear VR devices (and Samsung smartphones) to 17 participants. In feedback collected from diaries after use for a few weeks, participants reported technological issues when using the equipment, including audio difficulties, and issues concerning the wearability of the headset (heat/weight issues). It was reported that these issues are not prohibitive to the use of the headset but did affect the participants' immersion. The participants reported that the primary barrier to use of the equipment was the inability to move naturally. These issues highlight both the weaknesses of 3DoF tracking and the potential effectiveness of this technology.

Since 2019, the release of the Oculus Quest potentially marks the start of a new wave of VR devices. These new devices are completely "untethered", meaning they are capable of running standalone without the use of a high-performance PC and make use of "inside-out" 6DoF tracking, meaning they do not require external tracking hardware. Such a compact tool is, therefore, much more feasible to deploy in the home, as set-up complexity is kept to a minimum. An example of this is the Oculus Quest 2, which internally runs on an Android-based operating system. The Oculus Quest 2 is also relatively inexpensive at £299, which is far more accessible to most users compared with the £1000+ cost of PC-based VR. The Oculus Quest addresses these barriers by being entirely self-contained, incorporating its own power supply, storage and processing capabilities. It also features inside-out tracking, meaning external hardware is not required for the headset or controllers to be tracked, and it is completely wireless. This, as well as its relatively low cost, makes it far more accessible to a wider range of users. Further, the immersive experience of the user can be monitored by using the "casting" feature to a nearby display device, so that therapist can easily monitor usage if required (see Fig. 1.3).

In a recent review, 19 papers on the use of VR for the rehab of lower limb and 52 papers for the upper limb were reviewed, with the majority focused on stroke populations (Keijsers et al., 2021). This review reported that many studies now recognise VR and game-based stroke rehabilitation to be useful. However, another extended study and review found that use of VR and interactive video gaming were not more beneficial than conventional therapy approaches in improving upper limb function. VR may be beneficial in improving upper limb function and activities of daily living

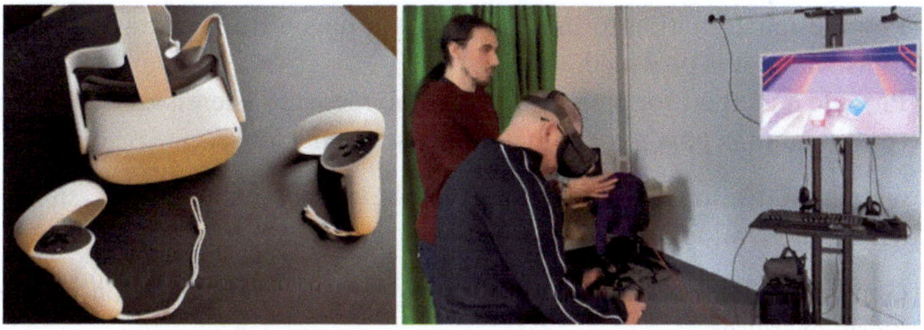

Fig. 1.3 Oculus Quest untethered headset for immersive experience of virtual reality (left). Casting of the immersive experience monitored on a display screen (right)

function when used as an adjunct to usual care (to increase overall therapy time). Thus, it should be noted that the advancements in VR technology show it could be used in combination with existing therapy to improve morale, build motivation, encourage repeated exercise, provide feedback, create challenge and improve the overall rehabilitation experience of stroke patients. Through the analysis of these reviewed technologies, we have seen that different technological solutions present unique challenges and requirements when applied to a home deployment scenario. We have been able to speculate on the suitability of COTS systems because of their well-known characteristics but still make some assumptions about available play area and environmental set-up. Bespoke systems designed for home deployment seem to have favoured the all-in-one approach of a self-contained system confined to a desk space. This has practical implications, as it is a relatively small space footprint and requires little interaction with the user beyond the intended use of the device.

Based on an analysis of current, and the requirements for, computer-assisted stroke rehabilitation systems, the following framework provides criteria for assessing the effectiveness of such a system:

- Potential for independent use: The level of independence a user can reach with the system is important, potentially allowing the use of the system without requiring a therapist's intervention. This could increase the time a patient can spend exercising, particularly important for the initial recovery phase for the best chance of regaining motor control. Research suggests that patients could recover movement in affected limbs by performing hundreds of daily repetitions (Alankus, 2011) and thus independent use is therefore an important factor.
- Elicit appropriate movements: For effective upper limb rehabilitation, the activity must promote reach, grip and manipulation exercises, as well as exercises that combine multiple movements to form an activity.
- Provide opportunities to practise not limited by distance, cost and availability of services. Low-cost systems could provide an opportunity for use in patients' homes to:
  - Allow earlier discharge from hospital whilst allowing the recovery process to continue.
  - Allow the patient to rehabilitate in a comfortable environment.
  - Provide rehabilitation to those who might have difficulty travelling to locations where it is provided.
  - Provide a method for patients to continue recovery exercises in the long term (past 6 months post-stroke) that do not strain health service resources.
- Provide a motivational context. For example, game rehabilitation systems could provide a motivational context for patients:
  - Gameplay can foster interest and engagement and be based on simple real-world exercises.
  - Player engagement techniques could be borrowed from conventional games, such as achievement trophies for reaching key milestones.

  - Fitness games like Wii Fit motivate the player by tracking performance over time and highlighting improvements to the player. A similar system could be utilised for stroke recovery.

- Capturing and displaying useful metrics. It is important that the system can provide useful feedback to a therapist and patient on the patient's performance, for example:
  - Real-time skeletal feedback
  - Graphics displaying improvement in range of motion over time
  - Frequency and time of use
  - Highlighting of compensatory movements
- Affordable. Whether the approach uses a COTS or bespoke system, systems must be cost-effective.

Summary

As we have seen through our review of the current state of the art, research has focused on testing different input methods to control VR games. Whilst all input methods share the common feature that they are operated through the user's motion, games are designed to utilise these motion controls providing a context for the user to engage with the system. Games are also designed so that the motions required to perform well in the game match the movements required for effective rehabilitation.

Whilst there are several studies using different motion input devices, all appear to show advantages to the rehabilitation process when VR games are used to complement a traditional course of therapy. However, the main focus has been on identifying different hardware solutions to provide a range of advantages compared with other systems. This includes evaluating low-cost hardware for home use, markerless tracking for maximum usability and the utility of commercial game systems. After a new hardware set-up has been developed for a new set of rehabilitation-based requirements, it will then usually be tested to see if it is clinically effective.

As a result, a wide range of hardware set-ups have been identified as having a beneficial impact when used for stroke rehabilitation. Performing a study to test clinical effectiveness is a very resource-intensive process. Willing stroke survivors are required to participate over a period of time and therapists are needed to perform examinations of the patient's clinical progression. This has left us with many systems that show promise but not enough clinical evidence to make informed decisions to see whether the different input methods presented in the literature exhibit different levels of clinical effectiveness.

To properly address this issue, we will need to review longer-term studies, with larger populations than current projects are using or evidencing. This will allow us to see what effect VR-based game rehabilitation has over a longer term. It could also offer insights into evaluating their potential for use after the end of conventional therapy.

An alternative study that could give similar insights, but with less clinical results, would be to perform a shorter study that incorporates several different hardware and game systems to directly compare them with each other. Measuring the user's ability and performance of these systems over a few user sessions would be required rather than looking for clinical progression over weeks or months.

This approach could also be used to capture qualitative information from stroke user groups regarding their enjoyment and user experience to investigate which hardware set-ups provide a better user experience. This type of study would provide a useful precursor to an in-depth clinical study on effectiveness in developing, or maintaining, motor control post-stroke.

Looking to the Future

As we have seen from the review of the current state of the art, many promising rehabilitation systems are in an early stage of development. There are several areas open for further investigation.

The cost of depth-sensing hardware is falling. Future systems will be less intrusive to the user than current hardware configurations, and algorithms will be more robust than existing computer vision approaches. The latest VR technologies are now composed of compact hardware, available to users at costs lower than ever before, and facilities increasingly accommodative of stroke rehabilitation needs, such as monitoring users' position through inbuilt cameras and sensors. As more detailed tracking methods become increasingly available, they could be used to provide more complex systems that can monitor the user's skeletal pose more accurately. This will allow more complex, and a greater range of, exercises to be used in rehabilitation; this could potentially have a positive impact on recovery, as it would involve a greater range of motion providing effective rehabilitation.

Our review of the state of the art includes hardware used as a driver to control game applications. The user is then given feedback regarding their performance usually through in-game scores. Whilst the score can show an improvement over time, it cannot be conclusively linked to an improvement in upper limb motor control. Other factors could contribute here, such as the user becoming more familiar with, and better at the game, within the confines of their current range of motion. However, this could be overcome by employing robust action recognition models that are capable of determining correct and compensatory movements, which is an important aspect for independent rehabilitation.

By employing better tracking methods and/or additional sensors, information could be captured about the user's range of motion, spasticity and exertion. This information can then be used to give a direct overview of the patient's clinical progression over time. These additional sensors may not be used to drive the game input at all.

Research into the field has currently focused almost entirely on the creation of systems that encourage user interaction through motion control. However, the games that are used as a motivating context for use are very rudimentary and missing most game design principles that are currently applied to commercial games. Particularly in the context of home use or systems that are intended to be used independently, games that have a higher level of enjoyment and engagement could be significantly more effective as they would provide a motivational factor for the patient and thus potentially lead to more frequent use. Research into adaptive rehabilitation systems (Burke et al., 2009) has taken steps in this direction by developing games that utilise the well-known game design principle of a difficulty curve. This adjusts the game difficulty based on the user's performance to keep the user challenged but still able to successfully play the game. Keeping the patient appropriately challenged may help them stay motivated over a longer period of time. However, there is still more to be done in applying game design principles to stroke rehabilitation games.

A key motivating factor in COTS gaming systems designed for improving the player's fitness has been to track and graphically represent their improvement over time. In the game Wii Fit, the use of the Wii "balance board" allows the player's weight to be tracked. This information can then be fed back to the player showing improvements, thus increasing player satisfaction and motivation. Games designed for stroke rehabilitation could employ similar strategies to help stroke survivors become more satisfied with their recovery and motivate them to further their rehabilitation gains.

By using more advanced sensing devices and algorithms capable of upper limb tracking, systems can potentially gather clinical level data to monitor important recovery information, such as increases in the patient's range of motion. Other secondary sensors could be used with the gaming system to gather additional clinical information, including skin temperature maps, muscle response, breathing patterns, blood pressure and heart rate. This rich set of clinical data could provide a highly motivational feedback loop when offered to the patient in an appropriate format. These data can be used for the purposes of remote health monitoring by communicating this information over the Internet to a therapist, presenting opportunities for remote tele-health.

References

Adamson, J., Beswick, A., & Ebrahim, S. (2004). Is stroke the most common cause of disability? *Journal of Stroke and Cerebrovascular Diseases: Official Journal of National Stroke Association, 13*, 171–177. https://doi.org/10.1016/j.jstrokecerebrovasdis.2004.06.003

Alankus, G. (2011). *Motion-based video games for stroke rehabilitation with reduced compensatory motions* (p. 239).

Alankus, G., Lazar, A., May, M., & Kelleher, C. (2010). Towards customizable games for stroke rehabilitation. In *Proceedings of the 28th international conference on human factors in computing systems – CHI '10. Presented at the 28th international conference*. ACM Press, p. 2113. https://doi.org/10.1145/1753326.1753649

American Association of Neurological Surgeons (AANS). (2022). *The grants register 2023* (pp. 49–50). Palgrave Macmillan. https://doi.org/10.1057/978-1-349-96053-8_16447

Brockmyer, J. H., Fox, C. M., Curtiss, K. A., McBroom, E., Burkhart, K. M., & Pidruzny, J. N. (2009). The development of the game engagement questionnaire: A measure of engagement in video game-playing. *Journal of Experimental Social Psychology, 45*, 624–634. https://doi.org/10.1016/j.jesp.2009.02.016

Brusco, N., Voogt, A., Nott, M., Callaway, L., Mansoubi, M., & Layton, N. (2022). Meeting unmet needs for stroke rehabilitation in rural public Health: Explorative economic evaluation of upper limb robotics-based technologies through a capabilities lens. *Societies, 12*, 143. https://doi.org/10.3390/soc12050143

Burke, J. W., McNeill, M. D. J., Charles, D. K., Morrow, P. J., Crosbie, J. H., & McDonough, S. M. (2009). Optimising engagement for stroke rehabilitation using serious games. *The Visual Computer, 25*, 1085. https://doi.org/10.1007/s00371-009-0387-4

Carregosa, A. A., dos Santos, L. R. A., Masruha, M. R., Coêlho, M. L. D. S., Machado, T. C., Souza, D. C. B., Passos, G. L. L., Fonseca, E. P., Ribeiro, N. M. D. S., & Melo, A. D. S. (2018). Virtual rehabilitation through Nintendo Wii in Poststroke patients: Follow-up. *Journal of Stroke and Cerebrovascular Diseases, 27*, 494–498. https://doi.org/10.1016/j.jstrokecerebrovasdis.2017.09.029

Csikszentmihalyi, M. (1978). Intrinsic rewards and emergent motivation. In *The hidden costs of reward* (pp. 205–218). Psychology Press.

Dobkin, B. H. (2004). Strategies for stroke rehabilitation. *Lancet Neurology, 3*, 528–536. https://doi.org/10.1016/S1474-4422(04)00851-8

Domínguez-Téllez, P., Moral-Muñoz, J. A., Salazar, A., Casado-Fernández, E., & Lucena-Antón, D. (2020). Game-based virtual reality interventions to improve upper limb motor function and quality of life after stroke: Systematic review and meta-analysis. *Games for Health Journal, 9*, 1–10. https://doi.org/10.1089/g4h.2019.0043

Fitzsimons, C. F., Nicholson, S. L., Morris, J., Mead, G. E., Chastin, S., & Niven, A. (2020). Stroke survivors' perceptions of their sedentary behaviours three months after stroke. *Disability and Rehabilitation, 44*, 382–394. https://doi.org/10.1080/09638288.2020.1768304

Galeoto, G., Iori, F., Santis, R. D., Santilli, V., Mollica, R., Marquez, M. A., Sansoni, J., & Berardi, A. (2019). The outcome measures for loss of functionality in the activities of daily living of adults after stroke: A systematic review. *Topics in Stroke Rehabilitation, 26*, 236–245. https://doi.org/10.1080/10749357.2019.1574060

GestureTek Health. (n.d.). GestureTek Health IREX white paper [WWW document]. http://www.gesturetekhealth.com/sites/default/files/general/irex_concept_note_0.pdf. Accessed 15 Jan 2021.

Google Cardboard – Google VR [WWW Document]. (n.d.). https://arvr.google.com/cardboard/. Accessed 6 May 2021.

Habgood, J., & Ainsworth, S. (2011). Motivating children to learn effectively: Exploring the value of intrinsic integration in educational games. *The Journal of the Learning Sciences, 20*, 169–206. https://doi.org/10.1080/10508406.2010.508029

Herpich, F., & Rincon, F. (2020). Management of acute ischemic stroke. *Critical Care Medicine, 48*, 1654–1663. https://doi.org/10.1097/ccm.0000000000004597

Hocine, N., Gouaïch, A., Cerri, S. A., Mottet, D., Froger, J., & Laffont, I. (2015). Adaptation in serious games for upper-limb rehabilitation: An approach to improve training outcomes. *User Modeling and User-Adapted Interaction, 25*, 65–98. https://doi.org/10.1007/s11257-015-9154-6

Intercollegiate Stroke Working Party. (2016). *National clinical guideline for stroke* (5th ed.). Royal College of Physicians.

Johansson, B. B. (2011). Current trends in stroke rehabilitation. A review with focus on brain plasticity. *Acta Neurologica Scandinavica, 123*, 147–159. https://doi.org/10.1111/j.1600-0404.2010.01417.x

Keijsers, N., Aärts, P., Grisoni, L., Müller, K., Wellburn, S., Martin, D., & Green, D. (2021). Virtual reality and rehabilitation: Review of reviews. In *13th international conference on disability, virtual reality & associated technologies*, pp. 1–8.

Kissela, B. M., Khoury, J. C., Alwell, K., Moomaw, C. J., Woo, D., Adeoye, O., Flaherty, M. L., Khatri, P., Ferioli, S., De Los Rios La Rosa, F., Broderick, J. P., & Kleindorfer, D. O. (2012). Age at stroke: Temporal trends in stroke incidence in a large, biracial population. *Neurology, 79*, 1781–1787. https://doi.org/10.1212/WNL.0b013e318270401d

Krakauer, J. W. (2006). Motor learning: Its relevance to stroke recovery and neurorehabilitation. *Current Opinion in Neurology, 19*, 84–90. https://doi.org/10.1097/01.wco.0000200544.29915.cc

Laver, K. E., Lange, B., George, S., Deutsch, J. E., Saposnik, G., & Crotty, M. (2017). Virtual reality for stroke rehabilitation. *Cochrane Database of Systematic Reviews*. https://doi.org/10.1002/14651858.CD008349.pub4

Lewis, G. N., Woods, C., Rosie, J. A., & McPherson, K. M. (2011). Virtual reality games for rehabilitation: Perspectives from the users and new directions. In *2011 international conference on virtual rehabilitation. Presented at the 2011 international conference on virtual rehabilitation*, pp. 1–2. https://doi.org/10.1109/ICVR.2011.5971842.

Luengo-Fernandez, R., Violato, M., Candio, P., & Leal, J. (2019). Economic burden of stroke across Europe: A population-based cost analysis. *European Stroke Journal, 5*, 17–25. https://doi.org/10.1177/2396987319883160

Ma, M., McNeill, M., Charles, D., McDonough, S., Crosbie, J., Oliver, L., & McGoldrick, C. (2007). Adaptive virtual reality games for rehabilitation of motor disorders. In C. Stephanidis (Ed.), *Universal access in human-computer interaction* (Ambient interaction, lecture notes in computer science) (pp. 681–690). Springer. https://doi.org/10.1007/978-3-540-73281-5_74

Malone, T. W. (1981). What makes things fun to learn? A study of intrinsically motivating computer games [WWW document]. https://www.researchgate.net/publication/234608112_What_Makes_Things_Fun_to_Learn_A_Study_of_Intrinsically_Motivating_Computer_Games. Accessed 28 Nov 2020.

Microsoft Handpose: Fully Articulated Hand Tracking. (2014). https://www.microsoft.com/en-us/research/video/handpose-fully-articulated-hand-tracking/. Accessed 4 Nov 2023.

Moustafa, F., & Steed, A. (2018). A longitudinal study of small group interaction in social virtual reality. In *Proceedings of the 24th ACM symposium on virtual reality software and technology, VRST 18*. Association for Computing Machinery, pp. 1–10. https://doi.org/10.1145/3281505.3281527

Paiva, D. M. B., Freire, A. P., & Fortes, R. P. D. M. (2021). Accessibility and software engineering processes: A systematic literature review. *Journal of Systems and Software, 171*, 110819. https://doi.org/10.1016/j.jss.2020.110819

Pareto, L., Johansson, B., Ljungberg, C., Zeller, S., Sunnerhagen, K. S., Rydmark, M., & Broeren, J. (2011). Telehealth with 3D games for stroke rehabilitation. *International Journal on Disability and Human Development, 10*. https://doi.org/10.1515/ijdhd.2011.062

Patel, A., Berdunov, V., Quayyum, Z., King, D., Knapp, M., & Wittenberg, R. (2020). Estimated societal costs of stroke in the UK based on a discrete event simulation. *Age and Ageing, 49*, 270–276. https://doi.org/10.1093/ageing/afz162

Rand, D., Kizony, R., & Weiss, P. L. (2004). Virtual reality rehabilitation for all: Vivid GX versus Sony PlayStation II EyeToy. In *Proceedings of the 5th international conference on disability, virtual reality & association technology*, pp. 87–94.

Rodgers, H., & Price, C. (2017). Stroke unit care, inpatient rehabilitation and early supported discharge. *Clinical Medicine, 17*(2), 173

Rogers, J. M., Jensen, J., Valderrama, J. T., Johnstone, S. J., & Wilson, P. H. (2020). Single-channel EEG measurement of engagement in virtual rehabilitation: A validation study. *Virtual Reality*. https://doi.org/10.1007/s10055-020-00460-8

Rutten-Jacobs, L. C., Larsson, S. C., Malik, R., Rannikmäe, K., Sudlow, C. L., Dichgans, M., Markus, H. S., & Traylor, M. (2018). Genetic risk, incident stroke, and the benefits of adhering to a healthy lifestyle: Cohort study of 306 473 UK Biobank participants. *British Medical Journal*, k4168. https://doi.org/10.1136/bmj.k4168

Samsung Gear VR with Controller [WWW Document]. (n.d.). *Official Samsung Galaxy Site*. http://www.samsung.com/global/galaxy/gear-vr/. Accessed 6 May 2021.

Samsung Mobile Press [WWW Document]. (2014). https://web.archive.org/web/20140906045517/http://www.samsungmobilepress.com/2014/09/03/Samsung-Explores-the-World-of-Mobile-Virtual-Reality-with-Gear-VR-1. Accessed 12 May 2021.

Sarsfield, J., Brown, D., Sherkat, N., Langensiepen, C., Lewis, J., Taheri, M., Selwood, L., Standen, P., & Logan, P. (2019). Segmentation of exercise repetitions enabling real-time patient analysis and feedback using a single exemplar. *IEEE Transactions on Neural Systems and Rehabilitation Engineering, 27*, 1004–1019. https://doi.org/10.1109/TNSRE.2019.2907483

Schrier, K., & Gibson, D. (Eds.). (2011). *Designing games for ethics*. IGI Global. https://doi.org/10.4018/978-1-60960-120-1

Shires, L., Battersby, S., Lewis, J., Brown, D., Sherkat, N., & Standen, P. (2013). Enhancing the tracking capabilities of the Microsoft Kinect for stroke rehabilitation. In *2013 IEEE 2nd international conference on serious games and applications for health (SeGAH)*. IEEE. https://doi.org/10.1109/segah.2013.6665316.

Silva, E. C. G., Lange, B., Bacha, J. M. R., & Pompeu, J. E. (2020). Effects of the interactive videogame Nintendo Wii sports on upper limb motor function of individuals with post-polio syndrome: A randomized clinical trial. *Games for Health Journal, 9*, 461–471. https://doi.org/10.1089/g4h.2019.0192

Snyder, S., & Sheehan, R. (1992). The Rasch measurement model. *Journal of Early Intervention, 16*, 87–95. https://doi.org/10.1177/105381519201600108

Stroke statistics [WWW Document]. (2018). Stroke Association. https://www.stroke.org.uk/what-is-stroke/stroke-statistics. Accessed 20 Mar 2023.

Stuck, R. A., Marshall, L. M., & Sivakumar, R. (2014). Feasibility of SaeboFlex upper-limb training in acute stroke rehabilitation: A clinical case series. *Occupational Therapy International, 21*, 108–114. https://doi.org/10.1002/oti.1369

Tamayo-Serrano, P., Garbaya, S., & Blazevic, P. (2018). Gamified In-home rehabilitation for stroke survivors: Analytical review. *International Journal of Serious Games*, 5. https://doi.org/10.17083/ijsg.v5i1.224

Unibaso-Markaida, I., & Iraurgi, I. (2021). Effect of the Wii sports resort on mobility and health-related quality of life in moderate stroke. *Behavioural Neurology, 2021*, 1–7. https://doi.org/10.1155/2021/6635298

Wee, S. K., Hughes, A.-M., Warner, M., & Burridge, J. H. (2014). Trunk restraint to promote upper extremity recovery in stroke patients. *Neurorehabilitation and Neural Repair, 28*, 660–677. https://doi.org/10.1177/1545968314521011

Westera, W. (2015). Games are motivating, aren't they? Disputing the arguments for digital game-based learning. *International Journal of Serious Games, 2*. https://doi.org/10.17083/ijsg.v2i2.58

Chapter 2
A Framework for Designing Tabletop Games in Group-Based Motor Rehabilitation

Jonathan Duckworth, Nick Mumford, Jessica D. Bayliss, and Peter H. Wilson

Principle Supporting Therapeutic Design in Movement Rehabilitation

One of the best predictors of change in motor rehabilitation is time on task or the intensity of physical therapy. However, many individuals with neuromotor disabilities find it difficult to engage in therapy and experience it as monotonous, which can reduce motivation to progress in therapy. As such, designing therapeutic tasks and environments that can be presented in a meaningful and stimulating way is one of the key challenges facing therapists. Presentation of tasks in a game context can be a valuable adjunct to more traditional therapy, capturing attention, encouraging playful participation, and augmenting treatment effects.

The physical and cognitive impairments that result from brain trauma and conditions affecting the motor system are often associated with a set of secondary issues including higher rates of depression and anxiety and low self-concept. In turn, these issues present a psychological barrier to engaging in rehabilitation, daily activities, and recreation (Esbensen et al., 2003). This vicious cycle of inactivity and

J. Duckworth (✉)
School of Design, College of Design and Social Context, RMIT University, Melbourne, VIC, Australia
e-mail: jonathan.duckworth@rmit.edu.au

N. Mumford · P. H. Wilson
School of Behavioural and Health Sciences, Faculty of Health Sciences, Australian Catholic University, Melbourne, VIC, Australia
e-mail: peterh.wilson@acu.edu.au

J. D. Bayliss
School of Interactive Games and Media and Computer Science, Rochester Institute of Technology, Rochester, NY, USA
e-mail: jdbics@rit.edu

E. Brooks, D. J. Brown (eds.), *Virtual Reality Games for Rehabilitation*, Virtual Reality Technologies for Health and Clinical Applications,
https://doi.org/10.1007/978-1-0716-3371-7_2

impairment is strongly predictive of longer-term psychosocial problems (House & Hosker, 2013; Starkstein & Pahissa, 2014). These psychosocial problems often include isolation, low self-esteem, reduced social support, and chronic anxiety and depression, which are often part and parcel of a broader pattern of psychopathology later in life (Rutter et al., 2006; Taylor et al., 2011). The strong presence of psychosocial deficits among people with neurological impairments highlights a need for design solutions in therapy that encourage social interaction and a more playful orientation to participation in rehab.

Group-Based Solutions in Movement Therapy

Group-based rehabilitation that is playful in nature, thematically appropriate, and engaging to the client group has been shown to enhance participation. Importantly, this provides more opportunity for the development of both movement skills and social competencies, ameliorating the psychosocial impact of the conditions in question (Green et al., 2013). For example, the group-based Breathe Magic program, founded in the United Kingdom, is designed to encourage children with hemiplegia to learn (bimanual) magic tricks involving assorted props (like cards), culminating in a magic show after the 3-week program (Green et al., 2013). This program has demonstrated significant improvements in motor function (Green et al., 2013) and, based on child and parent reports, improved interaction with typically developed peers and family members at home.

Another recent group-based approach is the Pirates program of Aarts et al. (2012). This program is based on the fundamental premise that play is the primary means by which children interact, learn, and derive meaning in their world. Here children dress as pirates and are encouraged to role-play scenarios that involve bimanual and locomotor activity. The Pirate groups consist of six children who are guided by between four and six therapists. The therapy space is set up as a "pirate island" with a range of thematic props like a treasure chest, plastic swords, deck tools, "booty," etc. The program also incorporates several weeks of constraint-induced movement therapy (CIMT) wherein the child is told that their arm has been "injured" during some pirate activity and needs rest. Pilot case study data have shown gains on the AHA and ABILHAND assessment tools measuring upper-limb function, with very positive parent reports on the translation of skill to the home environment. Taken together, playful interaction and role-play provide opportunities for peer modeling, cooperation, and friendly competition, all of which provide a fulcrum for goal-related activity and practice. Indeed, the rehabilitative effect of the environment is regarded almost as an incidental outcome of the play itself and, as such, is not seen as an added burden on the child's time and energy.

Participation and Social Engagement: The ICF Framework

One critical advantage in using games and play in a group rehabilitative context is the potential to design and customize environments and interfaces to foster participation and social engagement. Based on the International Classification of Functioning, Disability, and Health (ICF), the standard for conceptualizing levels of function and planning rehabilitation, participation refers to a person's involvement in physical, recreational, and social life situations (WHO, 2001). Critically, participation is more than merely being physically present in life situations but includes a sense of belonging and involvement in these social settings (Granlund, 2013). As shown in Fig. 2.1, the ICF model proposes a bidirectional relationship between reduced participation and negative personal outcomes (see Rosenbaum & Stewart, 2004, Granlund, 2013, Duckworth et al., 2019 for further discussion on participation). Conversely, it is the task of the therapist to design and implement therapeutic environments that provide opportunities for the patient to use their affected limbs and to develop functional skill (Eliasson et al., 2003). Put another way, the structure of therapeutic tasks should encourage participation, expand the movement repertoire of patients, and, in so doing, develop personal resilience and a sense of self-efficacy and achievement. These reciprocal effects are illustrated in the ICF framework.

The ICF framework provides a vital reference point for therapists and researchers assessing the health status of patients and developing therapy solutions that address their needs. For example, the design of a therapeutic task involving

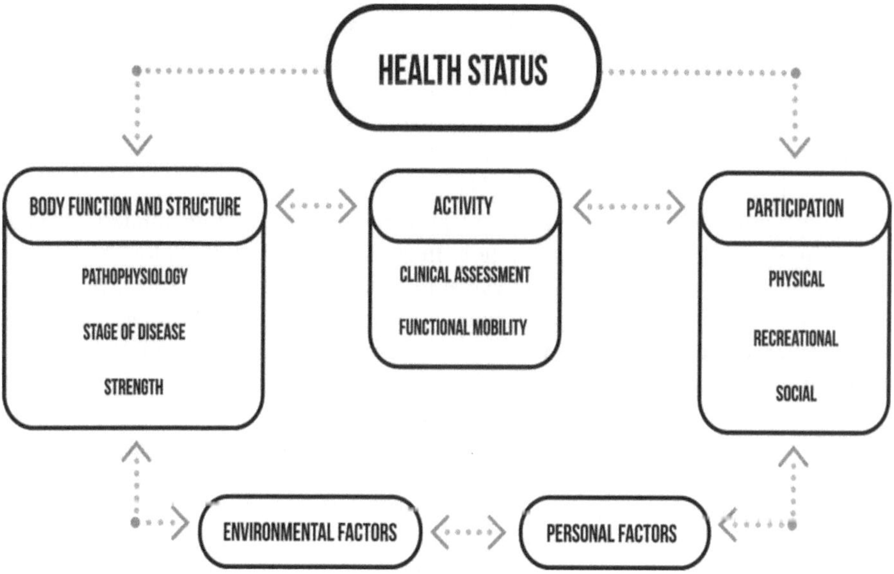

Fig. 2.1 The ICF model of functioning and disability

collaboration between a number of patients may improve psychosocial function, enhancing self-esteem and movement confidence. The ability to match task levels and challenges to the individual capabilities of the patient could promote a sense of competency, with flow-on effects for participation. Computer games that require physical movement together with social interaction may improve the physical, social, and recreational aspects at the participation level in the ICF model and reduce both motor and psychosocial deficits. Moreover, integrating principles from computer games and human-computer interaction (HCI) with the ICF framework may provide new design avenues for therapists and researchers developing novel therapeutic solutions for group environments.

Human-Computer Interaction Meets the ICF Framework

The way computers can mediate and support work in a group environment is a research domain of computer-supported cooperative work (CSCW), a sub-field of human-computer interaction (HCI). The advent of large-format interactive walls and tabletop displays heralded the potential of computers to facilitate the work practices of small teams co-located around the same physical interface (Dietz & Leigh, 2001; Wellner, 1993). In particular, tabletop displays can support face-to-face multi-user interaction through the physical affordances of the horizontal interface or the users' mental models of working around traditional tables (Scott et al., 2003). Tabletop displays can support a broad range of user interactions such as multi-finger touch, hand gesture, and simultaneous manipulation of physical objects (Han, 2005; Ullmer & Ishii, 1997; Wu & Balakrishnan, 2003), lead to collaborative learning in a group setting (Kharrufa et al., 2010), (Rick et al., 2011), and foster multimodal communication between users (Fleck et al., 2009). For example, tabletop computer games have been shown to support social competence training for children with autism spectrum disorder (Giusti et al., 2011). Here children are encouraged to solve a navigation task by manipulating different features of the environment, but only through cooperative activity can the problem be solved.

Use of games that involve groups of players using tabletop technology is relatively unexplored in motor rehabilitation. In this chapter we will explore how social aspects of group interaction and physical affordances of tabletop displays may be exploited to enhance the design of game environments for rehabilitation. We consider game design research, social psychological literature on group-based interaction and group environments in CSCW to build a framework of design principles. We embed the design principles from these domains within the ICF framework to forge an integrated view of the possibilities of co-located interactive games. In particular, we discuss the advantages of tabletop interfaces as a playful medium for rehabilitation and identify areas of potential development.

The Advantages of Tabletop Interaction for Rehabilitation

Our rehabilitation system called EDNA™ (formerly known as Elements) provides a useful model for designing interactive tabletop environments that enhance upper-limb rehabilitation for traumatic brain injury (TBI) patients (Duckworth & Wilson, 2010). At the heart of the EDNA system is a tabletop graphics display and four soft graspable objects used by the patient [i.e., tangible user interfaces (TUIs)]. A suite of interactive software applications provides the patient with tasks geared toward reaching, grasping, lifting, moving, and placing TUIs on the tabletop display. Real-time audiovisual feedback is designed to reinforce to the patient their position in space and effect of their movements, helping them refine movements over time. Patients can also manipulate the computer-generated feedback to create unique audiovisual outcomes. For example, in one environment the patient can experience the creative pleasure of being able to mix and manipulate sound and colorful graphics in an aesthetically pleasing way (Fig. 2.2).

The overall system design of EDNA provides tactility, texture, and audiovisual feedback to encourage patients to move in response to external cues or in a self-directed way. The various feedback mechanisms provided by the system assist patients and therapists to monitor their progress and plan for improvement over time. Our early evaluation research shows that EDNA is a viable adjunct to conventional physical therapy in facilitating motor learning in patients with TBI (Mumford et al., 2010, 2012) and acquired brain injury (Rogers et al., 2019). Importantly, we observed that interactive tabletop displays offer several unique advantages for motor rehabilitation that are specific to the medium that are explored below.

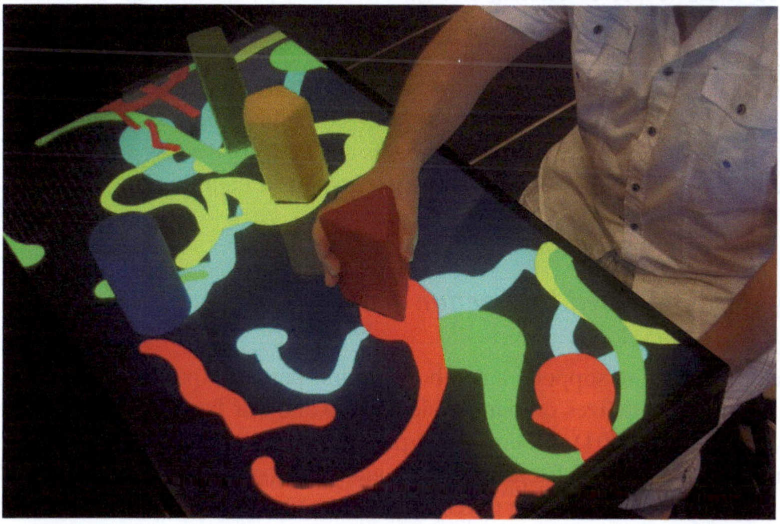

Fig. 2.2 An individual using the EDNA system explores the functions of several soft graspable tangible user interfaces to draw and paint digitally

Supports Upper-Limb Interaction

Tabletop displays naturally support upper-limb interaction as the main form of user input. Approximately 85% of brain-injured patients suffer acute impairment to their upper body, and most patients regard the return of upper-limb function as a high priority (McCrea et al., 2002). This is no surprise as activities for daily living and self-care, such as feeding, grooming, toileting, and dressing, all require object manipulation using the arms. The EDNA tabletop interface is configured to enable the user to reach, grasp, lift, and place physical objects (or TUIs) in an interactive environment. The horizontal display and TUIs logically constrain user movement within a defined (planar) area above the table. The task constraints include the ways in which the TUIs can be held, moved, and stabilized in relation to the environment projected on the tabletop display and reinforced by audiovisual feedback. By reducing the number of alternative actions that can be performed by the patient in the early phase of recovery, we make explicit the functionality of the user interface to perform a certain task or function. Varying the task and environmental constraints is designed to increase the patient's ability to plan and initiate movements over time. For example, in some tasks the size, distance to, and shape of target locations are variable, as is the nature of the response goal (touch or avoid).

Supports Multimodal Communication

Tabletop environments support multimodal forms of communication between co-located users (Piper & Hollan, 2009). For example, the configuration of EDNA enables a close visible relationship between the patient and the therapist. The therapist can supervise the patient's activities and provide feedback, encouragement, and prompts. Patients can explore, learn, and share how new movements can be performed and validate these actions in direct communication with the therapist. In addition, as performance improves, patients can actively discuss and select with the therapist the environments they wish to use as part of their therapy.

Supports Embodied Interaction

Tabletop interaction supports an embodied, first-person experience of user interaction, one that capitalizes on our physical skills and our familiarity with real-world objects (Dourish, 2001). An embodied perspective of human interaction with computer technology is consistent with ecological approaches to movement rehabilitation. The term "ecological" in psychology refers to the view that behavior or action can only be fully appreciated by understanding the nature of the interaction between the individual, the task at hand, and the structure of physical and social environment

(Gibson, 1979). In rehabilitation, an ecological approach refers to the degree of relevance or similarity that a therapeutic activity has relative to the "real" world and in its value for improving a patient's everyday functioning (Rizzo, 2005). A key feature of tabletop displays is their capacity to integrate and support the manipulation of physical objects such as TUIs in ways that are natural to the user's body and their environment (Ishii, 2008). TUIs placed on the tabletop are the primary means for users to control features and events within the EDNA virtual environment. The shape and physical weight of each TUI offers the patient varying perceptual motor cues for action. For example, the TUI design assists patients to relearn perceptual motor skills akin to lifting a cup, tumbler, or similar-sized object and refine control while moving it. These simple actions offer some element of real-world human experience through the ways one might manipulate real-world objects.

Design Characteristics of Tabletop Interfaces for Group Rehabilitation

Supporting a game design framework for group rehabilitation, this section considers related work on tabletop interface design for co-located interaction in shared workspaces. We identify the socio-physical characteristics of co-located environments that designers should consider when developing rehabilitation applications. More specifically, we explore constructs and sub-themes from interactive tabletop research that may influence the design of co-located systems for rehabilitation, (1) physical space, (2) group awareness, (3) territoriality, and (4) interaction simultaneity (Fig. 2.3), and consider how each construct and their sub-themes can be expressed in particular design solutions for rehabilitation of ABI in a group setting.

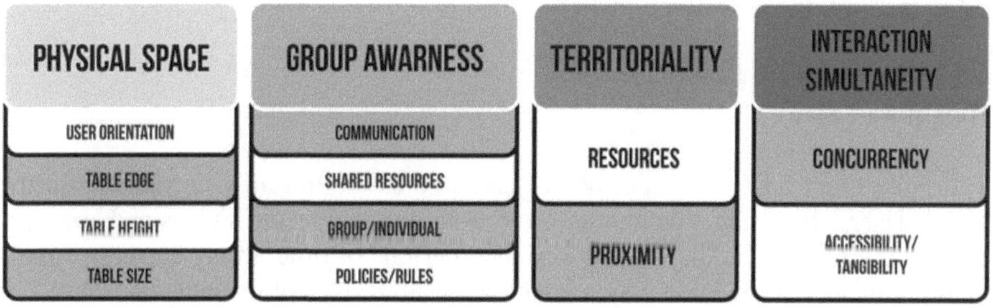

Fig. 2.3 Four characteristics and sub-themes defined within interactive tabletop research

Physical Space

The physical space surrounding tabletop displays can influence the dynamics of co-located interaction. More specifically, the arrangement of users and table ergonomics (height, size, and table edge) has basic implications in the design of applications for tabletop interfaces.

User Orientation

The spatial orientation of users around tabletop displays has been shown to influence how individuals comprehend information, coordinate actions between one another, and communicate in a collaborative setting (Kruger et al., 2003). Tasks may support the arrangement of users sitting side by side, but other tasks may support users sitting opposite one another depending on the orientation of the information displayed. Other findings have shown user position affects the level of participation across a tabletop surface (Rick et al., 2009). The level of participation is partially dependent on how well a participant is able to physically reach across the table (Toney & Thomas, 2006). Also there is a generalized preference for users to interact within the region of the display closest to their body (Scott & Carpendale, 2010). This has basic implications for the design of tabletop interfaces that enhance group cohesion and provide space for collaboration. The software design will affect how groups of participants partition the tabletop display and whether this is scaled optimally to the physical ability of the users.

Table Edge

Other physical attributes such as the shape and width of the non-interactive edge surrounding the display can assist how interactivity is managed (Muller-Tomfelde & O'Hara, 2010). For example, the size of the rim around the tabletop display can enable users to rest their arms without interfering with the interactive area of the display. The rim can also influence how physical resources (e.g., papers, TUIs) are arranged and selected for use both on and off the display during performance (Muller-Tomfelde & O'Hara, 2010).

Height and Size

The table must have sufficient height and size to comfortably accommodate the group. Users should be able to maneuver around the table and sit or stand comfortably facing toward the display for extended periods of time. Many current systems incorporate technology that may render one or more sides of the table unusable. For a detailed review of these systems, see Muller-Tomfelde & Fjeld, 2010. For easy access, active sides of the table should be free of encumbrances such as rear projection equipment or display attachments. Accessibility is a common issue for ABI patients who may have postural difficulty in sitting and standing. Physical obstructions may impact on their level of comfort and interfere with their interactions with others.

Group Awareness

Awareness is regarded as the first step in self-regulation and plays an important role in skill development (Ravizza, 2010). Group awareness is the degree to which people perceive and understand others' existence and activities in a shared task (Nacenta et al., 2010). The ability of interactive tabletops to support awareness of others' actions is often cited as one of the main benefits of collaborative face-to-face learning (Rick et al., 2011). Participants can observe and learn from how others are directly manipulating objects. Awareness of what others in a group are thinking and doing is also essential in coordinating collaborative learning and achieving common goals around a shared tabletop. Such learning is effective when the tabletop is a shared resource, participants using gesture and moving icons to communicate their ideas and understanding to others (Fleck et al., 2009).

Communication

Communication patterns in co-located groups, including the use of gesture, have been examined in various ways (Beattie & Shovelton, 1999), (Goldin-Meadow, 2003). Both communication and participation increase when groups interact around a tabletop display (Rogers & Lindley, 2004). Tabletop games have been used effectively to develop social skills and foster collaboration in children and adolescents, including those with autism spectrum disorder (Battochi, 2009; Piper et al., 2006).

Shared Resources

Providing shared access to physical and digital artifacts can help maintain group focus and facilitate group awareness (Rogers et al., 2009). Moreover, tabletop interfaces can be designed to enable more equitable participation and sharing among members of the group (Battochi, 2009; Harris et al., 2009; Marshall et al., 2008); Piper & Hollan, 2009), although sometimes groups work well together when one person dominates the action (Rick et al., 2011).

Groups/Individual and Policies/Rules

Differences in the way tabletop interactions are designed affect individual and group processes and thus participants' experiences. Nacenta et al. considered three perspectives in the design of tabletop interactions (Nacenta et al., 2010). The *action perspective* refers to whether local space or shared space is used to provide input for the technique and display the action's output. The *person perspective* differentiates physical and virtual embodiments for people in shared workspaces. The *group perspective* deals with policies and rules that govern interactions and provide support for those participating. The elements of these three design perspectives have differing effects on the criteria used to evaluate interaction techniques. Nacenta et al. found higher levels of awareness when input and output are in shared space; objects are manipulated through direct-input techniques such as touching, dragging, and lifting; and participants are represented by their physical body.

Territoriality

The notion of territoriality has its roots in both ethology and more recently in evolutionary psychology and ecological psychology. In essence it refers to the spatial area that an individual or group lays some claim to (Hall, 1966). Related to this is the notion of peripersonal space, which is the perceived boundary within which personal actions are performed (Previc, 1998), as distinct from those of others. These spatial frameworks bias our behavior according to the location of objects in the environment relative to the self and their reward or resource value to the species. Put another way, territorial behavior is bound up with the notion of resource and its proximity.

Resources

These resources are traditionally environmental (like food sources or nesting sites) but can also be other valued commodities like a site where a valued object is situated (like a cache of money or jewels) (Hinsch & Komdeur, 2010). Importantly, in advanced human behavior, resources can be purely symbolic (like a token that can be exchanged later for some reward). This capacity of the human mind enables resources and the experience of reward to be extended in time; that is, the physical object does not need to be physically present to elicit territorial behavior. However, the symbolic value of a resource can be highlighted by the use of salient physical cues.

Accordingly, a range of nonverbal factors influences territoriality and the notion and experience of personal space. Edward T. Hall delineated at least six such factors that influence how humans and non-humans position themselves in relation to each other: visual, touch, kinesthetic, voice loudness, thermal, and olfactory (Hall, 1963).

This approach has some useful implications for interaction design insofar as some combination of these cues can be manipulated using the display and user interfaces to alter the performer's perception of personal space and territory.

In the sphere of virtual rehabilitation, for example, these nonverbal factors can be manipulated in strategic ways to compensate for the impaired processing capacities of the patient, post-injury. For example, sound pitch and/or loudness might be used to signal a form of interaction with a tangible interface, perhaps inviting manipulation on the one hand or signaling that an approach might infringe on the territory and resources of another person. This scenario can also be imbedded within the context of a game where permitted actions are defined by both physical and symbolic cues.

Proximity

Research also suggests that the physical size of the tabletop display can impact the social interaction and working strategies among groups of users (Ryall, 2004). For example, physical size may engender a particular style of interaction when there is a clear perception of personal and/or group territory (Scott & Carpendale, 2010). The table size directly impacts the physical proximity between individuals around a display, which can change how they collaborate when performing individual and group tasks. A smaller table ensures all users can reach every part of the table, which may encourage them to negotiate and collaborate. By comparison, partitioning the display environment and orientating parts of the graphics to each user may support both personal and group spaces on the table and transitions between personal and group work (Scott et al., 2003).

Territoriality can be used as an organizing principle in the design of rehabilitation tasks. The proximity of users should be considered carefully so that interactions within a person's intimate or peripersonal space do not feel socially awkward. The location of the patients and the scale of the workspace, considered together with rules of interaction and the number of resources, can define how a co-located space is utilized and explored in rehabilitation. Depending on the rules by which resources are collected and distributed, different modes of interaction may be afforded, some cooperative, some playful, and some competitive. Each mode of interaction may achieve slightly different therapeutic ends in the realm of motor rehabilitation. For example, competition for resources in a discrete space, under time pressure, may enhance the reward value for patients while also encouraging faster actions. Although little is known about how groups of patients with brain injury interact with each other in rehabilitation, tabletop displays may offer ways for patients to relearn social skills and sense of personal space that may be adversely affected as a result of their injury.

Interface Simultaneity

Unlike single-user interfaces such as desktop computers, tabletop technology can support multiple interfaces for collaborative work. TUIs can be selected, passed around, manipulated, and shared by groups of users (Rogers et al., 2009). With groups of users comes the possibility for individuals to interact simultaneously with others and the tabletop interface.

Concurrency

Concurrent interaction among groups enables a wider variety of collaboration styles, including working in parallel, working sequentially in tightly coupled activities, working independently, and working in assumed roles (Scott et al., 2003). Scott et al. suggest concurrent interaction enables the user to focus on the task at hand rather than monitoring others in order to tell when the system is available. Rogers et al.'s findings indicate that shareable interfaces promote more group participation, highly coordinated forms of collaboration, and verbal communication when tabletops support multiple points of interaction. Importantly, they suggest more tangible and accessible interfaces may consequently encourage greater participation from people who normally find it difficult to communicate verbally or those who simply find contributing in a group setting socially challenging.

Accessibility/Tangibility

A key advantage of tabletop displays is that the technology supports tangible interaction using multiple physical input devices and multi-touch input (Muller-Tomfelde & Fjeld, 2010). Conventional interfaces like keyboard and mouse tend to neglect the intrinsic importance of body movement and tangible interaction (Djajadiningrat & Matthews, 2007) and limit opportunities for relearning movements among brain-injured patients. Physical input devices or TUIs, however, can exploit multiple human sensory channels otherwise neglected in conventional interfaces and can promote rich and dexterous interaction (Ishii & Ullmer, 1997).

The development of these naturalistic interfaces for user interaction is essential to optimize performance and improve access for patients with cognitive and motor impairments (Rizzo, 2005). The form factor of the interfaces should take into account the deficits experienced by patients. Brain-injured patients frequently suffer perceptual difficulties in auditory and visual functions, perception of objects, impaired space and distance judgment, and difficulty with orientation. High-contrast colors and simple graspable shapes, for example, were used in the design of the EDNA system to assist a visually impaired user to individuate each interface and ease cognitive overload.

Game Design Characteristics for Group-Based Motor Rehabilitation

Building upon the design characteristics of group work environments, co-located game-orientated rehabilitation may provide patients with a more comprehensive social experience that is playful and engaging. Indeed, rehabilitation game design that supports social co-located play has been shown to evoke stronger social engagement and increased levels of enjoyment (Gajadhar et al., 2009). To develop rehabilitation tabletop games, developers and designers need to be aware of the patient's particular needs, deficits, the characteristics of group social interactions, and how these relate game mechanics particular to tabletop interfaces. Recent findings suggest the principles of game design relevant to acquired brain injury rehabilitation include meaningful play that translates into learning outcomes; handling the level of failure in game play so as to maintain patient engagement; setting adaptable challenges, rules, and goals appropriate to the abilities of the individual user; and the setting of game reward structures to assist in motivation and tracking the progress of the patient over time (Burke et al., 2009). Furthermore, the social aspects of gaming such as shared user interfaces may provide patients with other important avenues for learning (Xu et al., 2001). As shown in Fig. 2.4, we consider how these game design elements might be used for brain injury rehabilitation in a co-located group context using tabletop interfaces.

Feedback

Feedback is a central feature of most games that is provided to the player in response to some action. Typically, this involves the player performing an action that has some causal effect within the game. The feedback then informs how the next action can be performed to progress in the game.

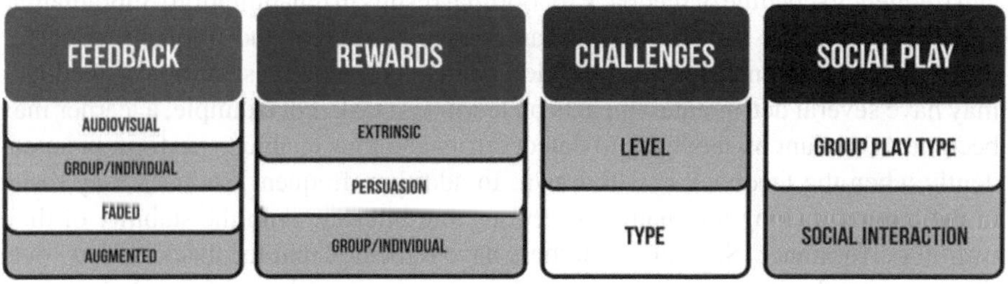

Fig. 2.4 Four characteristics and sub-themes of computer game design

Audiovisual Feedback

In movement rehabilitation contexts, audiovisual feedback provides the patient with additional functions that revolve around understanding the nature of their movement and overall performance. Feedback provides patients with additional knowledge of the outcomes of their actions to refine decision-making and movement planning over time (Wilson, 2012). The audiovisual feedback can also direct the patient to focus their attention on the external effects of their movement, rather than the internal biomechanics of the movement itself. A review of motor learning techniques indicates that internally focused movement can result in slow, consciously controlled movement that disrupts performance (Wulf & Prinz, 2001). Wulf et al. emphasize that externally focusing the user's attention on the anticipated effects of movement may enhance learning. They observe that an external focus and extrinsic feedback lead to more rapid, natural, and autonomous actions (van Vliet & Wulf, 2006).

Augmented Feedback (AF)

Augmented feedback (AF) in rehabilitation refers to the provision of additional sensory information paired with movement [e.g., changing the pitch of a sound based on the speed of arm movement (Duckworth & Wilson, 2010)] and is generated by the system to reinforce the patient's sense of position in space. In motor learning theory, feedback is provided to the learner about their movement patterns or knowledge of performance (KP), as well as feedback about the outcome of the movement or knowledge of results (KR). For example, a therapist's (post-performance) feedback to a learner about their movement trajectory is a form of KP. Feedback provided by the system itself in real time is regarded as concurrent AF (Wilson, 2012).

Faded Feedback

The use of KP and KR in game design can provide task-related information about the skill being learned. However, there is limited evidence to support the amount and frequency schedule of feedback for optimal results in rehabilitation (Subramanian et al., 2010). While modern digital games give consistent and frequent feedback, this may be detrimental for rehabilitation games. Frequent presentation of feedback may have several detrimental impacts on learning a task. For example, a learner may become too reliant on feedback to detect errors and thus unable to perform independently when the feedback is withdrawn. In addition, frequent feedback may result in the learner making too many corrections that interfere with the stability of their overall performance. Several researchers have indicated that feedback "faded" over time compared with a continuous schedule may be more beneficial to longer-term retention and learning (Hemayattablab & Rostami, 2010; Winstein & Schmidt,

1990). However, more research is required to establish how the frequency and intensity of feedback in games can best be utilized to enhance real-world outcomes.

Our initial discussion with therapists suggests that complete therapist control over the presentation of KP, KR, and concurrent AF (i.e., augmented audiovisual feedback) is desirable. As such, in EDNA, from a default (off) setting, the therapist can select a variety of feedback options (Fig. 2.5). In this way, the therapist can adapt the frequency of the feedback and task variables to the appropriate level to suit the client and their progress.

Group/Individual Feedback

Tabletop media offer unique instances of how feedback can be presented to the patient, particularly in a group setting. Feedback may be targeted to an individual, the group or both. For example, private feedback in a shared environment context can be provided in a user's local space directly in front them. Depending on the size of the tabletop display, a local space may not be easy for other users to see or reach. Morris et al. report that in a shared learning environment private feedback assisted in reducing potential embarrassment over incorrect actions by not highlighting them to the entire group (Morris et al., 2006). This can be used to highlight the different roles for users in a shared game environment.

Activities on tabletop displays are generally designed for shared activities. Individual feedback that others can see as well as feedback on the group performance on a shared task can be designed to facilitate awareness of others' actions (Nacenta et al., 2010; Rick et al., 2011). In this way, participants might learn by

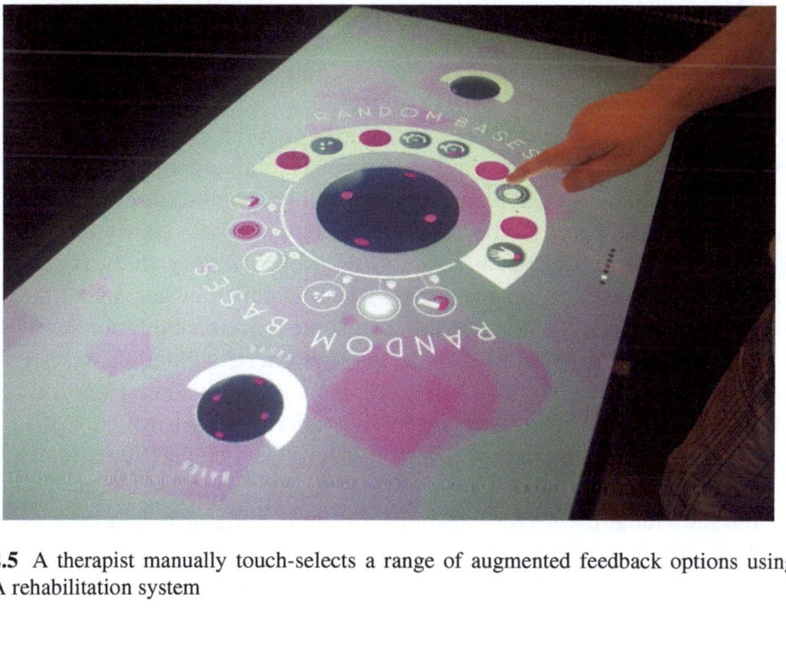

Fig. 2.5 A therapist manually touch-selects a range of augmented feedback options using the EDNA rehabilitation system

observing and imitating others' performance, thereby enlisting higher levels of attention and concentration in users.

Reward Structures

Reward structures in games are designed to intrinsically motivate engagement in game challenges and increase expenditure of effort (Wang & Sun, 2011). Intrinsic motivation refers to a person's free will of doing an activity for its inherent satisfaction rather than for some consequence external to the individual or activity (Przybylski et al., 2010). Game-related rewards can take many different forms including experience points, resources, item unlocks, achievements, and feedback messages (Wang & Sun, 2011). These incentives might lead to increased enjoyment that in turn motivates the player to complete a particular task and reach certain goals.

Extrinsic Rewards

The purpose of a reward may be to allow players to experience challenge as well as demonstrate mastery and is understood to be extrinsically motivating. In movement rehabilitation contexts, reward structures may be linked to performance accomplishments. For example, movements of different complexity or time engaged in play may be rewarded using a scoring mechanism. Rewards might occur on multiple levels, from moment-to-moment to cumulative rewards based on overall performance. Game rewards such as scoring can help the performer assess their own capability to perform a certain task and can foster feelings of autonomy and self-efficacy (Burke et al., 2009). In general, extrinsic rewards in games can provide a means of self-assessment and comparison that satisfy the innate desire for competence and self-determination (Burke et al., 2009).

In a recent study, use of operant conditioning in a rehabilitation game targeting manual action was found to increase participants' motivation to play longer (Shah et al., 2014). A combination of parameters including reward scores, activity bonuses, and aversive stimuli that reset the game to the beginning was shown to increase the level of enjoyment and player motivation. However, further study is required to evaluate whether operant conditioning in games can translate into longer-term acquisition of motor skills. It is possible that short-term rehabilitation rewards may need to be different from those meant for longer-term rehabilitation. Rewards given semi-randomly may be an optimal solution to enhance motivation (Deci et al., 1999).

As a note of caution, strategies that focus primarily on extrinsic rewards to control behavior may undermine intrinsic motivation (Deci et al., 1999). Such rewards (particularly tangible ones like money) tend to quell self-regulation, or in other words the individual taking responsibility for motivating or regulating themselves (Deci et al., 1999). Extrinsic rewards may inadvertently impose values on behavior and status, may not be well understood, and are not universally appreciated (Antin

& Churchill, 2011; Salen & Zimmerman, 2003). Having said this, the effects of extrinsic game rewards such as player achievements, trophies, and badges are not well understood in the context of game-orientated rehabilitation. The mainstream literature would suggest that these rewards may reduce intrinsic motivation over time (Deci et al., 1999).

Persuasion

Other than operant conditioning rewards, verbal persuasion that provides encouragement or information about performance may be of benefit. For example, in EDNA we provide short positive messages as a form of reward at the end of each task. These messages are generally encouraging and humorous in tone and we are careful not to introduce value judgments. In the case of severe brain injury, it may be desirable to reward all engagement with success in the initial stages of game play. By doing so, failure is dealt with in a positive way rather than highlighting the player's impaired capabilities.

Group/Individual Rewards

Rewards in a group setting add social dimensions that may motivate game play, foster social relationships, and encourage social interactions between players. Many games require players to work together cooperatively to complete a goal such as collecting resources. Rewards that show group achievement can enhance feelings of belonging and team building. In the case of rehabilitation, team rewards may add a social component that enables the player to feel strongly committed to remain in the game and work together with other players to develop strategies to maximize the reward. The social aspects of game rewards may enable players with severe impairments to find new ways to increase communication and social support related to their health issues. Indeed, recent surveys with stroke patients indicate that the opportunity for social interaction as part of rehabilitation is a key motivation to participate in therapy (Lewis & Rosie, 2012).

Game Challenges

The level of challenge in games is a primary mechanism to increase player engagement with the game. In general, the level of difficulty in a game is designed to gradually increase as the game progresses to maintain a level of challenge for the player.

Challenge Level

In motor rehabilitation it is unlikely that designers will know the skills and capabilities of players in advance. A range of movement tasks may seem trivial for some patients while challenging (and often painful) for many others. For optimal player engagement, games should present an ideal level of challenge for each individual player that is neither too difficult that it becomes frustrating nor too easy that the player loses interest (Salen & Zimmerman, 2003). Dynamic difficulty adjustments are of particular importance in games for rehabilitation.

Games for rehabilitation should be designed so that the therapist can always set the level of difficulty according to their assessment of the patient's capabilities. Typically, video games use levels to structure difficulty. For example, new game levels are made available to the player on completion of the previous ones. As the game progresses, each successive level builds upon the skills and knowledge acquired by the player, requiring the acquisition of new skills or fine-tuning of existing skills as the difficulty increases with each new level. Challenges used in this example allow the player to progress only after once they understand enough of the game play.

Challenge Type

There are many different types of challenges in games. Chris Crawford provides a list including cerebellar, sensorimotor, and spatial reasoning, pattern recognition, sequential reasoning, numerical reasoning, resource management, and social reasoning (Crawford, 2003). Within rehabilitation game design, the preferred challenges are based on sensorimotor skills, which are the skills used to throw a balled-up piece of paper into a waste paper basket. Placing a TUI accurately onto an onscreen target used in the EDNA system is a good example of this. These skills may be mixed with other types of challenges such as spatial reasoning and pattern recognition.

Spatial reasoning is commonly used in puzzles such as Tetris and when combined with sensorimotor learning can create a variety of potential rehabilitation games. It is possible to create puzzles that can enhance sensorimotor learning. Pattern recognition is useful for *boss* fights, an enemy-based challenge usually at the end of a video game level. In order to overcome the *boss*, game players may need to learn its attack patterns in terms of both attack frequency and movement. This may be useful in rehabilitation contexts where a specific movement may need to be learned repeatedly.

Social Play

Social play can be categorized into collaborative, cooperative, and competitive play (Crawford, 2003). These types of game play can be designed to influence a range of social interaction between players.

Group Play Type

In rehabilitation games, competitive play may be a poor design choice as the existence of competition means that there are winners and losers. Losers may experience reduced motivation to continue with therapy, which is undesirable. In addition, it may be difficult to match players with similar skills and abilities due to the diversity of impairments experienced by individuals with brain injury. Restricting or enhancing game features to carefully balance the abilities of each player with others may provide a strategy in creating a level playing field.

In contrast, in both collaborative and cooperative game play, individuals play a game together to achieve a desired outcome. In collaborative game play, individuals form a team that obtains the game's objective. In cooperative game play, individuals may choose to form a team, but each will receive their own benefits from their cooperation. Group play in general is seen as beneficial and may facilitate vicarious learning when individuals can observe and imitate each other's behavior. Observing others' success in accomplishing certain tasks provides a sense of self-efficacy to the observer that they might also have the ability to accomplish the task.

One of the guiding factors in encouraging true collaborative play is to encourage selfless decisions by bestowing different abilities or responsibilities upon the players (Crawford, 2003). In rehabilitation games this is beneficial since different individuals will likely have different strengths and weaknesses. This also reduces the tension involved in a group setting where individuals may see each other's abilities and compare themselves to the other participants (Aarts et al., 2012).

Social Interaction

Most co-located video games direct players to focus attention on a common wall-mounted screen but not on other players. This configuration hinders social interaction and reduces opportunity for more complex interpersonal communication. Tabletop display interfaces offer several advantages in this regard by offering a shared workspace where users can clearly observe the actions of others face-to-face, communicate in a collaborative setting, and coordinate activities between each other. Furthermore, studies indicate that co-located face-to-face play provides additional fun, challenge, and perceived competence in games (Kruger et al., 2003). Studies indicate that co-located play increases player enjoyment through shared attention, increased motivation, higher arousal, and performance contingent on the social context of the game setting (Gajadhar et al., 2009).

The ability to give players different roles in a shared game environment also enhances the ability for players to play the game many times. By changing roles players can experience the same game but from a different perspective incorporating unique challenges and rewards specific to the character. This is partially what makes role-playing fantasy games playable over long periods of time.

Discussion: A Game Design Framework for Tabletop Motor Rehabilitation

We have discussed eight key design parameters in the context of developing multi-user rehabilitation games for tabletop displays. We maintain that tabletop rehabilitation activities that incorporate game design challenges, judicious rewards, meaningful feedback, and co-located social play afford a powerful therapeutic tool to engage individuals with brain injury socially in rehabilitation and motivate them to persist in therapy. A critical predictor of success in therapy is time on task, together with high levels of user engagement and investment in the activity (de Kort et al., 2007). For designers, the critical task is to find a balance between these key ingredients.

Figure 2.6 shows the ICF model combined with the design parameters discussed in this chapter. This framework may be used for developing co-located games that support participation and social engagement within motor rehabilitation contexts. The framework may be useful for analysis and conceptual guidance for design of interactive environments for movement learning. The framework is organized on three levels of abstraction. Themes on the first (top) level are derived from the ICF model. The second and third levels are derived from concepts in game design and the social dimensions of human-computer interaction research, respectively. They provide analytical tools to guide the design process. The framework is not prescriptive and thus may need to be interpreted, expanded, and otherwise made appropriate for other therapeutic contexts.

This model highlights the design principles developers may consider and how they might be applied to create games in a group therapeutic setting. With respect to activity, both the level of challenges and mode of interaction will determine the design of the task as well as the level of participation. Users must be fully engaged in the activity, which presupposes some discretion or independence in selecting game attributes and the level of challenge.

Environmental factors are important in a therapeutic context where patients may initially be hesitant about working in a group of people they do not know and reluctant to reveal their level of disability. This is particularly relevant when players can see the performance feedback of others. The challenge for the designer is to consider carefully how, when, and in what form feedback (both real time and in

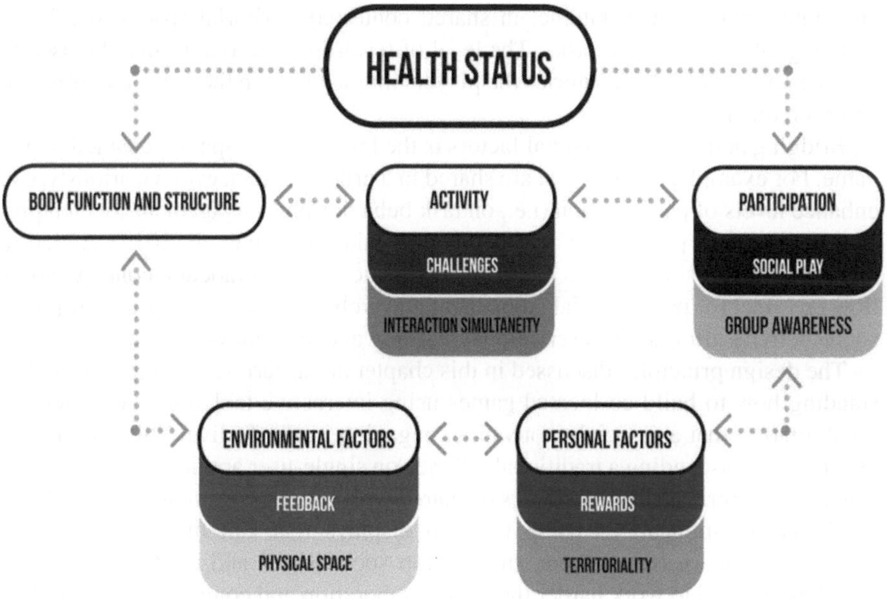

Fig. 2.6 The ICF model integrated with the design parameters

summary) is supplied to the performer and reduce potential cognitive overload. Indeed, the take-home message is "more is not always better." A good example of this is the use of Nintendo Wii Fit games in rehabilitation where the effects of repeated failure are made apparent in the game avatar combined with discouraging comments (de Kort et al., 2007). Related to this point, a shared physical space can be structured in ways that assist a patient group to develop an alliance and shared agenda. For example, a simple tabletop game can be set up that requires the group to work together and compete against the computer to score points. How patients will collaborate with each other and the possible consequences of participation are less predictable. For the practitioner, the ability to manipulate the physical workspace (and territories) can, in turn, cater to patients with different needs and skill levels.

Embedding appropriate reward structures and facilitating space for players required to interact effectively in the game environment relate to personal factors. To facilitate user engagement, designers and therapists should consult clients during the research and development phase to ensure that game rewards are presented in an appropriate format or in a way that is motivationally significant. It is important that both extrinsic and intrinsic forms of reward be considered and how these are integrated over different time scales – short term and longer term. Short-term rewards may promote persistence in the game and enable users to learn basic game rules. But this does not necessarily translate to persistence over extended time, from session to session and month to month. Combined with rewards is the personal space required to interact comfortably with other co-located players. To achieve rewards and status, players may interact in shared contested territorial spaces to achieve certain goals and perform tasks. The level of reward and resources may be used to balance and control the territories the players interact with in the game environment and each other.

Bridging activity and personal factors is the level of participation enabled by the game. For example, rewards that are shared in a group context, even vicariously, can enhance levels of participation (i.e., on task behavior plus engagement), which predicts longer-term persistence and therapeutic gains (Lange et al., 2012). Added to this are (i) the positive effects of social engagement in a therapeutic context and its flow on effect for psychosocial adjustment and well-being and (ii) the opportunities social activity affords for observational learning and awareness of others.

The design principles discussed in this chapter are a starting point toward understanding how to build co-located games using interactive tabletops for movement rehabilitation that are social, motivating, engaging, and effective. This presents an avenue for transcending a traditional reliance on single-user applications. By understanding the intrinsic characteristics of shared workspaces, we aim to develop therapeutic group applications using tabletop displays that can maximize patients' potential to "learn from others," to develop social skills and confidence, and to instill motivation to work harder through collaboration and competition with fellow patients. Our principled approach to interface design that supports groups of patients will hopefully make brain-injured individuals more willing to persist in rehabilitation, ultimately speeding their recovery.

Acknowledgments This work is supported by an Australian Research Council (ARC) Linkage Grant LP110200802 and Synapse Grant awarded by the Australia Council for the Arts.

References

Aarts, P. B., et al. (2012). The pirate group intervention protocol: Description and a case report of a modified constraint-induced movement therapy combined with bimanual training for young children with unilateral spastic cerebral palsy. *Occupational Therapy International, 19*(2), 76–87.

Antin, J., & Churchill, E. F. (2011). *Badges in social media: A social psychological perspective* (CHI 2011). AMC.

Battochi, A. (2009). *Collaborative puzzle game: A tabletop interactive game for fostering collaboration in children with Autism Spectrum Disorders (ASD)* (ITS '09) (pp. 197–204). AMC Press.

Beattie, G., & Shovelton, H. (1999). Do iconic hand gestures really contribute anything to the semantic information conveyed by speech? An experimental investigation. *Semiotica, 123*, 1–2(1).

Burke, J. W., et al. (2009). Optimising engagement for stroke rehabilitation using serious games. *The Visual Computer, 25*(12), 1085–1099.

Crawford, C. (2003). *Chris Crawford on game design*. New Riders.

de Kort, Y. A. W., et al. (2007). *People, places, and play: A research framework for digital game experience in a socio-spatial context*. DiGRA.

Deci, E. L., et al. (1999). A meta-analytic review of experiments examining the effects of extrinsic rewards on intrinsic motivation. *Psychological Bulletin, 152*(6), 627–668.

Dietz, P., & Leigh, D. (2001). DiamondTouch: A multi-user touch technology. In *Proceedings of the 14th annual ACM symposium on User interface software and technology* (pp. 219–226). ACM.
Djajadiningrat, T., & Matthews, B. (2007). Easy doesn't do it: Skill and expression in tangible aesthetics. *Personal and Ubiquitous Computing, 11*, 657–676.
Dourish, P. (2001). *Where the action is: The foundations of embodied interaction*. MIT Press.
Duckworth, J., & Wilson, P. H. (2010). Embodiment and play in designing an interactive art system for movement rehabilitation. *Second Nature, 2*(1), 120–137.
Duckworth, J., et al. (2019). Interactive arts and disability: A conceptual model toward understanding participation. In *Interactivity, game creation, design, learning, and innovation* (pp. 524–538). Springer.
Eliasson, A.-C., et al. (2003). Clinical experience of constraint induced movement therapy in adolescents with hemiplegic cerebral palsy–a day camp model. *Developmental Medicine & Child Neurology, 45*(05), 357–360.
Esbensen, A. J., et al. (2003). Reliability and validity of an assessment instrument for anxiety, depression, and mood among individuals with mental retardation. *Journal of Autism and Developmental Disorders, 33*(6), 617–629.
Fleck, R., et al. (2009). *Actions speak loudly with words: Unpacking collaboration around the table*. Its '09, New York.
Gajadhar, B., et al. (2009). Rules of engagement: Influence of co-player presence on player involvement in digital games. *International Journal of Gaming and Computer-Mediated Simulations, 1*(3), 14–27.
Gibson, J. J. (1979). *The ecological approach to visual perception*. Houghton Mifflin.
Giusti, L., et al. (2011). *Dimensions of collaboration on a tabletop interface for children with autism spectrum disorder* (CHI 2011). AMC Press.
Goldin-Meadow, S. (2003). *Hearing gesture: How our hands help us think*. Harvard University Press.
Granlund, M. (2013). Participation–challenges in conceptualization, measurement and intervention. *Child: Care, Health and Development, 39*(4), 470–473.
Green, D., et al. (2013). A multi-site study of functional outcomes following a themed approach to hand–arm bimanual intensive therapy for children with hemiplegia. *Developmental Medicine & Child Neurology, 55*(6), 527–533.
Hall, E. T. (1963). A system for the notation of Proxemic behavior. *American Anthropologist, 65*(5), 1003–1026.
Hall, E. T. (1966). *The hidden dimension*. Garden City, Double Day.
Han, J. F. (2005). *Low-cost multi-touch sensing through frustrated total internal reflection* (p. 2005). UIST.
Harris, A., et al. (2009). *Around the table: Are multiple-touch surfaces better than single-touch for children's collaborative interactions?* (CSCL '09). ISLS.
Hemayattablab, R., & Rostami, L. R. (2010). The effects of feedback on the learning of motor skills in individuals with cerebral palsy. *Research in Developmental Disabilities, 31*, 212–217.
Hinsch, M., & Komdeur, J. (2010). Defence, intrusion and the evolutionary stability of territoriality. *Journal of Theoretical Biology, 266*(266), 606–613.
House, A., & Hosker, C. (2013). Emotional disorders in neurological rehabilitation. *Neurological Rehabilitation: Handbook of Clinical Neurology, 110*, 389–398.
Ishii, H. (2008). *Tangible bits: beyond pixels* (TEI '08) (pp. xv–xxv). AMC Press.
Ishii, H., & Ullmer, B. (1997). Tangible bits: Towards seamless interfaces between people, bits and atoms. In *SIGCHI conference on human factors in computing systems, Atlanta, GA*. ACM Press.
Kharrufa, A., et al. (2010). *Digital mysteries: Designing for learning at the tabletop* (ITS 2010). AMC Press.
Kruger, R., et al. (2003). *How people use orientation on tables: Comprehension, coordination and communication* (GROUP '03). AMC Press.
Lange, B., et al. (2012). Designing informed game-based rehabilitation tasks leveraging advances in virtual reality. *Disability and Rehabilitation, 34*(22), 1863–1870.

Lewis, G., & Rosie, J. A. (2012). Virtual reality games for movement rehabilitation in neurological conditions: How do we meet the needs and expectations of the users? *Disability and Rehabilitation, 34*(22), 1880–1886.
Marshall, P., et al. (2008). *When the fingers do the talking: A study of group participation with varying constraints to a tabletop interface* (TABLETOP '08). IEEE Computer Society.
McCrea, P. H., et al. (2002). Biomechanics of reaching: Clinical implications for individuals with acquired brain injury. *Disability and Rehabilitation, 24*(10), 534–541.
Morris, M. R., et al. (2006). Mediating group dynamics through tabletop interface design. *IEEE Computer Graphics and Applications, 26*(5), 65–73.
Muller-Tomfelde, C., & Fjeld, M. (2010). Introduction: A short history of tabletop research, technologies, and products. In C. Müller-Tomfelde (Ed.), *Tabletops – horizontal interactive displays* (pp. 1–24). Springer.
Muller-Tomfelde, C., & O'Hara, K. (2010). Horizontal interactive surfaces in distributed assemblies. In *Tabletops – horizontal interactive displays* (pp. 435–456). Springer.
Mumford, N., et al. (2010). Upper limb virtual rehabilitation for traumatic brain injury: Initial evaluation of the elements system. *Brain Injury, 24*(5), 780–791.
Mumford, N., et al. (2012). Upper-limb virtual rehabilitation for traumatic brain injury: A preliminary within-group evaluation of the elements system. *Brain Injury, 26*(2), 166–176.
Nacenta, M. A., et al. (2010). Individual and group support in tabletop interaction techniques. In C. Müller-Tomfelde (Ed.), *Tabletops – Horizontal interactive displays* (pp. 303–333). Springer-Verlag.
Piper, A. M., & Hollan, J. D. (2009). *Analyzing multimodal communication around a shared tabletop display* (ECSCW 2009). Springer.
Piper, A. M., et al. (2006). Sides: A cooperative tabletop computer game for social skills development. In *Proceedings of Computer-Supported Cooperative Work (CSCW)* (pp. 1–10).
Previc, F. H. (1998). The neuropsychology of 3-D space. *Psychological Bulletin, 124*, 123–164.
Przybylski, A. K., et al. (2010). A motivational model of video game engagement. *Review of General Psychology, 14*(2), 154–166.
Ravizza, K. (2010). Increasing awareness for sport performance. In J. M. Williams (Ed.), *Applied sport psychology: Personal growth to peak performance* (pp. 189–200). McGraw-Hill.
Rick, J., et al. (2009). *Children designing together on a multi-touch tabletop: An analysis of spatial orientation and user interactions*. IDC.
Rick, J., et al. (2011). *Beyond one-size-fits-all: How interactive tabletops support collaborative learning*. IDC.
Rizzo, A. A. (2005). A SWOT analysis of the field of virtual reality rehabilitation and therapy. *Presence, 14*(2), 119–146.
Rogers, Y., & Lindley, S. (2004). Collaborating around vertical and horizontal large interactive displays: Which way is best? *Interacting with Computers, 16*, 1133–1152.
Rogers, Y., et al. (2009). Equal opportunities: Do shareable interfaces promote more group participation than single user displays? *Human-Computer Interaction, 24*(1–2), 79–116.
Rogers, J. M., et al. (2019). Elements virtual rehabilitation improves motor, cognitive, and functional outcomes in adult stroke: Evidence from a randomized controlled pilot study. *Journal of Neuroengineering and Rehabilitation, 16*(1), 1–13.
Rosenbaum, P., & Stewart, D. (2004). The World Health Organization international classification of functioning, disability, and health: A model to guide clinical thinking, practice and research in the field of cerebral palsy. *Seminars in Pediatric Neurology, 11*(1), 5–10.
Rutter, M., et al. (2006). Continuities and discontinuities in psychopathology between childhood and adult life. *Journal of Child Psychology and Psychiatry, 47*(3–4), 276–295.
Ryall, K. (2004). *Exploring the effects of group size and table size on interactions with tabletop shared-display groupware* (CSCW 2004). AMC.
Salen, K., & Zimmerman, E. (2003). *Rules of play: Game design fundamentals*. MIT Press.
Scott, S., & Carpendale, S. (2010). In C. Müller-Tomfelde (Ed.), *Theory of tabletop territoriality* (pp. 357–385). Springer.

Scott, S., et al. (2003). System guidelines for co-located, collaborative work on a tabletop display. In *Proceedings of the 2003 eighth European conference on computer-supported cooperative work.*

Shah, N., et al. (2014). Design parameters in multimodal game for rehabilitation. *Games for Health Journal, 3*(1), 13–20.

Starkstein, S. E., & Pahissa, J. (2014). Apathy following traumatic brain injury. *Psychiatric Clinics of North America, 37*(1), 103–112.

Subramanian, S. K., et al. (2010). Does the provision of extrinsic feedback result in improved motor learning in the upper limb Poststroke? A systematic review of the evidence. *Neurorehabilitation and Neural Repair, 24*(2), 113–124.

Taylor, S. E., et al. (2011). Early adversity and adult health outcomes. *Development and Psychopathology, 23*(Special Issue 03), 939–954.

Toney, A., & Thomas, B. H. (2006). Considering reach in tangible and table top design. In *First IEEE international workshop on horizontal interactive human-computer systems (Tabletop '06)*. IEEE Computer Society.

Ullmer, B., & Ishii, H. (1997). *The metaDESK: Models and prototypes for tangible user interfaces* (UIST 1997) (pp. 223–232). ACM Press.

van Vliet, P. M., & Wulf, G. (2006). Extrinsic feedback for motor learning after stroke: What is the evidence? *Disability and Rehabilitation, 28*(13–14), 931–840.

Wang, H., & Sun, C. (2011). *Game reward systems: Gaming experiences and social meaning.* DiGRA 2011 Conference: Think Design Play.

Wellner, P. (1993). Interacting with paper on the digital desk. *Communications of the ACM, 36*(7), 87–96.

WHO. (2001). *The international classification of function, disability and health (ICF).* World Health Organization.

Wilson, P. (2012). Developmental cognitive neuroscience perspective on motor rehabilitation: The case for virtual reality-augmented therapy. In *Proceedings of the 9th international conference on disability, virtual reality and associated technologies.*

Winstein, C. J., & Schmidt, R. A. (1990). Reduced frequency of knowledge of results enhances motor skills learning. *Journal of Experimental Psychology: Learning, Memory, and Cognition, 16*(4), 677–691.

Wu, M., & Balakrishnan, R. (2003). *Multi-finger and whole hand gestural interaction techniques for multi-user tabletop displays* (UIST 2003) (pp. 193–202). AMC Press.

Wulf, G., & Prinz, W. (2001). Directing attention to movement effects enhances learning: A review. *Psychonomic Bulletin & Review, 8*(4), 648–660.

Xu, Y., et al. (2001). Chores are fun: Understanding social play in board games for digital tabletop game design. In *The fifth international conference of DiGRA.*

Chapter 3
The Role of VR Simulation and Game Technology in the Understanding and Treatment of Visual Impairments

James Lewis

Introduction

Visual impairments are the most common class of disability to effect society. Their impact can vary widely from the afflicted individual being virtually unaware of any problem, through to the complete loss of all vision. Some impairments such as colour blindness are untreatable lifelong genetic conditions which a person is born with. Others, for example, diabetic retinopathy, are acquired impairments that are becoming increasing prevalent in society as a result of lifestyle changes. A large number of impairments, in particular macular degeneration, cataract and glaucoma, are age related. Set against a context of an ageing population increasingly dependent upon visual communication channels such as television and the Internet, it is likely that the treatment and accommodation of visual impairments will become an increasingly significant global issue.

VR has a clear role to play in the training and education of the medical professionals who will be called upon to assist in the clinical treatment of the eye diseases that cause impairment. The sheer number of such operations, together with the impact that a surgical error could have upon an individual's quality of life, creates a significant demand for virtual simulators that can be used to train and rehearse these clinical processes in risk-free way.

For many visual impairments, early treatment can have a significant impact upon overall success. It is therefore unfortunate that one of the key factors likely to delay an individual from seeking treatment is a lack of awareness of the symptoms of visual impairments. There is a recognised need for the development of effective approaches to educate the wider public about how certain visual impairments will present themselves and to raise awareness of the importance of seeking early

J. Lewis (✉)
Nottingham Trent University, Computer Science, Nottingham, UK
e-mail: james.lewis@ntu.ac.uk

E. Brooks, D. J. Brown (eds.), *Virtual Reality Games for Rehabilitation*, Virtual Reality Technologies for Health and Clinical Applications,
https://doi.org/10.1007/978-1-0716-3371-7_3

treatment in order to ensure the optimal long-term outcome. This need to raise awareness does not only apply to individuals who already have or are at risk of developing a visual impairment.

A wider understanding of the nature of some visual impairments can increase the possibility of a carer or friend recognising a treatable condition and highlighting the need for treatment. Moreover, people who need to care for or work with visually impaired people can more effectively serve their needs if they have a clearer idea of how their visual impairment affects their perception of the world. This aspect of serving the needs of visually impaired people applies also to people who provide goods or services to them, to the architects who design the public spaces around which they are expected to move, the designers who layout print publications and web pages, the people who invent products which they are expected to operate and the marketeers who would seek to attract their business through advertising campaigns.

Virtual reality simulation and computer game technology can perform a variety of roles that can help to solve these problems. Games have been employed as preventative medicine to raise awareness of the diet and lifestyle choices that can lead to diabetes (DeShazo et al., 2010). Virtual reality technology can perform a valuable role as assistive technology, enabling visually impaired people to more easily understand and experience the world around them (Cooper & Taylor, 1998; Evett et al., 2009; Yu & Brewster, 2002). VR simulations have been developed to assist with the acquisition of the surgical skills required by significant numbers of medical staff, enabling them to carry out delicate procedures on a large segment of society with the aim of preserving or restoring visual acuity. Virtual reality simulations and image processing techniques can also be used to enable people with normal vision to begin to understand the impact that various visual impairments have upon how visually impaired people see the world. This chapter will review these approaches and highlight the role that virtual reality simulation and computer game technology can perform within the field of visual impairments.

Nature of the Impairments

Glaucoma

Glaucoma refers to a collection of conditions that are often related to a problematic increase in pressure within the eye. Glaucoma can go unnoticed for many years as visual symptoms often do not appear until the condition is well established. The increased intra-ocular pressure results in the degeneration and death of the ocular nerve cells, and it is this nerve damage that compromises vision. As the nerves are degraded, there is a reduction in the visual field, initially impacting upon the peripheral vision. A gradual reduction of peripheral vision can go unnoticed or be ignored as it does not have a profound impact upon day-to-day function. However, as the disease advances, the visual field is reduced to tiny islands and eventually, if untreated, vision loss becomes complete. Glaucoma has a prevalence of around 1 in 200 people under the age of 50, rising to 1 in 10 above the age of 80. Worldwide it is the second most frequent cause of blindness.

Cataracts

A cataract is an opaque discolouration affecting the crystalline lens of the eye. In general, they will develop in both eyes, though one eye may show more advanced symptoms than the other. Its development may be promoted by multiple causes including exposure to ultraviolet and infrared light and as a side effect of diabetes and hypertension. It is however more commonly associated with the ageing process. A loss of visual acuity is the first indication of cataract, as the opacity increases contrast sensitivity is reduced and colour vision will become less vivid, with a particular reduction at the blue end of the spectrum. Light scattering caused by the cataract can also create an impression of glare, exacerbating the problems. Cataract is the leading cause of blindness worldwide affecting 18 million people. Its incidence rate rises with age, affecting more than 90% of people aged over 75.

Age-Related Macular Degeneration

The macular region is a small area of colour-sensitive cells near the centre of the retina. The macular region is responsible for central, detailed vision. Age-related macular degeneration (AMD) takes two forms, the "wet" and "dry" forms of the disease. The dry form causes the cones in the macula to atrophy, thinning their density, and is generally regarded as untreatable. The wet form is caused by the growth of pathologic blood vessels behind the retina. It is the growth of these blood vessels that leads to bleeding, protein leaking and scarring, ultimately damaging the photoreceptors and leading to a loss in sensitivity. If treated early the growth of these blood vessels can be halted and even reversed with a subsequent recovery of vision. Left untreated the condition can result in a complete loss of central vision, making tasks such as reading, watching television or recognising faces impossible, though the residual peripheral vision can remain useful. The earliest signs of AMD are distortions in the visual field and straight lines can appear wavy. This is likely to be accompanied by a loss of visual acuity. People with the condition may also notice shadows or obstructions (scotomas) in their visual field.

Diabetic Retinopathy

Diabetic retinopathy is caused by elevated levels of sugar in the blood. These elevated sugar levels result in damage being caused to the blood vessels at the back of the retina. Sugar take-up can also cause swelling of the crystalline lens resulting in temporary myopia. The onset is gradual but often irreversible because many afflicted individuals delay seeking treatment until their vision is significantly impaired. The visual symptoms of diabetic retinopathy can include small dots or scotomas appearing in the visual field along with blurred vision.

Hemianiopia

Also known as hemianiopsia or hemianiopsis, this is a form of impaired vision that affects half of the horizontal or less frequently vertical field of view. It is a curious impairment that can cause a form of blindness to light, colour or form. It most commonly occurs following a stroke, and its effects can be complicated by the perceptual implications of unilateral neglect.

Diplopia

Diplopia, or double vision, occurs when the brain perceives the same object to be located in different spatial positions. This is often related to the ability of the extraocular muscles to properly converge both eyes upon an object. There can be many causes for diplopia, alcohol intoxication for one; however it is also associated with multiple sclerosis, brain tumours, cranial nerve palsies and thyroid eye disease. Because of the mismatch between where the eyes are pointing and what the brain is seeing, the same object can appear to be located in two different positions in the visual field.

Colour Blindness

Colour blindness is generally a result of genetic factors that make discriminating between two or more colours difficult. The most common form is protanopia, which is caused by the absence of red retinal photoreceptors. Deuteranopia is a colour vision deficiency in which the green retinal photoreceptors are absent, and tritanopia is associated with the absence of blue retinal receptors. More commonly, people who experience difficulties with red/green discrimination are anomalous trichromats, meaning that although all three colour photoreceptors are present, one of the types has a shifted spectral sensitivity. A related condition is achromatopsia, perception of the world only in shades of grey, which can have a variety of causes, both in the receptors of the eye and in the way that information from the eye is processed by the brain.

VR Simulation for Clinical Training

Pioneering early work involving the simulation of the human eye for surgical simulation was undertaken during the early 1990s (Sagar et al., 1994). Sagar's graphical system used simple polygonal geometry and Gouraud shading to produce a smooth curved appearance to a virtual model of the human eye. The complex appearance of the iris was represented either with two layers of vertex painted "fibres" made from geometric polygons of six or more vertices or alternatively a simpler geometric disk textured with a digitised photograph. They system selected which model to utilise depending upon the level of manipulation required. Non-uniform rational B splines (NURBS) were used to represent the facial areas surrounding the eye and biquadratic patches used to construct individual eyelashes. The graphical rendering of this simulated eye pushed the currently available hardware to its limits, with typical refresh rates of around five frames per second on the Silicon Graphics workstation used to develop the simulation.

The system developed by Sagar was however more than just a simple visualisation tool. The simulator was coupled to a finite-element model of corneal tissue, enabling the surfaces to deform and allowing stress field information to be calculated. This software was coupled to a real-world interface, the actual tools used in an operating theatre for robot-aided microsurgery. Through this approach a trainee surgeon was able to interact with the eye model, seeing the virtual simulation rendered in real time on a stereoscopic display, whilst forces applied to the virtual eye using the virtual tools could be haptically fed back in an appropriate and accurate way to the operator of the microsurgical robot.

Sagar's simulation pushed the envelope of what was achievable at the time; subsequent years however saw a multitude of simulation-based approaches developed for opthalmological training. In 1998 at the University of Illinois in Chicago, Paul Neumann et al. created a simulator designed as a training aid for vitrectomy, a surgical procedure for correcting retinal detachment (Neumann et al., 1998). Neumann developed a soft body simulation that was able to respond to cuts made in the material of the virtual eye. A set of virtual tools such as pick, blade and laser were incorporated into the simulator to enable surgical skills to be practised.

Further work on vitrectomy simulators has been undertaken by Shen et al. (2008) and by Lam and Sundaraj (2010). These simulators take the haptic feedback concept pioneered by Sagar et al. (1994) and improve upon the fidelity of the haptic interface. Both implementations are based upon the Phantom Omni device developed by SensAble Technologies. The Phantom offers a motorised stylus that is capable of applying force feedback along *x*, *y* and *z* axes. The device is capable of allowing the operator to experience tactile sensations when operating upon the virtual eye using a set of virtual tools. Once selected the virtual tools could be manipulated with six degrees of freedom and tactile sensations such as pressure, texture, puncture, softness, wetness, friction and slip can be fed back to the user to simulate the nature of the material that the virtual tool is being applied to.

Both implementations can be considered prototypes, and of the two, Shen's simulator appears the most developed. Three display paradigms were deployed: traditional 2D display, 3D autostereoscopic and large-scale immersive. Their physics implementation fed back through the haptic device supports gravity, deformation and cutting (Shen et al., 2008). By comparison, the Lam and Sundaraj simulator is much less developed; at the time of publication, it was reported that the appropriate physical characteristics were still being calibrated with the assistance of opthalmological professionals. It is also acknowledged that many of the characteristics developed by the previous generation of simulators, such as an accurate deformable mathematical model representing the eye surface and the representation of cutting actions with changes in the virtual topology, were not implemented (Lam & Sundaraj, 2010).

There appears to be no evaluation of whether the simulator devised by Lam and Sundaraj was actually effective in achieving its aims. Shen's simulator however was trialled with a small group of eye surgeons. Test subjects were asked to rate the simulations by giving them a mark out of five. The results of this, though highly subjective, appear to show a lukewarm response to the fidelity of the phantom as an input device in terms of how well it represented the surgical tools, with a mean rating of 2.7 out of 5. Satisfaction scores for the fidelity of the haptic feedback provided by the device were somewhat better with a rating of 4 for cornea incision, 3.5 for tissue deformation and 3.8 for tissue pulling (Shen et al., 2008).

One of the most common visual ailments requiring surgical intervention is cataract. As an age-related ailment, the incidence in the wider population is liable to increase from its current frequency, which is approaching 1/100 inhabitants/year (Soderberg et al., 2005). The most common surgical procedure used to treat cataracts is a process called phacoemulsification, and several simulations have been developed to help surgeons train for the procedure (Agus et al., 2006; Choi et al., 2009).

Phacoemulsification is a two-handed procedure, and the virtual reality simulators developed to train in the process reflect this. Choi et al.'s system was based upon a pair of phantom haptic devices enabling trainee surgeons to practise whilst utilising both hands. They returned to the "mass spring" physics simulation proposed by Neumann et al. to facilitate tissue deformation as forces were applied. They went to great lengths to improve upon the simulation of tissue cutting developed by the preceding simulators. For the initial stages of simulating the clinical operation, the eye model was considered as a volumetric mesh, rather than a simple surface model. The route of a cut across the surface of the model was used to subdivide the mesh, and the mesh topology regenerated to reflect the progressive modification of the surface resulting from the cut. Furthermore the tension applied by the mass spring model serves to pull apart the virtual cut edges. This characteristic of their simulation also serves to simulate the tearing process used during the capsulorrhexis stage of the phacoemulsification process (Choi et al., 2009).

To simulate phaco-sculpting, a process of removing parts of the clouded cataract lens using ultrasound energy to form a cross-shaped trench, the relevant part of the virtual eye was represented by a dense arrangement of 14,300 tetrahedrons. A hierarchical octree was used to partition the space to optimise performance, and a collision detection algorithm based upon a bounding sphere utilised to identify the tetrahedrons touched by the virtual probes' collision sphere. Tetrahedrons that intersected the collision sphere were removed from the simulation, and by modifying the size of the sphere, it was possible to simulate the level of ultrasound energy. The complexity of representing this process can be noted in the frame rate of only ten frames per second, and it is the hardware capability that ultimately restricts the realism of this simulation (Choi et al., 2009).

Despite the many innovate techniques developed for this simulation, there remain several key limitations. The physics system used to model tearing is not based upon the actual characteristics of the eye material, so will behave in a slightly different way to an actual eye. The tetrahedral approach is enforced by the processing limitations of the hardware and results in a visibly jagged surface, where a smoother finish would be desirable. Additionally, no arrangement is made for binocular vision, though it is noted that this facility could be added if the increased cost of hardware warranted it.

Simulators for the development of clinical practice may have a significant role to play; however they are only of value to a relatively limited number of people. When it comes to raising an awareness of the nature of visual impairments, the potential audience, and possible impact upon society, is arguably much larger.

Simulating the Appearance of Visual Impairments

In clinical practice, the nature of visual impairments is generally descriptively oversimplified, reduced to a pair of numbers representing the Snellen acuity, a figure derived from an individual's ability to resolve a letter of given size on a monochrome chart viewed from a specific distance. Yet the experience of seeing the word encompasses a much wider range of sensory experience. Contrast sensitivity, colour vision, movement sensitivity, field of view and stereo acuity are all part of the smorgasbord of sensations that feed into the visual psychosensory experience. The complex interplay between all of these characteristics makes painting a verbal picture of exactly how an impaired individual sees the world an impossible task.

The nature of human vision, or more specifically visual perception, and, in particular, the way in which this can vary between individuals is very difficult to explain using verbal or written communication methods. This is partially due to the difficulty in comprehending that what the optical and sensory systems of the eye actually detect is subsequently interpreted by the brain in order to form the "picture", the impression that a person gets of the world. It is perhaps worth considering a distinction that could be drawn between "vision", what the eye actually sees, and "perception", what the brain interprets the signals from the eyes to mean. Science can tell us a lot about what the eye can detect. Ophthalmological tools can quantify the objective measures of aberrations in the optical system and from this make deductions about how this will affect vision. However, there is no way of objectively measuring the way in which the brain can utilise alternative cues such as sound and memory in order to be able to fill in these gaps, mitigating the apparent effect of the impairment, and meaning that perception is perhaps better than objectively measured vision may suggest.

Notwithstanding this major limitation, there has been a long-standing deliberate attempt or inadvertent oversight that communicates the nature of these effects to a wider audience. The blurry impressionist paintings of Renoir and Cezanne may owe much to their own visual impairments. According to Trevor-Roper (1957, p. 724), the distortions of colour and form evident in Cezanne's work are:

> …the product of a 'realistic' vision, which took into account the eye's unconsciously guided movements that the static realism of his fore-runners had neglected. And his myopia could well have provided an incentive or 'short-cut' to his especial awareness of the true shapes and hues in the peripheral field.

Renoir tended to paint more detail into objects close to him than those in the distance, a style that became more marked as he aged; it is also known that the artist would step back, moving the subject out of his near range of clear vision to give the painting a more impressionistic effect (Dan, 2003).

There is also plentiful evidence that anomalous colour vision has found its way into the visual representations made by the great artists. It has been suggested (Trevor-Roper, 1957) that the brown hues generally used by Constable when painting trees, even in springtime scenes, are easily explained if Constable is considered a partial protanope. Evidence of colour shift attributable to cataract has been widely discussed, perhaps incorrectly in the case of Turner (Lanthony, 2009) but more convincingly in the case of Monet, whose use of a duller colours and more yellow palette in his later works can be linked with his known development of bilateral cataract. The hypothesis that this colour shift was not deliberate, but a representation of how Monet saw the world may be reinforced by the retouching he did to some paintings after an operation to restore his sight (Ravin, 1994). John Singer Sargent, an artist known to have astigmatism, reportedly saw a red or green line around white objects. Frequently this chromatic border was incorporated into his artwork (Mills, 1936).

More recently the approach has evolved to using photographs that have been digitally manipulated to distort and adjust the appearance of the represented scene. However, it is a reasonable hypothesis to suggest that because the artists' impressions and photographs traditionally used are in no way immersive, they lack many of the cues used by the brain in perception of the real world. It therefore stands to reason that though they may provide a reasonable impression of how a photograph looks to a visually impaired person, they are unlikely to be very effective in allowing somebody else to understand how visually impaired people actually experience the world. The real potential value therefore of visual simulators are the possibilities that they open up for people to engage in real-world activities. Through this process of experiential activity, a constructivist learning paradigm is enabled, which should enable a deep level of understanding.

Physical Intervention to Modify Vision

Significant work has been undertaken using physical intervention approaches to simulate impaired vision. They will be discussed over the following pages in order to provide a clear understanding of what can be achieved without the use of a computerised VR system. Some of the earliest work in this field was undertaken by Joel Zuckerman. He determined that it was possible to simulate the effect of cataract on the optical system by spotting petroleum jelly onto a photographic lens and measuring the reduction in contrast and acuity on the resulting image. Although the purpose of this simulation was to provide a mechanism for evaluating the relationship between severity of cataract and loss of visual sensitivity, Zuckerman was able to show that this apparently simple method provided a realistic simulation of the effect of cataracts (Zuckerman et al., 1973).

More recently Fine and Rubin (1999) have utilised acetate film as a media for creating visual impairments. Their methods included the use of lightly frosted acetate to simulate cataract and printing a solid black circle on clear acetate film to simulate the effect of scotoma in the central visual field. Fine and Rubin did not accurately measure the way in which their acetate scattered light, and it is unlikely that a central vision scotoma would be perfectly circular; however they did demonstrate similarity in contrast loss through the acetate. The results from Fine and Rubin's simulator served to illustrate that acuity measurements made by reading words or identifying letters is not a good measure of visual ability. This theme is also found in the results of some studies based on simulator spectacles.

Simulation spectacles are glasses that have been modified to adjust how light passes through them. They are designed to recreate the most common visual impairments, though there is no standardised measure of severity between the various vendors, so they can be variable in their effect.

Elliott et al (1996) evaluated a variety of light scattering media and found that the lenses of the Vistech cataract simulation spectacles scattered light with an angular distribution very similar to actual cataracts. After this validation of the media, they went on to evaluate the impact that this scattered light had upon three real-world activities, these being face recognition, reading speed and mobility orientation. Through using the simulation spectacles, Elliott discovered that there was relatively little loss of visual acuity under normal lighting conditions. However low-light, low-contrast and glare conditions can have a very disabling effect due to wide angle light scatter. Through simulating the effect of the impairment on otherwise normally sighted people, Elliott was able to support the assertion that measurement of visual acuity is not a reliable indicator of visual ability in cataract patients and that a patient's reported visual disability will:

> probably depend on the percentage of time that they spend under low contrast and/or low luminance and/or glare conditions, such as walking or reading in dim illumination, night driving and walking or driving in fog or heavy rain... Contrast sensitivity and glare tests may be better representatives of these patients' vision than visual acuity (Elliott et al., 1996 p. 803).

Wood and Troutbeck (1994) used a set of goggles designed to simulate the effects of cataract, visual field restriction and monocular vision. Their study was designed to investigate the degree to which impaired vision accounts for reduced driving performance in elderly drivers. Measuring the performance in a series of driving tasks, both with and without the impairment glasses, the researchers were able to quantify the impact of reduced vision on performance. Wood and Troutbeck were able to demonstrate that performance was significantly degraded when the simulation goggles were worn. It is interesting that the severity of impairment simulated was within the permitted acuity limits for holding an Australian driving licence. They note the limitations of a Snellen-type chart as a tool for measuring visual perception due to its inability to assess issues of colour perception, contrast sensitivity and glare.

A study conducted on 99 social work students (Shuldberg, 2005) utilised simulation spectacles to develop awareness of visual impairments with the goal of tackling ageism. The study followed a qualitative methodology with theme analysis based upon certain keywords to evaluate the effectiveness of the simulated activities. The set of spectacles used simulated cataract, AMD, glaucoma, hemianopsia and yellowing of the lens. Indications of the research were that the use of simulation kits "led to greater self-awareness and critical reflection on ageism and discrimination". Students reported being "surprised by the difficulties" that a variety of impairments could cause. Although the study was designed to develop goals for advocacy, the most significant theme, noted by 40% of participants, was increased compassion.

Another study (Rousek et al., 2009) also used a similar set of simulation spectacles, to impair the vision of normally sighted people in order to identify hospital wayfinding difficulties. Through the use of the simulation glasses, Rousek was able to identify that design elements like lighting, shiny tiles or changing patterns in floor surfaces present problems. He acknowledges that the participants of the experiment would not have developed the coping mechanisms that many visually impaired people have, a limitation that all studies of this type have to accept. Looking at his research from a different perspective, it is notable that 2 of the 50 participants stumbled during the task, highlighting the potential safety risks of allowing a normally sighted person to experience the world with impaired vision.

So, simulation specs are an effective tool. They can be produced relatively cheaply and a wide range of activities can be devised to enable the wearers of them gain a greater appreciation of the difficulties faced by visually impaired people. They have some significant constraints in that the nature and level of the impairment cannot be customised. They are also not suited to demonstrating the progression of a visual impairment as the severity of the simulation is fixed. Because of the health and safety implications, activities involving simulation specs are usually restricted to relatively static exercises to minimise risk of injury, which limits their use as tools for constructivist learning.

2D Computer Simulation of Impaired Vision

In terms of employing computer technology to enable people to enhance their understanding of visual impairment, a series of software tools for processing images and web pages have been developed. For the most part, these simulators arose as a facet of the web accessibility initiative and have predominantly been designed as tools for improving the accessibility of web pages. A designer (Kentaro et al., 2006) is a software tool designed to help Internet developers to ensure that web pages they design are accessible for visually impaired people. It supports the evaluation of page layouts in terms of their usability for people who are blind or have low levels of functional vision. A designer does not give the designer an impression of how the page would look to a visually impaired person; rather it provides guidance regarding levels of colour contrast on the page, impacts that the design has on the ability of a user to adjust the font size and the provision of alternate text for images. An alternative approach, illustrated by The WebAIM Low Vision Simulator (WebAim, 2012), provides users with the opportunity to experience a web page as a user with visual disabilities. The simulation is not particularly accurate, and it can only impair a single mocked-up web page; however it enables designers to begin to comprehend some of the issues associated with macular degeneration, cataract and glaucoma.

2D simulations that offer greater versatility than these packages have been developed. ColorDoctor (Fujitsu, 2012) and Vischeck are simulators that can check colour selection for design issues, enabling the layout to be visualised from the perspective of somebody with a colour impairment. Both are able to transform the colours found on a web URL into a set of colours that represent the view that somebody with protanopia, deuteranopia or tritanopia would have of the content. ColorDoctor also utilises a greyscale to present an impression of monochromacy. As well as enabling web content to be transformed into impaired colour versions, Vischeck also enables images to be uploaded from a user's computer for transformation, whilst ColorDoctor is even more versatile, as when operating in its "Transparent" mode in which the four conversion filters can be overlaid over a wide variety of screen content to enable presentations or multimedia content to be evaluated.

The visual impairment simulator (VIS) for Microsoft Windows is another 2D screen modification simulator tool that enables glaucoma, cataract, macular degeneration, colour blindness, diabetic retinopathy, retinitis pigmentosa and hyperopia to be simulated (iCITA, 2012). A drop-down menu is used to enable the impairments, which then operate on the user's desktop. Cambridge University has developed a vision impairment simulator that is included in the inclusive design toolkit (Clarkson et al., 2007). The vision simulator modifies a digital image to show what the image might look like when viewed with a variety of different vision conditions.

Each condition can be applied with different levels of severity, controlled via a slider.

In a clinical context, a computer simulation developed by Crabb et al. at University College London was designed to improve the assessment of a glaucoma patient's field of view (Crabb et al., 1998). Measurement of monocular fields of view of glaucoma patients is a routine clinical process that plays an essential role in the detection and management of glaucoma. In contrast binocular assessment is of little value clinically; however, it provides the closest approximation indication of a patient's actual field of view, which is a more useful measurement underpinning their real-world functional capability. Crabb et al.'s simulation algorithm combined the left and right Humphrey field data, and the results were compared with the binocular Humphrey Esterman visual field test. It was found that the simulation results closely agreed with measurements made using the binocular test and that the simulator could be used as a clinically useful indicator for determining visual field requirement to drive in the UK.

Simulation of Visual Impairments Using a VR System

The first notable attempt at using VR to simulate visual impairment was undertaken by the University of Chicago, beginning with the simulator developed by Ai et al. (2000). A virtual reality model of an apartment, visualised through a stereoscopic display, was developed as the foundation of the system. The first version of the simulator contained virtual representations of diplopia, macular degeneration and cataract, and it was later enhanced (Jin et al., 2005) to incorporate an implementation of colour impairment. The simulator also contained a more traditional pedagogical component, with a 3D model of the eye itself used to explain the causes and treatments of the visual impairments. Both Jin and Ai asserted that representing impairments through an immersive VR simulator was able to have a profound impact upon users, and they maintained that their simulator was suitable as a tool for practitioner training.

Another significant attempt at using VR to recreate the effects of visual impairments can be seen in the work of Maxhall et al. (2004). The simulator developed by Maxhall et al. approaches the problem from the particular perspective of helping carers to understand the impact that stroke has had upon the people they care for. It is therefore based upon an interesting VR interface where the environment is experienced from the perspective of a head-mounted display and the environment is navigable using a specially modified wheelchair as the input device. Interactivity was facilitated through a set of magnetic motion-tracking sensors, tracking the head, hands and body, whilst pinch-sensitive gloves were used to enable virtual objects to be grasped. Due to its bias towards visual anomalies associated with stroke, the types of impairment represented are atypical of the broader field. The simulation utilised blurring and camera movement as devices to represent dizziness and nausea. It also attempted to represent the manifestation of hemianopsia by selectively hiding objects on the left-hand side of the visual field. The apartment supported three interactive virtual tasks: reading a newspaper, filling a glass with water and putting toothpaste on a toothbrush.

The results gleaned from observations and interviews suggest that this simulator was effective in influencing caregivers empathy; it was noted that "this stroke simulator is usable for training caregivers empathy for stroke patients, possibly creating an increased understanding for stroke patients daily problems" (Maxhall et al., 2004, p. 229). The researchers noted similar behaviours as would be expected from a stroke patient, including problems with orientation and dizziness, not using the left hand for interaction and feelings of frustration and anger. From the context of visual impairment, it is impossible to separate the effect of the simulated visual impairments on caregiver empathy from the effect of the simulated disability through the wheelchair. However, the evidence of strong sympathetic reaction noted in Jean Schulberg's SimSpecs study (Shuldberg, 2005) would support a hypothesis that the simulated visual impairment was a very significant factor in the positive results reported by this study.

There are two key criticisms that can be levelled at both of these simulators. The first is the degree to which the effectiveness of the simulators has been evaluated. It is clear that given the subtleties of understanding visual impairment, such evaluation is actually quite difficult to achieve; however, for Gin and Ai's simulator, a methodology based upon interview or questionnaire may have yielded valuable qualitative data that could have been utilised to guide the direction of the work that followed. For Maxhall's simulator, a methodology that was able to distinguish the effect of the VR interface from the effect of the impaired display would also have been valuable. For both of the simulators, it is clear that, despite utilising some of the best VR technology available at the time, it was still beyond the capabilities of the hardware and toolkits available to create a very realistic and interactive 3D environment.

The implications of this limitation are difficult to quantify. On the one hand, presenting an environment that is drawn through a computing process is, in itself, an impaired view of the space it seeks to recreate. The way in which light is reflected and diffused around the scene has to be simplified, the geometric nature of 3D curved surfaces is decomposed into an angular triangulated mesh and the impression of complicated surface details, colour and pattern has to be represented through photographic textures. Due to this overall lack of "normality", there must be an inherent ambiguity between the visual artefacts that the user is expected to attribute to the impairment being simulated and the visual artefacts that they are expected to disregard or ignore as they are due to the limitations of the simulation environment itself.

A second problem relates to the way in which the 2D image of 3D environment has to be drawn to a display in order for it to be viewed. The preceding systems have utilised a wide variety of display technologies as the visual interface to the virtual world, each of which comes with its own problems. Where systems have been developed that do not utilise stereoscopic display methods, they are removing a key perceptual sense. It seems reasonable to assume that depth perception provides a useful cue for object recognition within the first metre or so and taking this cue away may have the effect of exaggerating the effect of impairment.

Another key limitation relates to field of view. The only current practical method of creating a display surface that can enable a scene to be drawn that will match the angular field of view of the human visual system is to use a large-scale projection system akin to the CAVE developed for the University of Chicago (Cruz-Neira et al., 1993). The immersive nature of such display technology does allow environments to be drawn and experienced in a much more realistic way than a desktop monitor or head-mounted display; however, facilities like the CAVE are expensive and fairly permanent installations. One of the key issues is that they have traditionally been developed to run on bespoke hardware, necessitating a bespoke approach to the software development used to create the simulations displayed upon them. Ultimately, they have remained expensive testbeds for simulation software that would be difficult to deploy more widely in society once it has proven useful.

Even if the problem of visual fidelity and field of view are set aside, there remains another critical problem applicable generally to how 3D scenes are rendered but of particular prominence once considering vision realistic rendering and how a visually realistic scene would need to be adjusted to recreate realistic visual impairments. This is the problem of understanding exactly where on the display screen a person is looking. Visual acuity diminishes very rapidly with angle from the centre of focus. When looking at a monitor, or reading this text, for example, your optical system will only be able to resolve a handful of letters with a high level of acuity. It is only because of the way in which your eyes scan around, and the way in which the brain stores and uses this information to infill the lower-resolution parafoveal and peripheral field of view that our perception is of a richer visual field. This is of particular importance when simulating conditions, such as macular degeneration or diabetic retinopathy that can obscure central vision, to ensure that the simulator blocks the appropriate part of the screen relative to where the user is looking.

Now that we understand the background to the problem, the potential that simulation can offer and the limitations of the previous studies, the next section will propose the advantages that simulation methods based upon computer game technology can offer, leading to a discussion of recent visual simulation work that is trialling game technology for this purpose and laying out some key areas for further exploration.

The Relationship Between VR and Game Technology

It can be asserted that VR simulations and computer games have evolved symbiotically. Powerful and expensive rendering workstations and dedicated graphical cards had their development driven by investment in simulation technologies, whether this was from aerospace, engineering or the deep pockets of the military. However, the rendering methods and hardware design developed for these serious purposes did not take long to find their way into mainstream homes. Companies like Matrox and later Nvidia and ATI came to replace the old behemoth of '90 s rendering workstations Silicon Graphics. Of course, with mass market penetration came economies of scale and increased competition as each hardware platform sought to out-compete the other, reaching the point today where Nvidias Geforce GTX690 graphics card for hardcore gamers can perform a blistering 5.6 trillion calculations per second (gpureview.com, 2012).

This rapid evolution of computer hardware has been mirrored in the software developed to leverage the capabilities offered by the latest graphics cards. The billions of dollars up for grabs in the entertainment software market has seen a proliferation of software tools developed to speed up the process of game creation. Some of these tools have remained the private domain of the developers, utilising the capabilities of their own software and the commercial advantage it offers to power their own successes. Other software houses have recognised the economic value of the tools that they have developed and have been prepared to licence them for use by others in return for a one-off fee or a cut of the profits.

Current-generation computer games are often based upon sophisticated and realistic virtual environments. Players of games like Call of Duty expect the game environment to appear as, and behave like, the real world would. Not only does this mean that visual features like fire, smoke and water need to be simulated, but objects such as flags, clothing and dust need to move in response to gusts of virtual wind. Complex physics models are required to ensure that objects behave in accordance with Newtonian physics, falling with gravity or moving in response to impulse forces following the blast from explosions or being hit by moving vehicles. They need to support interactivity allowing the player to move within or act upon the world, and they need to support the behaviours of non-player characters within the world, autonomous agents able to operate to scripted behaviours or artificially intelligent controls. They will support a complex sound model, with three-dimensionally positioned sound sources being sent to particular speakers and attenuated according to distance.

Traditionally these individually complicated pieces of functionality were handed by collections of software tools. Often termed "Middleware", a selection of these software tools would be assembled by a game developer to meet the specific requirements of a particular game they were developing. In recent years some of these third-party tools have evolved into more complete game engines. Game engines can be considered to be specialised software development kits that are tailored to the creation of computer games. Notable examples today are the Doom engine by ID software, Valve software's Source engine and Epic's Unreal Developer Kit (UDK). Typically, a game engine of this sort has a generalised functionality capable of most of the tasks a virtual environment developer would need to accomplish. They will support the importation and display of geometric 3D objects, together with systems to configure the way in which the surfaces of the models are rendered, allowing shaders to be created with texture, opacity, specularity and luminance. These geometric objects can generally be given physical properties such as weight and friction and registered with the physics simulation so that they behave in a realistic manner. Engines will support complicated lighting models simulating direct and indirect light sources and take care of the shadowing and colour variations that will usually enable the importation, sequencing and positional location of sounds.

As well as the appearance of the world itself, the engines will generally enable interactive and temporal changes to occur within the virtual world, for example, through support for the sequencing of animations. There is also usually an underlying scripting language that can be used to simplify the programming of interactive features such as switches to turn lights on and off or open doors or to set up more complex goal-based interactions between players, objects and locations. If a project requires functionality beyond the generic capabilities of the engine, it is usually possible for the engine to be extended with additional programming.

Game Technology-Driven Research in the Field of Visual Impairment

In the context of visual impairments, there have been a handful of studies that have sought to leverage the power of game engines for simulation purposes. Sebastien Hillaire used ID software's Quake engine to attempt to resolve the problematic issue of representing foveal vision in a rendered 3D environment (Hillaire et al., 2008). Their system utilised eye-tracking software in order to ascertain what part of the screen a user was looking at. They then used a ray-testing approach to attempt to determine which object in the scene this related to and then applied a depth-based blurring to simulate the depth of field. The value of leveraging a game toolset in this context is that it would have already enabled the developer to quickly get a 3D environment up and running, avoiding the need to develop such content from scratch. In this example the free availability of the full Quake 3 source code would have meant that the rendering algorithms could be modified to utilise the input from the eye-tracking software and dynamically change the way the scene is drawn depending upon the target of focus.

Banks and McCrindle (2008) developed a visual eye disease simulator based upon Direct X and High-Level Shader Language (HLSL). The DirectX libraries, developed by Microsoft, are a particularly important codebase used in the development of computer games for the Windows and XBOX360 platforms. They operate at a lower level than the game engines previously discussed and generally require a significant amount of system development to be able to leverage their capabilities. By working in Direct X, Banks and McCrindle were able to utilise computer game technology without incurring the constraints that can sometimes be imposed by a commercial game engine. A key strength of Banks and McCrindle's approach is the use of HLSL. This language is designed to enable graphical effects to be programmed to run directly on the graphics card of a computer. Compared to the software processing employed by previous attempts, image processing using the dedicated specialism of the graphics processing units available on a graphics card dramatically speeds up the image processing necessary to simulate visual impairments in real time.

The system was capable of processing 2D content and could also render 3D models into a 2D image that could subsequently be fed into the impairment simulation. The authors also highlighted the possibility of using a video stream as an input, and in this context, the speed of HLSL would be critical to perform the complicated and computationally expensive calculations required in real time. The configuration of the way in which the impairments operated was retained within an XML file. This meant that it was possible to modify the way in which the impairments operated by changing the text values stored in the XML. Though this may not be a particularly intuitive approach, it highlights the advantage that a computerised simulation can offer over physical approaches, as Banks and McCrindle's system enables eye conditions of variable severity, or which combine several effects to be set up and saved for later reuse. It is this flexibility that is perhaps one of the most significant benefits that computer simulation offers.

Lewis et al. (2011) developed a simulator based upon the Unreal Tournament 3 Game. This can be regarded as a predecessor to the currently available UDK game development suite and the implementation aimed to investigate the degree to which a game mod would allow the impairments to be recreated. It was also an investigation into the timescales for producing a simple but realistic environment that could be impaired. The study was also notable in that it utilised a focus group, evaluated their baseline level of knowledge and obtained some strong preliminary indications of improved awareness and increased knowledge. Lewis and Mason's implementation was based upon a university cafeteria and used photographic textures and floor plans supported by tape measure survey to recreate an accurate representation of the room. Tables and chairs, partition screens food service counters, light fittings, noticeboards and posters were accurately recreated for the simulated environment, which was navigable using a keyboard and mouse using the same navigation style as first-person shooter games.

The game modification tools available with the Unreal 3 Engine were found to offer two key methods of modifying the visual display that would enable the impairments to be represented. The first of these methods were UI scenes. UI scenes are incorporated to enable the game developer to add menus and buttons to the screen; they can, however, be used to overlay any kind of imagery and they also support variable transparency through the alpha channel of the image developed.

In the simulator of Lewis et al. (2011), these masked images were used extensively, with fully opaque black splodges with feathered alpha edges representing the degraded central vision for macular degeneration and the floaters of diabetic retinopathy. A black opaque frame with a transparent centre was used to represent glaucoma. It was also found that the game modding tools offered access to the games "post-process chain", meaning that certain changes to the way in which the camera drew the 3D scene were possible. From the perspective of simulating visual impairments, the depth-based blur functionality allowed foreground to be selectively blurred, representing the reduced acuity of myopia, or the background to be selectively blurred, representing the reduced acuity of hyperopia. It was also found that the post-process chain could represent colour shift effects, utilised in this context to represent the yellowing effect of cataract, and for a simple implementation of monochromacy.

In terms of the advantages reported, utilising a game modification as the development platform for the investigation was able to speed up the development time, lower the development cost and improve the level of realism and level of accuracy conveyed by the simulation. In terms of speed, it was found that, even allowing for the steep learning curve required to develop familiarity with the Unreal toolset, the adoption of a game engine enabled a functional 3D simulation to be rapidly prototyped in just a few weeks. The game and its associated tools can be acquired at relatively low cost and development is possible on a typical midrange computer.

From the perspective of realism, all users that tested the simulator agreed that it conveyed realism successfully. The realistic appearance of the simulator can be attributed to a combination of high-quality 3D models and textures, as well as the sophisticated material and lighting model used by the game engine. This gave the models and textures a fidelity approaching photorealism. This is an important consideration required to create the illusion of reality in order to realistically replicate what the impaired person would see. This characteristic represents a significant advance upon the previous visual impairment simulators of Ai et al. (2000), Jin et al. (2005) and Maxhall et al. (2004).

In terms of the capability of the game engine to be able to simulate the impairments, it was found that the configurability of post-process effects and two-dimensional overlays offered by the game engine was suitable for the simulation of the visual impairments. The opinion of a visual impairment expert consulted as part of the study was that the representations were reasonably accurate simulations of the visual impairments. The study highlighted the possibility of varying the appearance of the impairment to reflect different degrees of severity; however such functionality was not implemented. Simulation of colour impairment was also set aside due to a lack of flexibility in the colour parameters of the games post-process effects. It was however made clear that it is relatively straightforward to represent a range of visual impairments using the software and that a deeper exploration of some of the more sophisticated capabilities of the game engine toolset would enable the techniques to be further refined.

Lewis et al. (2011) also highlighted that there are significant drawbacks that come from relying upon a game mod as a vehicle for software of this type. The first is that the mod requires the Unreal Tournament 3 game to be installed in order to load and run the simulation. Though the cost implications of this are not particularly significant, continuing availability of the game may be, and they recognise the issues concerning the installation of a violent "shooter" game rated for over 18 s could clearly become obstacles to the widespread deployment of a simulator, particularly on the corporate networks of schools, prisons and hospitals, for example.

In terms of educational effectiveness, the results of testing reveal some significant improvements in both reported and measured levels of understanding. Prior to using the simulator, only 5 of the 23 participants reported a "good" or "detailed" understanding of the symptoms of visual impairments. After using the simulator, nineteen participants described their understanding of the symptoms of visual impairments as "good" or "detailed". In terms of their awareness of the day-to-day difficulties encountered by people with visual impairments, the number of participants rating their understanding as "fairly good" or "detailed" rose from 4 to 18.

The authors acknowledge that these results were based upon the participant's own subjective reporting of their understanding and awareness, which is a significant limitation. However, it seems unequivocal that the participants themselves generally believe that they have learned something from the experience of using the simulator. The authors expressed surprise that the participants believed that their understanding had been so substantially improved after such a short period of simulator use. The high number of participants who also indicated that they would change their behaviour as a result of using the simulator may also suggest the learning is "deep" in its nature and perhaps indicative of an increasing empathy with people with a visual impairment. Again, it is important to acknowledge that this evidence should not be overstated but is worthy of future exploration utilising a less subjective means of assessment.

Lewis et al.'s (2011) work also highlights some of the difficulties of simulating human vision using a 2D screen. Only five of the participants described the simulation of hemianopia as the loss of vision on one side or loss of half the visual field. Seven others, scored as partially correct in the results, incorrectly interpreted the simulation as representing a loss of vision in one eye. Once more one could hypothesise that, if asked to picture the symptoms of hemianopia, the participant's recollection would be of the loss of half of the visual field, even if they did not describe their understanding of the symptoms thus.

One of the most encouraging results noted by Lewis et al. (2011) is the increase in the level of awareness and understanding of diabetic retinopathy. From a baseline of zero knowledge, 16 of the participants were able to describe the symptoms of this disease either substantially or partially correctly, and all 16 noted the interrupted vision caused by "floaters". This is important because early recognition of the symptoms and prompt treatment of this disease can prevent significant sight loss or blindness.

A second study (Lewis et al., 2012) extended the approach taken by Banks and McCrindle to utilise the versatility of HLSL to represent a range of impairments that were capable of being adjusted and configured in real time. Rather than base the implementation on Direct X, as Banks and McCrindle did, Lewis and Shires utilised Microsoft's XNA Framework. A managed code framework designed for the development of games that can operate across the PC, Xbox360 and Windows phone environments, XNA was found to interface easily with the shader code and allowed the rapid prototyping of a simple environment. Because the XNA libraries are designed to support a wide variety of game development tasks, the development pipeline was much less predetermined than would generally be the case if using a fully featured game engine. Subsystems for player input, navigation and interface design were all designed from the ground up and programmed using c#. This flexibility could certainly be useful, particularly to interface with non-standard input devices or to facilitate output onto unusual display screens such as a CAVE.

A feature of this prototype was an interface that would enable the impairments to be customised in terms of severity, and combined, so that, for example, the vision of somebody with cataract and protanopia could be demonstrated. From the qualitative results gained, it appears that the severity customisation was fairly successful in its implementation; however the range that could be simulated was found to be too limited, with the highest settings not restricting vision enough to accurately replicate a severe impairment. Overall it is suggested that the simulators accuracy is good enough for the application.

Lewis et al. (2012) used the open-source 3D modelling tool "Blender" as the software to construct the office environment developed for the simulation. In this context, Lewis et al. were employing a generalised 3D modelling tool to attempt to do many of the tasks that Unreal Ed, or other world-building packages attached to game engines, usually performs. In particular, the texturing and lighting of the environment proved to be more complicated tasks that would be the case if using a commercial game engine. Whilst this overhead remained manageable in the context of the spatially limited office environment that was developed, the time and cost of developing complex worlds comparable to a AAA computer game would suggest that XNA is not ideally suited to this role, at least until such time as a generalised 3D world-building tool and associated rendering libraries becomes available.

Lewis confirmed the utility of HLSL as a graphical system for the simulation of visual impairments, stating that it had "sufficient flexibility and computational efficiency to offer a great platform for the improvement and refinement of the shader algorithms" (Lewis et al., 2012). Lewis also points out that as the HLSL shader code is not specific to any particular application, it can potentially be integrated into a variety of applications, highlighting in particular the possibility of integrating the HLSL algorithms into the material system of UDK. This "best of both worlds" approach would harness the graphical prowess and simplified environment construction offered by the game engine whilst retaining the efficiency and flexibility of HLSL to modify the rendering and simulate the impairments. Lewis et al. (2012) also point out that a game engine's support for complex interactivity would help increase the level of immersion in the environment, suggesting that to achieve a comparable level of interactivity in XNA would take a huge quantity of development time over and above that already invested in the simple prototype.

A two-stage testing method was deployed for the Lewis et al. (2012) study; a first phase was aimed at validating the accuracy of the tool and a second to investigate its educational effectiveness. To achieve this a qualified optician was consulted to confirm the accuracy of the impairments and the potential utility of such a tool in her own professional practice. The optician's review provided some evidence in support of the hypothesis that increasing the amount of interactivity in a visual impairment simulator is an important factor in representing the impact of visual impairments.

> Moving around and seeing things come in and out of focus really highlights how your world is really in the first metre of your vision. We tried something similar with our website on images but interacting gives a better sense of having the impairment.

In addition to the large number of suggestions for improvement, the optician did give a very positive reaction to the simulation.

> It would be of huge help when trying to explain the effects of impairments to patients.
> Organisations like the RNIB are desperate for methods to inform the public about visual impairments and a program like this could really help.

By following the suggestions and increasing the accuracy and usability of the simulation, it seems that this tool could have serious potential for a real-world application. The results also highlight the utility of having an experienced vision specialist involved during the development process, as following an iterative development of refining the impairments based upon expert feedback could eventually lead to more accurate and nuanced implementations of impairments than a standardised "textbook" image.

The effectiveness testing of this simulator utilised questionnaires to establish the participant's level of awareness about visual impairments. The results of the effectiveness testing show a strong indication that the users had gained a good understanding of visual impairments through using the simulation tool. Seventeen users strongly agreed, and the other six agreed with the statement that "Using the visual impairment simulator has improved my understanding of visual impairments in general and how they affect the lives of the visually impaired". Eighteen users strongly agreed and five agreed that "Allowing movements around the environment provided a better sense of the impairments than looking at a still image".

Conclusion

Computer simulation approaches have already proved their value as training tools for surgical intervention. This success has been against a backdrop of expensive hardware, bespoke software and sophisticated technical approaches that squeezed the last drop of performance from the available technology. Despite the limitations of these first-generation approaches, the tools have continued to evolve and be further refined. There is also a trend of these simulators beginning to adopt technology such as autostereoscopic displays or simulated physics systems, the development of which owes much to the impetus provided by the widespread adoption of computer technology for gaming purposes.

When attempting to simulate human vision, the nature of perception itself limits the degree to which any simulation, no matter how advanced, can claim to be an accurate representation of the way in which an individual perceives the world. Historically the work of artists, and in particular artistic impressions, has offered a window into the perception of visually impaired people. Through this mechanism, and more recently modified photographs, the nature of the difficulties that visual impairments can begin to be seen and perhaps better understood. The three-dimensional nature of vision and perception however means that the approximation of visual experience offered by a 2D picture remains limited.

The utilisation of modified optical devices, the Sim Specs, overcomes many of these issues; however the impairments offered by such devices lack configurability, and they must present a rather generic archetype of the impairment they simulate, so they are not well suited to demonstrating the range of the impairments or how an impairment could progress over time. There is also a very real safety implication in allowing people with normal vision to experience the world with this kind of impairment. Without the coping mechanisms that visually impaired people have acquired over time, there is a danger that the hazards of the environment could cause actual injury unless the participant is carefully supervised or restricted in the range of activities they can undertake.

A viable alternative therefore is the use of virtual reality simulations. These enable participants to safely explore a virtual environment whilst the visual representation they are shown is modified to represent a range of visual impairments. Whilst early attempts at this approach were limited in terms of visual fidelity by the available processing power and software, more recent approaches have highlighted the opportunities to harness the advanced capability of modern computer game engines and recreational gaming hardware. As this approach continues to evolve, it is likely that simulators with increasing visual realism and more accurate and validated representation of visual impairments may come to be proven as educational tools for the public in the same way that surgical simulators have been for surgeons.

Furthermore, as the capabilities of mobile devices increase, again driven forward by the demands of processor-intensive gaming and graphical applications, the possibility of an augmented reality approach becomes more realistic. Whilst this would be encumbered by many of the same safety issues as Sim specs, the versatility and configurability of a software approach means that it would be possible to simulate the diversity and range of impairment types. Such information could be overlaid upon the highest fidelity visual representation possible. A place of infinite variability and configurability. The actual, real world, environment itself.

References

Agus, M., Gobbetti, E., Pintore, G., Zanetti, G., & Zorcolo, A. (2006). Real time simulation of Phaco-emulsification for cataract surgery training. In *Proceedings of the 3rd workshop in Virtual Reality Interactions and Physical Simulation "VRIPHYS"*. Madrid Spain.

Ai, Z., Balaji, K., Gupta, K., Rasmussen., Lin Y., Dech, F., Panko, W., & Silverstein, J. (2000). Simulation of eye diseases in a virtual environment. In *Hawaii International Conference on System Sciences* (HICSS-33). Wailea Maui. USA.

Banks, D., & McCrindle, R. J. (2008). Visual eye disease simulator. In *Proceedings of the 7th ICDVRAT with ArtAbilitation*, Maia, Portugal.

Choi, K., Soo, S., & Chung, F. (2009). A virtual training simulator for learning cataract surgery with phacoemulsification. *Computers in Biology & Medicine, 39*(11), 1020–1031.

Clarkson, P.J., Coleman, R., Hosking, I & Waller, S. (2007). *Inclusive design toolkit*. http://www.inclusivedesigntoolkit.com. Accessed 23 Nov 2012.

Cooper, M., & Taylor, M. (1998). Ambisonic sound in virtual environments and applications for blind people. In *Proceedings of 2nd ICDVRAT*. University of Reading.

Crabb, D., Viswanathan, A., McNaught, A., Poinoosawmy, D., Fitzke, F., & Hitchings, R. (1998). Simulating binocular visual field status in glaucoma. *British Journal of Ophthalmology, 82*(11), 1236–1241.

Cruz-Neira, C., Sandin, D. J., & DeFanti, T. A. (1993, August). Surround-screen projection-based virtual reality: The design and implementation of the CAVE. In *Proceedings of SIGGRAPH '93 Computer Graphics Conference*. ACM SIGGRAPH.

Dan, N. G. (2003). Visual dysfunction in artists. *Journal of Clinical Neuroscience, 10*(2), 168–170.

DeShazo, J., Harris, L., & Pratt, W. (2010). Effective intervention or child's play? A review of video games for diabetes education. *Diabetes Technology & Therapeutics, 12*(10), 815–822.

Elliott, D. B., Bullimore, M. A., Patla, A. E., & Whitaker, D. (1996). Effect of a cataract simulation on clinical and real world vision. *British Journal of Ophthalmology, 80*, 799–804.

Evett, L., Battersby, S., Ridley, A., & Brown, D. (2009). An interface to virtual environments for people who are blind using Wii technology – Mental models and navigation. *Journal of Assistive Technologies, 3*(2), 26–34.

Fine, E., & Rubin, G. (1999). Effects of cataract and scotoma on visual acuity: A simulation study. *Optometry and Vision Science, 76*(7), 468–473.

Fujitsu. (2012). *Color Doctor 2.1.* http://www.fujitsu.com/global/accessibility/assistance/cd/. Accessed 23 Nov 2012.

GPUREVIEW. (2012). *nVidia GeForce GTX690* [Online]. Available: http://www.gpureview.com/GeForce-GTX-690-card-668.html. 23 Nov 2012.

Hillaire, S., Lecuyer, A., Cozot, R, & Casiez, G. (2008). Using an eye-tracking system to improve camera motions and depth-of-field blur effects in virtual environments. In *Proceedings of the IEEE International conference on Virtual Reality (IEEE VR)*, Reno, USA.

iCita. (2012). *Visual impairment simulator for Microsoft Windows.* http://vis.cita.uiuc.edu. Accessed 23 Nov 2012.

Jin, B, Ai, Z, & Rasmussen, M (2005). Simulation of eye disease in virtual reality. In *Proc IEEE 27th Annual Conference on Engineering in Medicine and Biology. Shanghai.*

Kentaro, F., Hironobu, T., Junji, M., Shin, S., & Chieko, A. (2006). Web accessibility visualization and evaluation tool: aDesigner. *Konpyuta Sofutowea, 23*(4), 26–35.

Lam, C., & Sundaraj, K., (2010). Design and development of an eye surgery simulator. In *International Conference on Intelligent and Advanced Systems – ICIAS*. Kuala Lumpur, Malaysia.

Lewis, J., Mason, R. Brown, D. Cranton, W. (2011). Simulating visual impairments using the Unreal Engine 3 game engine. In *Proceedings of the IEEE 1st International Conference Serious Games and Applications for Health (SeGAH2011)*. Braga, Portugal.

Lewis, J., Shires, L., & Brown, D. (2012). Development of a visual impairment simulator using the Microsoft XNA framework. In *Proceedings of the 9th ICDVRAT.* Laval France.

Lanthony, P. (2009). *Art & ophthalmology: The impact of eye diseases on painters.* Kugler Publications.

Maxhall, M., Backman, A., Holmlund, K., Hedman, L., & Sondell, B. (2004). Participants responses to a stroke training simulator. In *Proceedings of the 5th ICDVRAT with ArtAbilitation,* Oxford, England.

Mills, L. (1936). Peripheral vision in art. *Archives of Ophthalmology, 16*(2), 208–219.

Neumann, P., Sadler, L., & Gieser, J. (1998) Virtual reality vitrectomy simulator. In *Proceedings of the First International Conference on Medical Image Computing and Computer-Assisted Intervention MICCAI98*, Cambridge MA, USA.

Ravin, J. (1994). Eye disease among the impressionists: Monet, Cassatt, Degas and Pissaro. *Journal of Ophthalmic Nursing & Technology, 13*, 217–222.

Rousek, J. B., Koneczny, S., & Hallbeck, M. S. (2009). Simulating visual impairment to detect hospital wayfinding difficulties. In *Proceedings of the 53rd Human Factors and Ergonomics Society Annual Meeting* (HFES 2009). San Antonio, USA.

Sagar, M., Bullivant, D., Mallinson, G., Hunter, P., & Hunter, I. (1994). A virtual environment and model of the eye for surgical simulation. In *Proceedings of the SIGGRAPH 94*. Orlando. USA.

Shen, X., Zhou, J., Hamam, A., Nourian, S., El-Far, N., Malric, F., & Georganas, N. (2008). Haptic-enabled telementoring surgery simulation. *Multimedia IEEE, 15*(1), 64–67.
Shuldberg, J. (2005). It's easy to make judgements if it's not familiar: The use of simulation kits to develop self awareness and reduce ageism. *Journal of Social Work Education, 41*(3).
Soderberg P., Laurell, C., Simawi, W., Nordqvist, P., Skarman, E., & Nordh, L., (2005). Virtual reality phacoemulsification: a comparison between skilled surgeons and students naive to cataract surgery. In *Proceedings of the Ophthalmic Technologies XV*, San Jose, CA, USA.
Trevor-Roper, P. (1957). The influence of eye disease on pictorial art. *Proceedings of the Royal Society of Medicine, 52*, 721–744.
WebAim. (2012). *WebAIM low vision simulation*. http://webaim.org/simulations/lowvision. Accessed 23 Nov 2012.
Wood, J. M., & Troutbeck, R. (1994). Effect of visual impairment on driving. *HumanFactors, 36*(3), 476–487.
Yu, W., & Brewster, S. (2002) Multimodal virtual reality versus printed medium in visualization for blind people. In *Proceedings of the 5th International ACM Conference on Assistive Technologies*. Edinburgh, Scotland.
Zuckerman, J., Miller, D., Dyes, W., & Keller, M. (1973). Degradation of vision through a simulated cataract. *Investigative Opthalmology & Visual Science*.

Chapter 4
Methodology for the Co-design of Shared VR Environments with Adults with Developmental and Intellectual Disabilities Using the Meta Quest

Matthew C. Harris, Pratik Vyas, James Lewis, David J. Brown, David Stewart, and Penny Standen

Introduction

This chapter proposes co-design as a methodology to elicit acceptable virtual environments with participants with intellectual disability (ID) within the context of a home-based application using current virtual reality (VR) technology. Significant developments in VR systems (such as the Oculus Quest 2) including "untethered" stand-alone devices and simplified set-up make home use of VR a realistic prospect for people with ID. The potential of VR to make a meaningful contribution to solving the real-world problems of participants with ID is now an opportunity worthy of serious consideration. Participants with ID have used VR in a lab setting with support (Harris et al., 2020), and by doing so, many problems they face can be studied. However, some problems can be better understood if investigation is moved to non-lab real-world settings. For example, in the use case given here aiming to reduce social isolation through VR-based social interaction, it is imperative to explore such interactions in the target context.

Furthermore, the predominant context where an individual with ID is going to experience social isolation is at home, and this is also the place where the equipment

M. C. Harris (✉) · P. Vyas · J. Lewis · D. J. Brown
Computing and Technology team, School of Science and Technology, Nottingham Trent University, Nottingham, UK
e-mail: matthew.harris@ntu.ac.uk; pratik.vyas@ntu.ac.uk; james.lewis@ntu.ac.uk; david.brown@ntu.ac.uk

D. Stewart
NICER Group, Oak Field School, Nottingham, UK
e-mail: d.stewart@oakfield.nottingham.sch.uk

P. Standen
Division of Rehabilitation and Ageing, School of Medicine, University of Nottingham, QMC, Nottingham, UK

E. Brooks, D. J. Brown (eds.), *Virtual Reality Games for Rehabilitation*, Virtual Reality Technologies for Health and Clinical Applications,
https://doi.org/10.1007/978-1-0716-3371-7_4

needs to be located in order to make a significant impact. Therefore, studying how participants with ID benefit from immersive technologies like VR when using them from home is critically important to evaluate the current potential of the technology. Out-of-lab experimentation increases the variables to be considered within a study and reduces the control of researcher on the observations made (Brown et al., 2011). The complex nature of a real-world setting warrants a detailed explanation and peer review of the research method itself.

To frame our approach to the research, we will describe how we strive to position participants with ID as co-designers. This means the research team acts as facilitator, observer, note-taker and organiser, while the decisions are taken by the participants themselves. This stems from the empathic design method proposed by Lee in "the behind stories of methods" (Lee, 2014) as well as "method stories" proposed by Hendriks et al. (2015), which help the researchers to understand their participant's experience, contextualising the use of technology, and explore the solution space "with" rather than "for" the participants with ID. Thus, in this article, we describe how our approaches work when co-designing with participants with ID, framed with the six key points for method stories.

This chapter does not provide the findings from the results of using this methodology. It focuses solely on developing a proposed methodology from existing research.

Co-design with Those with ID

Co-design treats the participants of research as "co-researchers". They are "experts by experience" (Sanders, 2005) in accessibility and disability issues and can provide valuable input. Thus, a co-design methodology treats the voices of those with intellectual disabilities as equally important and therefore must ensure that any barriers to this participation are eliminated. A good way to eliminate barriers is to give each individual the opportunity to have their voice heard. Another approach would be to systematically approach the development of questions and have the questions reviewed by experts in the domain so that co-researchers with ID are able to understand them.

The role of participant with ID has mostly remained one of iterating their experiences for the researcher to understand their perspective. Many studies utilise the expertise of carers of such participants to interpret the findings (Porter et al., 2001). This is valuable as it provides insights that carers have about the participants with ID and contributions which the participant themselves may have been unable to express. While this provides value, traditional researches with participants with ID still rely on the researcher to decide the objectives of study, device method of data collection, derive key findings from data and articulate the outcomes.

Before we can objectively study and replicate results in a scientific manner, we need clear understanding of the problem being studied. This can then determine the measurable aspects and the variables that can affect them including the intervention being studied. On the other hand, when studying the problem of social isolation of people with intellectually disability using VR interventions, we come across the need to measure aspects of social isolation as experienced by people with ID, but the problem is difficult to study for two reasons. The variety of disabilities and the variety of problems that associate with such disabilities are very diverse. Also, the problems as experienced are not categorised or measured in any objective format. For this reason, the need to co-design solutions with people with ID becomes important.

In co-design, the co-researchers are involved in *co-evolving* the understanding of the research problem and solution (Lawson, 2006). Understanding the problem space means questioning our underlying assumptions, challenging our understanding and rebuilding the framework of value propositions. When the problem is unclear, the development of solution is difficult, yet building solution can further enhance the understanding of problem itself. The *co-defining* of the study with the participants entails the participants devising what could be done during the study, how they will communicate and why they consider these decisions important. This not only provides structure stemming from experience but also ensures enthusiastic participation as the participants feel the ownership of the study. The *co-experience* during study can be very important as it encourages participants to share good practices and help each other overcome hurdles. This reduces the chances of experiment failure and can positively influence the participants' morale. When studying how VR can assist participants with ID, it is important that the participants and their carers and other participants generate the experience to address the problems like social isolation. The *co-sharing* process is where participants take charge of deciding not only what to share but also how to share it. Participants with ID and their carers could use a variety of effective techniques to enable communication. The participants can utilise these techniques to the extent as they see fit for themselves. These could include reliving through dramatisation, communicating through a variety of mediums or something different. The *co-verification* process could include the joint verification of the notes derived from data contributed. The participants further share their opinions on the experiences as well as contextualise it for documentation. The process could further utilise input from other researchers as well as experts such as carers of participants with ID. The *co-dissemination* is a critical part where the findings from the study are fed back to the community by the participants (Fig. 4.1). These could include integration of technology into their regular life, their community activities and even in educational institutions.

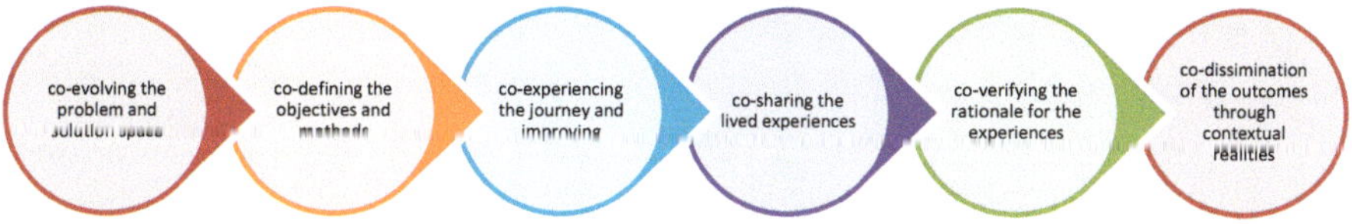

Fig. 4.1 The evolving co-design process

To give an example of where this methodology could be used, Serious Games for those with ID has received a lot of attention in research (Standen et al., 2006; Standen et al., 2009; Tsikinas & Xinogalos, 2019). Many of these games have been shown to be effective, though it is believed that a co-design could further aid here in creating games that are more appropriate, accepted and enjoyable to the target group.

Existing "Out of the Lab" Virtual Reality Studies

Few studies have placed significant focus on trialling VR systems in the home. While assessing the effectiveness of interventions in controlled conditions may be useful, it ignores the potential advantages that VR systems pose, e.g. not needing a dedicated facilitator to aid in learning new skills, and the ecological validity of such a study. In addition, eliminating the need to travel to take part in activities is another potential benefit. However, running VR studies outside of the lab introduces additional problems, which must be addressed, including the lack of control the researchers have over the participants' actions. Steed et al. (2021) discuss the challenges of conducting VR experiments outside the lab and state that "protocols have to be self-running, self-documenting and robust to user behaviour" in the context of using devices in non-lab settings. These qualities will be considered when developing the co-design method that is the subject of this paper.

Multiple studies (Huber & Gajos, 2020; Mottelson & Hornbæk, 2017) have found similar effects in unsupervised, online VR studies compared to lab-based VR experiments. When looking at the effect of embodiment illusion, Huber and Gajos (2020) found that effect sizes were smaller, so they point toward the importance of larger sample sizes when completing this kind of study. Thus, this will need to be considered when analysing the results of this study.

Rivu et al. (2021) propose a framework for running VR studies remotely, specifically using participant-owned HMDs. They identify two different types of remote VR study (both making use of the existing VR community). In the first type, participants completed the study independently, and in the second, participants completed the study with a virtually co-located experimenter present. They also discuss using an existing VR platform such as VRChat, RecRoom, AltSpaceVR or Mozilla Hubs as they share the advantage of being existing social VR platforms. While the framework focuses on recruiting existing VR users, many of the findings can be applied to a study distributing VR equipment to non-VR users such as this one.

Materials and Equipment

Virtual Reality Systems

The last 7–8 years marked the period in which high fidelity consumer-grade virtual reality systems first became widely available (Samsung Mobile Press, 2014). These systems are able to simulate a virtual environment through use of a "6 degrees of freedom" (6DoF) head-mounted display and controllers. 6DoF systems track the user's orientation and position in 3D space, allowing them to explore the virtual environment by walking around. They support much higher-resolution display of realistic environments compared to their predecessors. Examples of systems released around this time include the original HTC Vive and Oculus Rift (Fig. 4.2). However, these systems are required to be connected to a high-performance PC, which both increases the overall cost and adds to set-up complexity. They also require "base stations" that assist in tracking the headset and controllers' movement in space, further increasing set-up complexity.

Mobile phone-based VR systems were introduced as a response to these issues and often involve the user inserting their phone into a headset, which they use to drive the VR experience. Google cardboard (Google Cardboard – Google VR, n.d.) and Samsung Gear VR (Samsung Gear VR with Controller, n.d.) are examples of this kind of technology. These work well for simple 360 experiences such as viewing 360 videos; however, these systems are only capable of tracking the orientation (not position) of the headset. This is known as 3DoF tracking and limits the user's immersion somewhat. In a study exploring how geographically separated users could interact in social virtual reality, Moustafa and Steed (2018) distributed Samsung Gear VR devices (and Samsung smartphones) to 17 participants. In the feedback collected from diaries after use for a few weeks, participants reported technological issues when using the equipment, including audio difficulties, and issues with the wearability of the headset (heat/weight issues). It was reported that these issues are not prohibitive to the use of the headset but did affect the participants' immersion. The participants reported that the primary barrier to use of the equipment was the inability to move naturally. This highlights both the weaknesses of 3DoF tracking and the potential effectiveness of this technology.

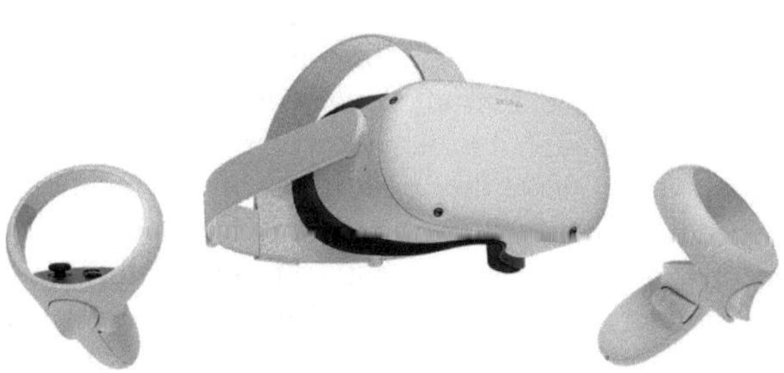

Fig. 4.2 Meta Quest virtual reality system

2019 saw the release of the Oculus Quest (since rebranded as the Meta quest) and potentially mark the start of a new wave of virtual reality devices. These new devices are completely "untethered", meaning they are capable of running stand-alone without the use of a high-performance PC and make use of "inside-out" 6DoF tracking, meaning they do not require external tracking hardware. Such a compact tool is, therefore, much more feasible to deploy in the home, as set-up complexity is kept to a minimum. This methodology will target the Meta Quest 2, which internally runs an Android-based operating system. The Meta Quest 2 is also relatively inexpensive at £400, which is far more accessible to most users compared with the £1000+ cost of PC-based VR.

In addition to the immersive virtual reality systems discussed above, VR CAVE systems in which projections on each of the surfaces in a room can also be used to create immersive virtual environments. Also, "mixed reality" and "augmented reality" platforms provide options for devices that could be used with this group. Modern smartphones can provide camera-based augmented reality to enhance the users' physical world with computer-generated input. Mixed reality takes this a step further through enabling the users to interact with both virtual and physical objects in their environment. A significant challenge of this co-design methodology will be communicating the benefits of each of these technologies so co-researchers are able to make informed design decisions.

Virtual Reality Software

The software used to facilitate the social interaction will depend on the study, although a range of social VR platforms exist that could be used as a starting point. Previous studies have used Oculus Rooms, VRChat (VRChat, n.d.), AltspaceVR (AltspaceVR, n.d.), vTime (vTime – Reality Reimagined, n.d.), RecRoom (Rec Room, n.d.) and Mozilla Hubs (Hubs by Mozilla, n.d.; Moustafa & Steed, 2018; Rivu et al., 2021; Yoshimura & Borst, 2020). The features these platforms provide vary, although common to all is the functionality that allows users to meet in various virtual environments, interact with these environments and embody an avatar. Rivu et al. (2021) points out that most of them also allow the creation of custom environments built on these platforms; however these can be more restrictive than standalone applications.

Rivu et al. (2021) also discuss the advantages of various other distribution methods for existing VR users. These include direct download, where the application file is downloaded and installed manually by the user. This gives the most development freedom, although it is the most complex to set up. An app store could also be used, which would make the application simpler for the participants to install, although depending on the app store platform the publishing costs might be prohibitive. This methodology will assume that the technical abilities of the participants will be limited; therefore an app store will be used to distribute and provide updates to the application. Meta have recently released their "AppLab" platform, which allows for free and easy distribution without the need for verification before publication on the Meta Store.

There are many potential use cases for VR for those with intellectual disabilities, e.g. creating a safe setting in which to practice skills including the development of independent living skills (Standen et al., 1998; Brooks et al., 2002), orientation (Standen et al., 2001), travel training (Brown et al., 2005) and vocational training (Michalski et al., 2020). Immersive virtual reality could also be used as a medium to communicate and socialise with one another remotely (which is especially relevant given the current global pandemic). Regarding the latter, services such as VRchat, AltspaceVR and Mozilla Hubs are all free and allow their users to meet together using immersive virtual reality in an online virtual environment.

VR-based rehabilitation has received a lot of attention in research literature, although less so in those with intellectual disabilities. While it may seem intuitively that this may be due to the level of cognitive and coordination skills required to use assistive technologies, it has been demonstrated that those with intellectual disabilities can use immersive VR technologies with varying degrees of assistance (Harris et al., 2020; Kongsilp & Komuro, 2019).

Method

A methodology specific for those with ID using immersive VR technology could be structured in a variety of ways. The lessons learnt from our previous research have indicated what worked well and what could be done better. This section explains the different aspects of the proposed research method.

Authors' Previous User-Centred Design Studies

This proposed methodology will draw from experience in completing two studies in reducing social isolation with adults with intellectual disabilities using AR and VR. Two studies with the "NICER" group will be discussed. NICER is a group of adults with disabilities including Down syndrome, Williams syndrome and moderate to severe intellectual disabilities. This group has been involved in various research projects for the last 20 years and were participants for both the studies being discussed here.

The first study (referred to from here as "study 1") used the "Mixed Reality" Microsoft HoloLens to investigate the use of augmented reality in combating social isolation conducted in 2019 (Harris & Brown, 2019). This field study began with an investigation of shared AR experiences to treat loneliness with adults with intellectual disabilities and applied some elements of user-centred design (Fig. 4.3). Feedback sessions took place at the group's monthly meetup at a local school, and the participants were invited to try the system for 5–10 min at a time.

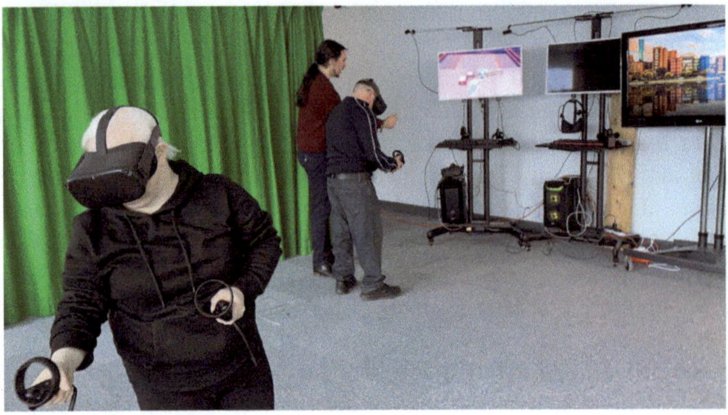

Fig. 4.3 Overview of the study 1 investigation of shared AR experiences

The aim of this study was to assess whether an application for the HoloLens could be used to reduce feelings of social isolation. The HoloLens was chosen initially due to its potential for "holoportation", where users can be virtually present in another's virtual space (Orts et al., 2016). Feedback sessions were held with the participants throughout and after the development of the system to obtain their views and evaluate the system, as well as raise any usability issues they found while using the system. This feedback session was recorded, and the participants' views transcribed and synthesised.

It was found that involving the individuals in the development process allowed the prototype to speak for itself, meaning the participants were more involved and invested in the outcomes of the project. However, the user-centred approach used had the researchers leading on design, which meant there could possibly be a gap between what the participants wanted and what the researcher interpreted.

It was identified that the use of a psychology-based questionnaire, though rooted in scientific enquiry, might not be appropriate to use with intellectually disabled adults to evaluate the system because the language used was deemed difficult to understand. Therefore the participants were also involved in discussion as to how the UCLA loneliness scale (Russell, 1996) could be adapted.

The second study (referred to from here as "study 2") in 2020 used immersive virtual reality (Oculus Quest) to assess the usability of VR with users with intellectual disabilities (Harris et al., 2020). The Oculus Quest was chosen here partly due to the gestures required to use the Microsoft HoloLens being difficult to perform for the participants and partly due to the lack of maturity of the HoloLens as a platform. While the Oculus Quest is also a relatively new technology, the software framework and the input media used to interact with the applications are much more mature.

Participants were invited to the university's VR lab to try the introductory activity "first steps" that comes preloaded on the Oculus Quest. The participants were advised that they could ask for help if they were stuck but were asked to complete the study independently where possible. After this, they took part in a focus group with semi-structured questions to discuss their experiences. They were introduced to the VR system without being told how it should be used to encourage unbiased contributions.

Prior to data collection taking place, a framework was developed, which would be used to assess the amount of assistance required by participants. This was validated by the participants and other stakeholders (including researchers familiar with working with this group). The amount of assistance required and the qualitative feedback given were used to assess usability.

It was found that those with ID can use the Oculus Quest with varying degrees of assistance. Most participants were engaged throughout. A few issues were raised that should be considered when developing virtual reality applications: The first was to keep the use of buttons (especially the grip button) to a minimum, and the second was to avoid complex gestures where possible. It was also suggested that VR applications not involving the use of the controllers could be effective. The results from this usability testing will be useful moving forward.

Neither of these studies invited the participants to help form the research aims, and those involved in both studies took on the role of participants rather than co-researchers. The methodology proposed here aims to empower the adults with intellectual disabilities involved as co-researchers, rather than participants.

Though relinquishing control can be very difficult, the research team experienced in the past studies that use of elements of co-design yielded unexpected, authentic feedback from the participants. In study 2, efforts were made both to not prime the participants on how the VR system should be used and to encourage independent use. Through this, it was made clearer what usability issues exist with that particular VR system.

Co-design

In study 1, participants only provided input on the software solution itself and the data collection measure. Everything else was left to the researcher to decide. This led to meaningful yet limited findings. In study 2, co-design was used to create the experimental methodology itself. The participants validated the coding framework that would be used to assess usability and contributed what they considered important. This study generated not only a greater number of contributions but also a variety of topics could be explored, some of which could not be predicted while planning the study such as the participants' use of the controllers. The benefits of researching "with" participants (or more accurately, co-researchers) with ID are now considered more important than researching "for" them. Therefore, this article proposes the use of co-design method to enhance co-researchers' contribution to the study.

In the feedback sessions in study 1, it was surprising to hear many participants give specific feedback on the functionality of the VR system during the focus group sessions. This helped the researcher understand what aspects of the system were important to the participants (such as voice chat). In this way the participants were able to help shape the system. However, the problem statement itself came from the literature, and in hindsight more effort could have been devoted to co-evolve the problem with the participants.

Initial feedback sessions in study 1 introduced the participants to the headset. These highlighted that while some of the gestures used to interact with the hardware were difficult to perform, most of the participants reacted positively to the AR system. By observing the participants using the system and involving them at such an early point in the project, it became clearer what kind of issues a system using this kind of device would need to address.

A basic initial prototype was then developed, with little functionality other than multi-user head tracking in mixed reality space. The participants were shown this, and many were quick to comment on new features they would like to see added (such as voice chat or full-body tracking functionality). This loosely fits into design for adapting spaces (Sanders, 2005), where the participants fill in an unfinished design artefact how they think it should look. This had the benefit of encouraging the participants to think creatively.

The participants were also able to co-experience the study not only through viewing their partner in VR but also by spectating the virtual environment through a (non-immersive) laptop set up nearby. The importance of this spectating was realised in this study and used more extensively in study 2 as it eliminated the need for the participants to describe what they were seeing.

The final evaluation session had the participants use the final version of the system and then discuss what issues they encountered in a focus group scenario. Use of an experienced facilitator familiar with the group here was key to promoting discussion. This took place at the group's monthly meetup; this relaxed environment promoted co-sharing of experiences. Valuable feedback was gathered from this meeting, although the nature of the session meant that the participants were using the system that was designed for online communication across the room from each other. In hindsight this did not help in communicating the purpose of the system to the participants. It would likely have been better to have the participants try the system on a more realistic deployment (e.g. from the homes) to better achieve this, and they then may have been prompted to impart more information on how they think it could have been improved.

A discussion was also held on how the final version of the system could be formally evaluated. The participants were encouraged to comment on how a pre-existing questionnaire-based measure could be adapted for use with people with intellectual disabilities. This was partially successful in that some suggestions were collected, though they largely came from other research staff and the aforementioned experienced facilitator. A potential benefit of this could have been to allow the participants to take ownership of the study.

The second study took place on the university campus to facilitate screen sharing more easily. Even though this was an unfamiliar location, many of the same research staff were present who the participants were familiar with. This helped the participants feel comfortable in providing feedback.

Co-evolving the problem involves working with the co-researchers to understand what social isolation means to them. Probes could be used, for example, in the form of a diary to help the co-researchers understand and communicate their issues and understanding of social isolation. This also has the effect of strengthening their role as experts by experience (as found in Spencer González et al. (2020)).

Helping the co-researchers understand how immersive virtual environments could be used to address these problems is key to co-defining the study. Workshops could take place which work to encourage the co-researchers' creative expression. Spencer González et al. (2020) point out that imaging desirable futures has proven to be difficult mindset to achieve for people with intellectual disabilities, as it requires speculative and abstract thinking.

Discussion

These elements from previous studies are considered in the current methodology. To begin with, focus groups will be held with the co-researchers to understand the issues relating to social isolation they face. From this, the problem statement can be formed, as can the project's objectives and scope.

After these have been defined, the co-creation of the system itself begins. The co-researchers have the VR equipment sent to their homes and are encouraged to try existing VR software to familiarise themselves with the technology. During this time, focus groups and one-to-one sessions can be held with the co-researchers to observe and gather feedback on how they use the VR equipment in order to aid development of a new VR software solution. These are flexible in nature depending on the objectives as defined in the earlier stage. Interpersonal process recall (Brown et al., 2016) sessions could also be held to help the co-researchers communicate their ideas more easily and reflect on their experiences using the VR software. Following this, focus group sessions can also be held on how the system is best evaluated.

Hendriks et al. (2015) propose a framework in which six key method stories are considered when carrying out co-design with co-researchers with intellectual disabilities (positioning the impairment, aiming for equivalence, balancing of viewpoints, dealing with ethical challenges, adjustment of co-design techniques and data collection, analysis and interpretation). The next sections will discuss how these have been addressed.

Positioning the Impairment

Initial Participant Selection

"Participants" in this study will in reality be treated as co-researchers and help co-design the virtual environment, and hence the term co-researcher is used consistently from now on.

Despite the benefits of using the latest virtual reality systems as discussed above, it has been noted that some intellectually disabled individuals have varying capacity to understand the technology on their own. These form an important part of participant selection criteria.

Intellectual disability is categorised based on intensity as mild, moderate, severe and profound (American Psychiatric Association, 2013). Those with mild and moderate intellectual disabilities were shown to have sufficient cognitive, coordination and communication skills to participate in the previous usability study (study 1), so long as use of controllers is kept to a minimum where possible (Harris et al., 2020). Those with severe or profound disabilities had more difficulty using the VR equipment and communicate their experience to the research team. For this reason, the study will work with adults with mild or moderate intellectual disabilities initially, with the view to expand the study to include co-researchers with severe and profound disabilities at a later date.

The technological literacy of those with ID varies, and those with experience with game consoles (e.g. some of the younger adults) might have better success in using the headset and controllers for VR study being proposed. It is important that the voice of both those who have this experience and those who don't are heard in studies of this kind.

Selection Criteria:

- Participant is able to give informed consent to take part in the study.
- Participant has mild or moderate intellectual difficulties initially, and then in future iterations of this study, participants with severe or profound disabilities will also be invited to participate.
- Participant's carer agrees to assist the participant with the VR device during the study.

Participants who are interested in research may be more likely to engage with the technology, and groups of individuals who have taken part in research projects before are ideally placed to take part and provide useful feedback. A governance meeting will be held with the participants and used as an opportunity to explain the purpose and the structure of the study. If the participants are to be treated as co-researchers, it is important they are offered help to shape the aims of the study and are supported in achieving this.

Facilitators/Carers

Those that care for individuals with intellectual disabilities have a good understanding of the special needs of such individuals. They can be considered the gatekeepers to the use of new technologies by intellectually disabled individuals, and including them in design increases the chance of uptake. It is important that the carers are included in the co-design process where possible.

The Oculus Quest 2 is a consumer-grade virtual reality headset, and the headset itself walks the user through much of the set-up. Despite this, in many cases intellectually disabled participants will need help to use it. Therefore, this responsibility falls to the participants' carers.

The carers are unlikely to have used the Oculus Quest or other virtual reality headsets before, and their technical literacy might be limited. This will mean that the carers will need to learn how to use the headsets themselves. The pre-installed training/tutorial software included on the headset should make this fairly straightforward, although the researchers may need to be able to provide further support.

Compared to other offerings, the Oculus Quest is relatively inexpensive. However, carers may be concerned about breaking/damaging the headsets. Therefore, the researchers will need to assume liability for the headsets; otherwise the carers may not wish to take part.

Aiming for Equivalence

To encourage valuable contributions from the co-researchers, they need to be made aware what is trying to be achieved with the technology. This information sheet should use clear, concrete language and be supported by symbols, and the information should be made clear through the study design itself. Accessibility can be achieved through careful choice of language and by taking time to explain what is meant. Therefore, the purpose of each session should be easily understood by the co-researchers.

Weighting the contributions from participants is a key part when a researcher is using user-centred design approach and designing for the people with ID rather than with them. However, in co-design, the contributions come from a shared experience and can be communicated by any participant. So an interesting experience by one participant (with good interaction with technology but not as good with communicating) could be explained by another participant, a group or a carer (someone better at explaining the details and recognising the valuable aspects). The community decides the valuable aspects in an organic way and communicates them through a variety of media (diary, act out, etc.). The researcher does not have to provide weights to any contributions or worry about everyone contributing. The data is co-shared.

Facilitating Discussion

Encouraging discussion is important to gather more detailed feedback from the co-researchers. Building relationships and having a familiarity with the group assists with this. This could be achieved through having prior experience in working with the group and collecting feedback over other activities. Co-researchers are more likely to be open with their thoughts on the system design if they feel confident and relaxed with the researchers.

An online focus group taking place within the virtual environment will be recorded as part of the data collection. Probes will be used to initiate conversation. It is hoped that this will remove the focus from the co-researchers and allow them to open up more. These probes will consist of elements (or even games) within the virtual environment. This has the additional benefit of helping the co-researchers become comfortable with the VR system. During these sessions the researchers, co-researchers and carers will all be expected to be virtually present and engage with the focus group discussion. Carers will also be used to help interpret feedback given by the co-researchers.

It is important that views of those with different impairments are listened to and considered, in a similar way to those expressed by academic-based researchers and carers. Academic-based researchers may have limited knowledge of the co-researchers' different needs. Therefore, an experienced facilitator will also be used to aid communication of ideas to the group. This individual has been working with the group with co-designers with intellectual disabilities for over 20 years. They are familiar with each of the group members and with each group member's disability and needs. They are also experienced in interpreting the limited spoken language from members of the group.

It is possible that big personalities may dominate the discussion during the focus group sessions. Therefore, in addition to these, one-to-one semi-structured interviews will also be held to further analyse design decisions. This is why carers should be introduced to the technology along with the adults with intellectual disabilities. The carers' understanding of the study could greatly aid them helping co-researchers as expected by the researcher.

Feedback will be carried out both within use of the VR-based intervention and post-immersion. The researchers will be virtually present during the use of the VR systems and will be encouraging the co-researchers to engage with the virtual environment, as well as record any issues raised.

Balancing of Viewpoints

It is possible that the viewpoints of the academic-based researchers, the co-researchers and the carers in the different design decisions may conflict. Hendriks et al. (2015) discuss situations in which the participants' views may conflict with the carers' views, and there is a risk that the researcher may rely too heavily on the input of carers. The need for co-verifying is important for balancing the viewpoints contributed by the community.

The semi-structured interviews can be recorded and reviewed not only by the researchers but also by the participants. "Interpersonal process recall" can be used to obtain further feedback by allowing the participants to view extracts of their recorded VR session, to allow them to recall further thoughts and feelings that they were not able to at the time (as used in Brown et al. (2016)). It's possible they may not be able to properly communicate feedback in the heat of the moment, so interpersonal process recall has the advantage of allowing them to effectively do this in following sessions and reflect on past co-design decisions. This aids in balancing viewpoints between those with less developed communication skills and those with more developed communication skills.

Dealing with Ethical Challenges

Consent

To take part in the study, the co-researchers need to provide informed consent. Effectively communicating the format of the study, the technology and the risks of the technology poses a significant challenge. Also, considering they are integral to the study, the co-researchers' carers also need to consent to taking part as well.

In the use case given previously, only those with mild to moderate intellectual disabilities will be asked to participate to begin with. This poses the issue of excluding those with severe or profound disabilities. This is regrettable, but based on the (limited) existing literature, those with severe or profound intellectual disabilities are much less likely to comprehend, understand and feedback on their experiences in using a VR headset and associated software. This group could be included in future iterations of this study if it were first trialled with other groups.

Since this is a co-design methodology, there is an increased importance placed on the co-researchers' understanding on the aims and objectives of the study. Therefore, the co-researchers need the information communicated to them as clearly as possible, which may require text alternatives such as pictures, video or Makaton (The Makaton Charity, n.d.).

Safety Concerns Using the Meta Quest in the Home

The Meta Quest is a virtual reality headset that is interacted with primarily through motion controls, so by definition it requires sufficient space (2 m × 2 m) to use safely and effectively. It is expected that the carers ensure that there is enough space (though it is anticipated that the room dimensions of a UK dwelling may create challenges here) (Threapleton et al., 2016). Also, the set-up process for the Meta Quest includes marking out a boundary that warns the user if they are in danger of crossing these boundaries. In addition to this, it also has pass-through cameras that are used in the set-up process, and it will identify objects that the co-researcher might be in danger of tripping over. Assuming the boundary is set up correctly (and no obstacles enter the boundary after set-up, such as pets), the risk to the user is manageable.

Another potential health and safety concern is that of virtual reality sickness. This commonly occurs after prolonged exposure to a virtual environment and causes symptoms similar to motion sickness (LaViola, 2000). Though the experience may vary, any motion sickness symptoms generally disappear shortly after removing oneself from the virtual environment. It is important carers and co-researchers are briefed on this and instructed to remove their headsets if symptoms are experienced. This information needs to be communicated in a sensitive manner to the co-researchers, as this may create a priming effect. In particular, the language used will need to be carefully chosen and verified by experts.

Additional support could be provided on top of the information documentation, to assist setting up and using the device. A member of the research team will be "on call" and available to the carers when the devices are in use. Assistance could be provided through video calls or similar.

Adjustment of Co-design Techniques

A virtual environment can be set up initially using Mozilla Hubs. The co-researchers can then visit the virtual environment using their Oculus Quests in a one-to-one session with one of the research team members. These sessions could be video and audio recorded using the software available on the headset, as can observations by the research team.

Discussion can be facilitated online with assistance from the experienced facilitator. Pre-recognised, open-ended questions will be used to obtain unbiased opinions from the co-researchers on their experiences and prompt natural discussion. These sessions can be held online both within the virtual environment and in person where possible. These can also be recorded for later analysis.

The feedback from these sessions will be collected and used to adjust the online environment based on feedback suggested by the co-researchers and academic-based researchers.

Data Collection, Analysis and Interpretation

Each co-researcher experiences the virtual environment in three types of session:

- *Virtual environment session*: A 10-min session with member(s) of the research team, in which they are asked to complete activities with a given focus for that week.
- *Focus group session*: A focus group session with the other co-researchers, in which questions are posed to the group to prompt discussion. These sessions take place on alternating weeks to the virtual environment sessions.
- *IPR session*: A one-to-one semi-structured interview, again with the research team. Interpersonal process recall will form part of these sessions to gain further feedback. These sessions take place every 4 weeks and prior to the virtual environment being updated.

These sessions take place alongside development of the virtual environment, and feedback is analysed to prioritise new features. As previously mentioned, all of these sessions are recorded. The focus group questions are reviewed by each of the team to remove bias. In addition to this, interpersonal process recall forms part of the interviews. Each co-researcher will be asked to review the recordings of the focus group sessions and the virtual environment sessions.

In the case where ambiguous statements have been made by the co-researcher, the experienced facilitator will be contacted to provide verification.

Anticipated Results

This methodology is considered successful if a virtual environment for people with intellectual disabilities can be created, which is tailored to their needs, as outlined by the co-researchers themselves and can be integrated within the community. The advantages afforded by co-design are a key to this. While most research methods have element of researcher bias, co-design method ensures that co-researchers co-design the process and co-experience it. The methodology aims to give co-researchers as much control over the design process as possible. It stands to reason that co-researchers who had a hand in creating a solution are more likely to enjoy using it more and that it is more likely to meet their requirements. Co-researchers should feel that they are involved in the process, have had a chance to collaborate and experience some ownership of the project. Thus, the measure of success for the co-design process is the acceptance by community of the outcomes of the research as it represents their own contributions.

Co-design focuses on designing for a purpose, rather than the designing of a product (Sanders & Stappers, 2008). The use of co-design to design for facilitating social interaction (rather than just simply designing a shared virtual environment) should promote the creation of a system that addresses social isolation. The research method will be used to investigate whether a VR environment can be used to reduce social isolation. The measurement of such feeling will be based on the experiences that the co-researchers illustrate. The criteria for success in such a study will evolve from the aspects of social isolation that the community considers to be most affecting them and the tool addressing the problem in one or more of these identified areas.

The application of the proposed research method will present experiences of working with adults with intellectual disabilities using VR and will allow other researchers and designers to learn from this. It will indicate to future researchers the advantages and risks of using co-design method for a VR-based study with individuals with intellectual disabilities.

The proposed methodology builds on both existing literature and the author's own experience investigating the uses of VR with individuals with intellectual disabilities. This study will further show the potential VR has to improve the lives of individuals in this group, if approached in a sensitive and inclusive way. The results will highlight design paradigms that can be used in future VR applications.

Further insights on methods used to evaluate VR systems from co-researchers' homes will help in designing studies run this way. Giving the co-researchers day-to-day access to the equipment to obtain collect data on how they use VR over the longer term is something that has not received as much attention in the literature.

References

AltspaceVR. (n.d.). *Be there, together*. In: AltspaceVR. https://altvr.com/. Accessed 22 Apr 2021.

American Psychiatric Association. (2013). *Diagnostic and statistical manual of mental disorders (DSM-5®)*. American Psychiatric Publishing.

Brooks, B. M., Rose, F. D., Attree, E. A., & Elliot-Square, A. (2002). An evaluation of the efficacy of training people with learning disabilities in a virtual environment. *Disability and Rehabilitation, 24*, 622–626. https://doi.org/10.1080/09638280110111397

Brown, D., Shopland, N., & Lewis, J. (2005). Design and evaluation of a flexible travel training environment for use in a supported employment setting. *International Journal on Disability and Human Development, 4*, 251–258.

Brown, B., Reeves, S., & Sherwood, S. (2011). Into the wild: Challenges and opportunities for field trial methods. In *Proceedings of the 2011 annual conference on Human factors in computing systems – CHI '11*. ACM Press, p. 1657.

Brown, D., Kettley, R., & Kettley, S. (2016). *Interpersonal process recall – A method for reflecting on co-design experiences* (p. 5).

Google Cardboard – Google VR. (n.d.). https://arvr.google.com/cardboard/. Accessed 6 May 2021.

Harris, M. C., & Brown, D. J. (2019). *Investigating the use of virtual reality in combating social isolation.docx*. Nottingham Trent University.

Harris, M. C., Lewis, J., Brown, D. J., & Vyas, P. (2020). Assessing the usability of current generation virtual reality in adults with intellectual disabilities. In *Proceedings of the 13th international conference on disability, virtual reality and associated technologies*, p. 9.

Hendriks, N., Slegers, K., & Duysburgh, P. (2015). Codesign with people living with cognitive or sensory impairments: A case for method stories and uniqueness. *CoDesign, 11*, 70–82. https://doi.org/10.1080/15710882.2015.1020316

Huber, B., & Gajos, K. Z. (2020). Conducting online virtual environment experiments with uncompensated, unsupervised samples. *PLoS ONE, 15*, e0227629. https://doi.org/10.1371/journal.pone.0227629

Hubs by Mozilla. (n.d.). Accessed 22 Apr 2021.

Kongsilp, S., & Komuro, T. (2019). An evaluation of head-mounted virtual reality for special education from the teachers' perspective. In *25th ACM symposium on virtual reality software and technology*. ACM, pp. 1–2.
LaViola, J. J. (2000). A discussion of cybersickness in virtual environments. *ACM SIGCHI Bulletin, 32*, 47–56. https://doi.org/10.1145/333329.333344
Lawson, B. (2006). *How designers think – The design process demystified*. Cambridge University Press.
Lee, J.-J. (2014). The true benefits of designing design methods. *Artifact, 3*, 5.1–5.12. https://doi.org/10.14434/artifact.v3i2.3951
Michalski, S., Ellison, C., Szpak, A., & Loetscher, T. (2020). *Using virtual environments to train work skills in people with neurodevelopmental disorders: A systematic review*.
Mottelson, A., & Hornbæk, K. (2017). Virtual reality studies outside the laboratory. In *Proceedings of the 23rd ACM symposium on virtual reality software and technology*. Association for Computing Machinery, pp. 1–10.
Moustafa, F., & Steed, A. (2018). A longitudinal study of small group interaction in social virtual reality. In *Proceedings of the 24th ACM symposium on virtual reality software and technology*. Association for Computing Machinery, pp. 1–10.
Orts, S., Rhemann, C., Fanello, S., et al. (2016). *Holoportation: Virtual 3D teleportation in real-time*.
Porter, J., Ouvry, C., Morgan, M., & Downs, C. (2001). Interpreting the communication of people with profound and multiple learning difficulties. *British Journal of Learning Disabilities, 29*, 12–16. https://doi.org/10.1046/j.1468-3156.2001.00083.x
Rec Room. (n.d.). In: Rec Room. https://recroom.com. Accessed 19 May 2021.
Rivu, R., Mäkelä, V., Prange, S., et al. (2021). Remote VR studies – A framework for running virtual reality studies remotely via participant-owned HMDs. *ArXiv210211207 Cs*.
Russell, D. W. (1996). UCLA loneliness scale (Version 3): reliability, validity, and factor structure. *Journal of Personality Assessment, 66*, 20–40. https://doi.org/10.1207/s15327752jpa6601_2
Samsung Gear VR with Controller. (n.d.). Official Samsung Galaxy Site. http://www.samsung.com/global/galaxy/gear-vr/. Accessed 6 May 2021.
Samsung Mobile Press. (2014). *Samsung explores the world of mobile virtual reality with gear VR*. https://web.archive.org/web/20140906045517/http://www.samsungmobilepress.com/2014/09/03/Samsung-Explores-the-World-of-Mobile-Virtual-Reality-with-Gear-VR-1. Accessed 12 May 2021.
Sanders EBN (2005) Information, inspiration and co-creation. In *Proceedings of the 6th international conference on european academy design*.
Sanders, E. B. N., & Stappers, P. J. (2008). Co-creation and the new landscapes of design. *CoDesign, 4*, 5–18. https://doi.org/10.1080/15710880701875068
Spencer González, H., Vega Córdova, V., Exss Cid, K., et al. (2020). Including intellectual disability in participatory design processes: Methodological adaptations and supports. In *Proceedings of the 16th participatory design conference 2020 – Participation(s) otherwise – Volume 1*. ACM, pp. 55–63.
Standen, P. J., Cromby, J. J., & Brown, D. J. (1998). Playing for real. *Journal of Mental Health Care, 1*, 412–415.
Standen, P. J., Brown, D. J., & Cromby, J. J. (2001). The effective use of virtual environments in the education and rehabilitation of students with intellectual disabilities. *British Journal of Educational Technology, 32*, 289–299. https://doi.org/10.1111/1467-8535.00199
Standen, P. J., Brown, D. J., Anderton, N., & Battersby, S. (2006). Systematic evaluation of current control devices used by people with intellectual disabilities in non-immersive virtual environments. *Cyberpsychology Behavioural Impact on Internet Multimedia Virtual Reality Behavioural Society, 9*, 608–613. https://doi.org/10.1089/cpb.2006.9.608
Standen, P. J., Rees, F., & Brown, D. (2009). Effect of playing computer games on decision making in people with intellectual disabilities. *Journal of Assistive Technologies, 3*, 4–12. https://doi.org/10.1108/17549450200900011

Steed, A., Archer, D., Congdon, B., et al. (2021). Some lessons learned running virtual reality experiments out of the laboratory. *ArXiv210405359 Cs.*
The Makaton Charity. (n.d.). https://www.makaton.org/. Accessed 21 May 2021.
Threapleton, K., Drummond, A., & Standen, P. (2016). Virtual rehabilitation: What are the practical barriers for home-based research? *Digital Health, 2*, 2055207616641302. https://doi.org/10.1177/2055207616641302
Tsikinas, S., & Xinogalos, S. (2019). Studying the effects of computer serious games on people with intellectual disabilities or autism spectrum disorder: A systematic literature review. *Journal of Computer Assisted Learning, 35*, 61–73. https://doi.org/10.1111/jcal.12311
VRChat. (n.d.). In: VRChat. https://hello.vrchat.com. Accessed 22 Apr 2021.
vTime – Reality Reimagined – vTime (en-GB). (n.d.). https://vtime.net/. Accessed 19 May 2021.
Yoshimura, A., & Borst, C. W. (2020). *Evaluation and comparison of desktop viewing and headset viewing of remote lectures in VR with Mozilla hubs*. The Eurographics Association.

Chapter 5
Amplifying Ability: Engaging Young People with Autism Spectrum Disorders Through Gesture, Movement and Sound Technologies

Wendy Keay-Bright

Introduction

> Our body applies itself to space like a hand to an instrument, and when we wish to move about we do not move the body as we move an object. We transport it without instruments as if by magic, since it is ours and because through it we have direct access to space. — Maurice Merleau-Ponty

In recent years the discipline of human–computer interaction (HCI) has shifted beyond studying the effectiveness of tools and functions to include more holistic experiences of emotions and senses. The affective relationship that humans have with interfaces has been of interest to artists for many decades. When a viewer appreciates a work of art, feelings of self-absorption arise from the colour, scale, degree of abstraction and representation, rather than physically manipulating the work. In this respect the viewer imagines the work to have some relationship to them (Vischer et al., 1994). Interactive artists began examining this affective relationship between users and technologies by using camera and projection technologies to permit users to disturb, distort and make a personal impression on virtual artworks. In 1969, computer scientist Myron Kruger (n.d.) used sensing floors, graphic tables and video cameras to enable participation using unencumbered, full-body action, which led to the term "virtual reality". His Videoplace[1] installation is one of the earliest references to interactive environment, as his projected artworks appeared to anticipate and respond to audience actions, acknowledging their presence. Hybridised systems of hardware and software have continued to excite artists,

[1] http://jtnimoy.net/itp/newmediahistory/videoplace/

W. Keay-Bright (✉)
Centre for Applied Research in Interactive Arts and Design (CARIAD), Cardiff School of Art and Design, Cardiff Metropolitan University, Wales, UK
e-mail: wkbright@cardiffmet.ac.uk

E. Brooks, D. J. Brown (eds.), *Virtual Reality Games for Rehabilitation*, Virtual Reality Technologies for Health and Clinical Applications,
https://doi.org/10.1007/978-1-0716-3371-7_5

who by nature explore assimilations of old and new techniques in order to push boundaries, provoke audiences and facilitate critical thinking.

Since their evolution in the 1970s, virtual environments have been exploited in therapeutic and medical contexts. Until recently, however, the cost and perceived complexity of virtual environments have inhibited their appropriation in mainstream practical settings. Now, the reduced cost and voracity for natural user interfaces, such as the Kinect 3D[2] motion sensing camera, have prompted the interest of researchers eager to resolve more day-to-day accessibility and communication problems for people with physical, developmental and cognitive disabilities. For the most part, research focuses on how to improve functionality through tangible, physical interaction, rather than considering how body movement and gesture are central to how humans experience the world. One of the key factors in this is that observing performance in relation to task can provide a source of objective, empirical data, whereas using the body for expressive purposes resists analysis; metrics for understanding creativity and expression are highly subjective and much more complex to quantify. However, we do know that when people feel good about themselves, when they feel happy and relaxed, they are more able to cope with challenge.

In response to these issues, the work described in this chapter has evolved through a conceptual approach to system development. We explore movement, gesture, rhythm and sound as the very essence of experience for all humans and take this as a starting point for discovering new possibilities for interactive collaboration. The interactive artworks we have created deliberately set out to appreciate any user responses and actions and to use these as the foundation for understanding how to engage young people with autism in meaningful ways. By adopting this position, we propose that artists, developers and end-user communities can be empowered to reshape the way in which we deploy technology systems to engage more people with disabilities.

A note on terminology. When discussing autism from a diagnostic perspective, we use the term autism spectrum disorders (ASD). However, in describing how our relationship with this audience influenced the design of the interfaces, we prefer to use autistic person as this is preferred by the major of participants in this research.

Structure of Chapter

Following a review of related literature, the chapter will describe work from a decade of creating software with young people diagnosed with autism spectrum disorders (ASD), their families and the professionals who support them. We make connections from the literature to support our methods of co-designing in authentic user contexts. The founding principle of co-design being that only users can bring their cumulative knowledge into the design process and make interaction a

[2] http://en.wikipedia.org/wiki/Kinect

meaningful extension of their experiences and interests (Desmet & Jan Stappers, 2011). Designing alongside young autistic people offers a highly relevant context for understanding how movement and sound may engage people with other complex cognitive, developmental, sensory and physical needs. In detailing our experience of developing two touch and camera input applications, ReacTickles and Somantics, we highlight some of the issues faced by researchers and designers interested in developing interactive systems. These are (1) how to facilitate a responsive design environment when the target population are diverse, possibly non-verbal and with complexities in sensory experience that can be overwhelming; (2) how to make any design outputs open enough to support experimental use and yet still afford meaningful outcomes in a range of settings; and (3) how can we learn from observations in order to improve the design of interfaces that have both therapeutic and educational impact.

Context and Related Literature

The section begins with an overview of the diagnostic criteria for autism spectrum disorders (ASD), with a focus on selective attention, stereotypical behaviour and sensory impairment. The purpose of this is to offer the reader a context for understanding how we have established design principles for software development in relation to these features. We continue to explore ideas related to the body by referencing key theoretical concepts from phenomenology, including the influence of gesture, mirroring and body schema, on how we perceive possibility for action through the senses. A short review of interactive arts is included in order to align our approach to current trends in interaction design.

Autism

Autism is defined as a developmental disorder in which a person demonstrates persistent deficits in (A) social communication and interaction across contexts, which impact on social-emotional reciprocity, non-verbal communicative behaviours and developing and maintaining relationships, and (B) repetitive patterns of behaviour and interests, which impact on speech, motor movements and object use. Recent updates to the diagnostic criteria now include hyper- or hypo-reactivity to sensory input or unusual interest in sensory aspects of the environment. This sensory dysfunction can manifest in adverse responses to sounds or textures, excessive touching and smelling, indifference to pain and a fascination with lights and violent movement (DSM 5, APA, , 2011).

Repetitive Patterns of Behaviour and Interests

Stereotypical behaviours tend to be utilised by a person with ASD as a way of coping with unpredictability in social situations. However, this issue is complex; these behaviours also occur as a consequence of sensory dysfunction; in some cases they are a way of creating sensory stimulation, but they may equally be a way of managing sensory overload (Leekam et al., 2011). Finding ways to manage these stereotypical behaviours effectively is essential as they can severely impact on a person's ability to turn their attention to new information, to concentrate over a sustained period of time and to interact creatively (Leekam et al., 2011). Furthermore, these behaviours can reinforce negative attitudes and in some cases become self-injurious (Nind & Kellett, 2002). When considering the relevance of movement in relation to engagement, it is important to note that the complexities associated with autistic sensory dysfunction can also mean that physical activity is a challenge. In addition to poor motor functioning (Koegel et al., 2001), difficulties in planning and self-regulation can all lead to low motivation for taking part in movement-related activity (Ozonoff et al., 1994; Renner et al., 2000).

There is a wide range of literature that discusses how rhythm-based strategies can promote the management of stereotypical behaviour, effective emotional regulation and social interaction in a variety of populations (Murray & Trevarthen, 1986; Wolf et al., 1967). Music therapy programmes and the playing of instruments have been reported as decreasing stereotypical, self-stimulatory behaviours (Muller & Warwick, 1993; Wimpory et al., 1995; Wylie, 1996). Other repetitive, rhythmic, physical exercises such as jogging (Kern et al., 1984) and horse riding (Jolliffe et al., 1992) have also been shown to reduce unwanted stereotypical behaviours. Stereotypical movements are not only associated with autism; studies have shown that there is likely to be an increase in repetitive behaviour in all humans during transition between key stages of physical development (Sharp & McGee, 2007). Examples cited are rocking and swinging legs when learning to sit. In relation to this, it has been suggested that rhythmic movements are a natural behaviour employed by humans to assist in mastering a new skill (Sharp & McGee, 2007).

Research exploring the impact of responding positively to stereotypical behaviour and restricted interest as a source of engagement is gaining support from educators and parents (Marans et al., 2005; Wetherby, 2006). Recent studies that use technology as a medium for incorporating restricted interests into an intervention programme have reported positive results when appropriately deployed (Jacklin & Farr, 2005; Morris et al., 2010). Murray, Lesser and Lawson have undertaken extensive research into the benefits of computers for autistic people; their work is universally cited and further acknowledged from the autistic perspective in blogs and discussion groups online (Murray, 1997; Murray & Aspinall, 2006; Murray & Lesser, 1997).

Positively rewarding computer interaction usually requires a user to direct their attention towards selected information in a confined space and to filter out distractions from other stimuli. The concept of selective attention, which refers to the tendency to focus on information that is meaningful and of interest, is of particular relevance as it is both a defining feature of autism (Murray et al., 2005) and a contributing factor for authentic involvement with interactive technologies (Bracken & Lombard, 2004; Steuer, 1992).

Selective Attention and Autism

Murray, Lesser and Lawson have used the monotropism theory to explain why being able to focus deeply and tightly on a narrow range of interests is one of the most defining differences between autistic and non-autistic people. For monotropic, autistic individuals, interests are highly aroused, meaning that all the available attention is attributed to one interest and they are unable to focus on other information. Non-autistic people, on the other hand, will have a polytropic tendency to focus more broadly on many things at one time. A highly aroused focus of attention that excludes anything that is not being specifically attended to can be a source of skill or excellence (Lawson, 2011). Computer interfaces tend to compliment the monotropic interest system, providing focus on task, filtering out extraneous detail and limiting interaction to one input attributed to one output.

Multi-modal technologies endeavour to incorporate more physically direct and emotionally expressive interaction. Having access to a richer sensory world has been cited as affording a more embodied, immersive experience. Embodied interaction requires deep focus, a sense of control, a self-absorbed flow of activity and a harmony of bodily and cognitive involvement (Dourish, 2001). However, there is little research that explores how people with sensory abnormalities, such as low-functioning autism, respond to such technologies.

Phenomenology and Human-Computer Interaction (HCI)

In phenomenological terms embodiment refers to the way in which the body engages with the world at hand in relation to its environmental aspects, through all the senses (Merleau-Ponty, 1962; Proffitt, 2006). Studies have shown that there is a direct relationship between the actions we are intending to perform, the effort required for such actions and the perception of the space (Proffitt et al., 2003; Witt et al., 2004). These facets of perception all contribute to our motivation to perform an action (Proffitt et al., 2003; Witt et al., 2004).

The term *affordance* refers to how a person uses conscious knowledge and perception for action when interacting with objects (Norman, 1988; Gibson, 1986; Overbeeke & Wensveen, 2003). For example, on seeing a cup, one knows to use the handle to grasp it and that it is possible to drink from it. In Gibsonian terms, this conscious understanding of possibility is not the product of high order cognition; rather it is derived from direct perception and corresponding sensory flow, without the need for any other form of informational processing (Gibson, 1986). According to Gibson's theory, it is not simply physical and sensory information that compels us to use an object; it is also our intentionality and the goals we perceive are possible. If we apply this reasoning to the spaces we encounter, for example, schools, then this explains why corridors and playgrounds are experienced as spaces to run in and classrooms are known for sitting still. For this reason, designers refer to the significance of affordances in reducing the amount of cognitive processing – and instruction – needed by a user in order to perceive the functionality of an object or interface (Overbeeke & Wensveen, 2003).

Maureen Connolly, a Professor of Physical Education and Kinesiology at Brock University, has developed therapeutic environments to help children with ASD to manage change and unpredictability. Through her research she has recognised that children with autism perceive information in their environment differently from their typically developing peers and that their sensory abnormalities can impact on how spatial-temporal information is processed. She has developed settings that can be customised through the use of colour and light; however, she points out that children may need habitual exposure to spatial-temporal change in order to reduce anxiety caused by sensory overload (Connolly, 2010). Habitual routines enable us to cope with the challenges of change through updated perceptions of possibility (Connolly, 2010; Seamon, 2012).

Body Schema

In the *Phenomenology of Perception*, Merleau-Ponty suggests that the body is constantly extending itself beyond the borders of the flesh and into the wider world, which it accesses through perception and reflection (Merleau-Ponty, 1962). Through perception the body reaches out of the physical or "objective" body; Merleau-Ponty calls this the phenomenal body (1945). If it were possible to visualise this body as a shape, it would be a continuously shifting and morphing shape (Seamon, 2012). Every posture, every gesture, every attitude and every pattern of thought would alter the shape in some way.

Body schema is understood to be an unconscious process used primarily as a means for organising one's body in relation to objects and the spatial environment. Head and Holmes first termed the *Body Schema* in 1911 to describe the unconscious mapping of the actuality of bodily experience in relation to the perceived possibility for experience (Head & Holmes, 1911). During body movement the body schema is continuously updated in relation to the configuration of limbs, the shape of the body surface and the integration of tools, actions and intentions (Holmes & Spence, 2004). Understanding the brain's representation of the body in relation to spatial-temporal awareness has important implications for people suffering from disabilities and disturbances of the body schema and is thus of relevance the design of virtual reality technology (Held & Durlach, 1993).

Mirrors

The use of mirrors as a schematic tool to extend the body's reaching space has been studied as a source visual and tactile stimulation for people with disabilities (Pavani et al., 2000). The studies suggest that the brain's representation of visuotactile peripersonal space can be modulated to *incorporate* mirror images, inanimate objects and tools held in the hand (Holmes & Spence, 2004). In a mirror, as in video representations, it is possible to see our body in one position while feeling it to be in another position through the proprioceptive sense (Held & Durlach, 1993). Mimetic activities that foster expression and musicality are not only a source of pleasure, but they are known to strengthen relationships and stimulate conceptual development or imagination and personal identity (Dissanayake, 2000; Foster, 2005).

In the design of responsive environments for people with ASD, we need to understand how the corporeal body is used in the process of interacting directly in space – through tools and through sensory perception (Connolly & Lathrop, 1997). Mirroring – either co-located or in representations of the body – may also a play key role in fostering engagement. The role of the body schema in affording such opportunities will be discussed later in the chapter in the discussions of the Somantics project.

Gestural Interaction

Gesture is a representational and observable form of body movement. As such, gesture can be understood to be both a response to whatever we perceive and an active contribution to our perception of the world (Goldin-Meadow, 2002; Goldin-Meadow, 2003). Gesture can be classified as being manipulative, based on physical, haptic contact (Miranda & Wanderley, 2006), and communicative, as semophoric sign or semiotic code (Quek et al., 2002). Other forms of gestural movement are not necessarily directly linked to semantic meanings and are more unconsciously expressive. An example of this is responding to rhythms and beats whereby people synchronise and move in resonance with the sounds and music (Godoy & Leman, 2010). When we sense that our movement is in time with the movements of others, this can lead to feelings of empathy and harmony with others (Godoy & Leman, 2010). Throughout history, moving and singing together have made collective tasks far more efficient, playing a profound role in creating and sustaining human communities (McNeill, 1995). Gesture has also been analysed by performance theorists as a medium for creating empathy between a performer and an audience (Foster, 2005). The dance critic John Martin proposed that not only does the dancer employ movement to express his ideas but also that while observing the dance the observer internally mirrors the movement in order to understand the meanings the dancer is trying to convey (Martin, 1965).

Neuroscientists have investigated the ways in which we relate to another's movement through the deployment of our own body movement. Research in this area shows that the mirror system is grounded in brain regions where the perception of action and the execution of action partly overlap. The mirror system offers a neuronal basis for understanding how people can understand each other's intentions without having to rely in building a mental representation or needing to construct a theory of mind (Gallese, 2005; Gallese & Goldman, 1998). Certain mirror neurons are thought to affect our capacity for visual/kinaesthetic recall, meaning that that action performed by one person can activate motor pathways in another's brain responsible for performing the same action. The second person understands what the first is doing because this mirror mechanism lets her experience it in her own mind (Rizzolatti et al., 2006).

These theories imply that interfaces that generate movement and rhythm may facilitate empathy between partners and groups without having to understand another person's intentions of feelings. In relation to people with autism, this is an important issue, as poor theory of mind is attributed to their perceived lack of empathy with others (Baron-Cohen, 2001).

Bodily Interaction with Technology

The introduction of consumer game platforms such as the Nintendo Wii and Microsoft Kinect, which allow for full-body input, led to the development of a range of interfaces that encouraged physical, sensory, social and emotional stimuli to increase attention, exertion and physical exercise.

Physical Exercise

A genre known as *exertion games* has emerged through virtual sport-type games (Mueller et al., 2010). While these tend to be outcome driven, they are of interest to our research as studies have shown that there is a direct correlation between the amount of physical effort required to perform effectively and the sense of immersion the player experiences. Studies of exertion games revealed that players associated meaning to their level of exertion actions, although this tended to be related to social context (Mueller et al., 2010). Significantly, Mueller et al. reported that exertion also elicited affective expressions from players and that verbal comments were supplemented by a gesture, such as throwing their hands in the air to indicate they had won.

However, not all gesture is communicatively expressive. We use gesture as an unconscious response to sensory stimuli such as music, rhythm and beat and how this might lead to the sense of autonomy, self-awareness and harmony. Before we bring this review of related literature to a conclusion, we reflect on the creative opportunities afforded by interactive arts applications that bring spontaneous, affective movements into consciousness.

Interactive Arts

Pioneering animators from the 1920s–1950s, such as Oskar Fischinger, Len Lye and Norman McLaren, used the frame-by-frame animation technique to create the illusion of moving artworks that synchronised with rhythm and music. These films enchanted audiences by offering a unique aesthetic experience that did not impose meaning through narrative or character. Audience appreciation of the films was facilitated through their perception of the synchronicity of light, colour, line, rhythm and beat. These films have no tools with which to physically interact, but the experience of watching them creates a bodily response that is similar to that of watching a dance performance (Wells, 2000).

The early pioneers of interactive artworks fashioned experiences with computers in which abstractions of light, colour, line, rhythm and beat appeared to be directly responsive to user input. More recently, with the availability of sensing input and projection output tools that accurately mirror body position, artists have been interested in mapping input to graphical and audio output data to create immersive interactive artworks. These interactive pieces do not impose meaning; instead, the user experiences a sense of presence by being able to exert control and modify the artworks. Examples of these techniques can be seen from the work of artists Golan Levin and Zachary Lieberman.[3] Software artists Scott Snibbe and Hayes Raffle describe the user experience of interaction with artworks as *socially immersive media* (Snibbe & Raffle, 2009). They have applied the concept of "using the person's entire body as the input device, unencumbered by electronics or props" to facilitate social interaction through projected museum exhibits. Audience participation enthusiasm and engagement in challenging and unfamiliar topics were reported to have increased as a result of the highly visceral interaction. The artists attribute the success of these exhibits to the fact that young visitors could discover engagement on their own terms through experiences that are emotional, social and physical (Snibbe & Raffle, 2009).

People without disabilities, and who are in good health, use their bodies unconsciously to attune to their environment; in this way they are able to carry out tasks and discover possibilities for actions without instruction. When there is a disability present, this natural ability becomes a challenge (Finlay, 2011). Concepts from phenomenology such as cause and effect, body schema, gestural interaction and mirroring can provide new ways of thinking about these challenges, but rather than thinking of disability, we can think more creatively about how humans attune to environments through their unique perceptual abilities. An arts-based approach provides an ideal medium for exploring the ways in which all humans, regardless of ability, find empathy through combinations of light, colour and rhythm.

To summarise, we have reviewed literature from a variety of perspectives that converges on the viewpoint that the body is central to our very being. Merleau-Ponty (1962) describes experiencing the world as perceived through the body as the

[3] http://www.tmema.org/mis/

foundation of all knowledge, for it is through the body that people gain access to actual and possible experiences of acting in the world (Connolly & Lathrop, 1997; Gunnar & Gapenne, 2009). In exploring the potential of technologies to enhance well-being for people with an autism spectrum disorder, we begin from these foundations. When bodily experience is expressed through movement, it indirectly communicates within the world in which it is situated. Rudolf Laban, through his theories and interpretations of movement, aimed to engage dancers and audiences through performing and observing the body's natural rhythms (Gunnar & Gapenne, 2009). Animators have similarly choreographed movement with abstract forms. In our approach designing interaction with technologies, we frame our work in the same way – as a mode of choreographing and observing authentic experiences of movement. In the following sections, we describe the software applications we have designed that have been informed by this literature but, most importantly, understood through practice.

From Theory into Practice: ReacTickles and Somantics

In this section we describe our observations of young autistic people engaging with two different software applications, ReacTickles Magic and Somantics. Each application has a different visual interface; however, they share the same ethos of encouraging movement and rhythm as both input and output. The challenge has been to understand how to *capture* interest and to *maintain* an enjoyable, immersive experience. In design terms we aimed to achieve this through temporal spontaneity and kinetics, visual simplicity and mirroring. The close harmony between bodily input and projected output establishes a visceral feedback loop between the user and interface, resulting in a cycle of dynamic bodily interaction. The amplification of self that occurs during the feedback cycle suggests that the graphical interfaces serve an important mediating role in interaction.

ReacTickles Magic and Somantics were co-created in special education settings: a school and a residential college for children and young adults with a diagnosis of autism and Asperger's syndrome. All design activities were conducted with the guidance of teaching professionals and focused on observing, documenting and reviewing the actions of young people as they explored prototypes over a period of time.

In view of our intentions to take a mindful approach to developing ReacTickles Magic and Somantics, we will describe the projects in two different ways. We will discuss ReacTickles Magic by drawing on studies with one group of autistic children undertaken over a 6-week timescale. Somantics has encompassed a wider range of user activity from the outset; therefore we will refer to early responses that were captured in a variety of settings. The purpose of this is to value first reactions as well as to appreciate the need to allow time for some young people to discover possibilities for action on their own terms. Firstly, we make reference to the original desktop version of ReacTickles to explain the origins of our recent work with sensing technologies.

ReacTickles

From 2005 to 2007, a project called ReacTickles included the design of a series of cause-and-effect applications in which shapes, patterns and colours responded playfully to interaction with a mouse, keyboard, microphone and interactive whiteboard. Throughout the development of the software, autistic children aged 4–7 years were involved in prototype iteration. Over the 2 years, teachers made many compelling videos that captured the engagement of children as they explored ReacTickles in the classroom. Research revealed that the key to unlocking communicative potential was to make the interface as uncluttered as possible, to strip out extraneous detail and to avoid semiotic references that may impose meaning. The cause-and-effect style of interaction was designed to shift attention focus from one fixed position. Inspired by phenomena such as elasticity, gravity and inertia, the first ReacTickles were based on circles that traced movement with a range of animated effects. As soon as the child disturbed the circles, they responded by moving around the screen or disappearing and reappearing, morphing and varying in luminosity. The circles appeared to have physical properties in that they could be pulled, pushed, stretched, dragged or tickled. The playfulness and predictability of ReacTickles was directly mapped to the affordances of the input device, for example, smoothing and circling the mouse, pressing and tapping the keyboard and stretching or smoothing across the interactive whiteboard. Repetitive actions were encouraged as a source of reassurance – enabling children to quickly gain control and mastery. This directness of the input-output feedback loop has remained the most defining feature of the software and has been embodied in an updated version, called ReacTickles Magic. For more detail on this early research, see publications (Keay-Bright, 2007–2011).

The iconic, universal design of ReacTickles has transferred well to other devices. The shapes lend themselves naturally into patterns, providing an ideal canvas for developing a sense of rhythm and harmony between the user and the interface or for co-located pairs or groups of users and observers. In describing how ideas for taking ReacTickles onto new platforms progressed, it is important to add that we were motivated, in part, by the widespread adoption of the iPad as a multi-touch surface and the Kinect 3D motion sensing camera, which permits unencumbered full-body movement. Both devices attracted the interest of software artists and programmers keen to use the hardware to engage audiences and users in expressive and interpretive experiences of interaction. With this in mind, we decided to name this new version of ReacTickles, ReacTickles Magic, taking MAGIC as an acronym for Musical and Gestural Interactive Communication.

ReacTickles Magic

ReacTickles Magic has been developed for iPad and Kinect motion sensing inputs. The interface perceptually maps body location, movement, sound and touch, but rather than the output being a pictorial image, a character or object, the outputs are colourful abstract shapes and repetitive patterns that are contrasted against a black background. These iconic shapes, mostly circles, are visually arresting in their simplicity and lack of surface detail. This means that they are easy to attend to and make little demand on cognitive resources. Interaction is entirely exploratory and therefore does not require a precise, predetermined action. By experimenting with different forms of movement, for example, jumping, dancing, spinning and even standing still, ReacTickles Magic will generate a corresponding colourful effect. Pressing, smoothing and tapping on the multi-touch surface of the iPad will create a graphical output that maps the pressure, movement and location of the touch. Any sound can impact on speed, size, position and so on. Furthermore, when the circles are presented as a repetitive pattern, they afford a visual rhythm. When the user touches a circle, cause and effect is experienced through the same sense; thus the bodily input and output are synchronised. When interaction occurs through sounds, the feedback loop is not as immediate – one sound directly maps to a response in the pattern of circles, and when another sound is made, this has a corresponding effect on the pattern, which tends to prompt another sound, and then another, and so on, eliciting a vocal or instrumental rhythm from the user. With movement inputs, again the mapping of input and output is not as direct as tactile manipulation, but because the circle follows the user, or the pattern changes according to user location, the user tends to move their body harmoniously with the graphics. Observing this highly visceral exchange between user input, interface and user output has enabled us to value the actions of our target population as a unique performance. When a projector is used to permit a large-scale rendering of action, the experience becomes more socially immersive as other people observing the action can mirror the actions of the user. This has been a notable discovery – other people appear to naturally join in.

Generative Research

As stated previously, ReacTickles Magic originated from a research project that set out to investigate whether everyday desktop and whiteboard technologies could be relaxing and playful for young children aged 4–7 years with ASD. In taking the project forward in new technological directions, we took the decision to work with an older group, aged approximately 15 years. Through previous connections with staff at a school in South Wales, in the UK, we were invited to locate our generative and evaluative design research activities at the school. We were offered a base room to situate our design activities, which would eventually become the setting where all pupils in the school could use the technology. The school provided specialist education for primary (4–11) and secondary (11–19) pupils.

We named the base room the Magic Room, which immediately served to give it a playful identity and enabled us to schedule activities within the school day without encroaching on other spaces. Having resolved the issue of where to situate the design activities and the technology, we then set about determining which pupils and staff would benefit from participating in the project. As we were aiming to create an application that could be used by pupils throughout the school, we began with a small sample group who experienced the most profound difficulties.

Participants

The core group of participants comprised of six pupils, all male and with an average age of 15 years. None of the boys used functional speech although two of them had single-word utterances. They were all noted to have very poor concentration and were generally passive and compliant. However, this was considered to be a problem as their teacher reported difficulties in finding meaningful activities to engage the pupils and each one required the support of a classroom assistant.

Design Lab

ReacTickles Magic evolved through collaboration with lead user stakeholders within the design research process (von Hippel, 1976). The first stage of *ideation* was organised as a *design lab*. The concept of the design lab has been cited as valuable to participatory design (Binder & Brandt, 2008) and can be useful as a short session for including stakeholders who have limited time to contribute (Westerlund, 2007). Our experience has been that the collaborative nature of a lab can inspire stakeholders to become involved in the longer-term strategic direction of the project (Keay-Bright & Lewis, 2011).

The Magic Room proved an ideal environment for the design lab. We set up a Kinect camera with a laptop computer and projector and worked in the room intensely over a period of 4 days, conducting short iterative cycles of prototyping. Activities were scheduled throughout this period during which children, teachers and classroom assistants contributed to the development of the software by exploring prototypes.

Ideas for ReacTickles Magic began with the circle. According to Jungian philosophy, the circle is a symbol of the self, expressing the "totality of the psyche in all its aspects, including the relationship between man and the whole of nature" (Jaffe, 1978, p.266). Arts theorist Rudolf Arnheim explains that the circle is the simplest possible shape available in the pictorial medium. Until shape becomes differentiated through perception, it does not stand for roundness, but for any shape at all and none in particular (Watts, 1977, p.60). Our vision was that the circle could afford a myriad of interpretations. We were concerned that we needed a starting point for inviting contributions from non-technical informants and suggested that as soon as the circle is subject to some kind of force – provided by user input – it may create some interest. We created a prototype in which a flock of coloured circles were attracted to the user's silhouette as they moved in front of the camera. The goal of this was to demonstrate how the technology worked and not to formalise any design features. When there was no movement, the circles disappeared. At the same time, we created a version that ran on the iPad in which the flocking circles appeared to attach themselves to the finger. We also projected this into the space, using the iPad as a controller. The flocking circles prototype provided the essential mechanism for gaining the confidence of staff, who quickly made suggestions, imagining how their pupils might respond. We documented their ideas using storyboards, which attempted to recreate the flow of user experience as a series of static images. This process of visualisation provided a shared vocabulary for capturing ideas without the use of technology. Hosting the lab over 4 days in the Magic Room meant that we could rapidly translate ideas into prototypes and immediately try them out with pupils and staff in an authentic setting. We were conscious that the ideas had come from adults and needed to evaluate these based in the experience of the children, so as soon as staff felt confident, we introduced ReacTickles Magic to the pupils.

Initial Observations

The Magic Room was initially an unfamiliar setting for the pupils, who consequently were anxious, but not upset, and found many things in the room distracting. As they walked into the room, the prototype of the flocking circles was projected on the wall. When the circles tracked their movement, they showed no interest. With so much new information in the room – people, objects, light and sounds – the projected shapes did not capture their attention. The light from the projector also distracted them and they appeared to seek out sources of sensory stimulation. To this effect, light switches were more compelling than the technology. The design team responded by rethinking the interface, reducing it to one shape that could be controlled by sound, replicating the idea of on/off.

During the lab we created prototypes that varied in complexity; the boys continued to come into the room, gradually relaxing and showing signs of interest. They wanted to use their hands to touch the shapes projected on the wall; however, the Kinect camera did not respond to touch. During an interview one of the teachers advised us that it had taken a long time for the boys to learn to use the interactive whiteboard; as a result it would be difficult for them to learn not to touch the projected graphical interface. It seemed that even though the adults were excited by motion capture, for the young people we were designing for, the relationship between body movement and projected effect was meaningless. Furthermore, only one of them had used an iPad and the device did not appear to interest them. They were unable to concentrate on the screen for long enough to create or observe any effects. In response to this, teachers encouraged the boys to use musical instruments as sound inputs that appeared to be more engaging, although there was little evidence to suggest that the cause-and-effect relationship between sound and image was being understood.

Next, five younger boys with Asperger's syndrome were invited to try the prototypes. This group was confident in articulating their experiences and very sociable. They enjoyed meeting the programmers and loved gaming. They knew immediately that Kinect would capture their movement and explored the prototypes without any need for instruction. They experimented with many different kinds of movement and showed no signs of concern at the lack of structure or goal. They very quickly realised that if they didn't move, the visual effects would disappear, rendering them invisible. They introduced challenge and turn taking, prompting one another to create different effects. These pupils were delighted to be interviewed and to critique the prototypes. As their feedback was entirely positive, we were motivated to ensure that we completed the lab with prototypes that could be explored over time, with different groups, and to continue to adapt and refine our ideas based on regular feedback.

By the end of the 4 days, we developed a ReacTickles Magic prototype interface with different icons providing access to eight different applications. A circle, or repetitive pattern of circles, provided the focal point for the applications, and depending on input – sound, movement or touch – it could cluster, spin, change shape or location, accelerate or decelerate. A summary of the ReacTickles Magic applications is provided below:

Expand: A circle changes to a cross on touch or sound input and increases in size, gradually filling the entire screen.

Flip: The screen is divided into two vertical symmetrical black and white rectangles; a circle attaches to touch or movement and flips the background colour as it moves.

Trail: A flock of circles create a trail around the finger or body as it moves. Sounds change the shape.

Cascade: Touch or movement releases a shimmering pattern of circles. Sounds change the shape.

Orbit: A clock-style pattern of circles is activated by sound or touch; on completion of a full circle, the shape and colour change.

Grid: On sound input circles replace a grid pattern of 24 squares.

Change: A screen of flat colour changes on sound, touch or movement input.

Follow: A circle gracefully follows the body or finger; when the movement stops, the size of the circle increases as if responsive to pressure.

Evaluating Experiences

Taking into account the features of the autistic condition, particularly in relation to sensory interest and attentional focus, it was crucial that we observed the system over time in order to appreciate any benefits. During the lab we had noticed that the boys in our main group had poor concentration and that they could be slow to react, or they could overreact, to a variety of stimuli. We had not yet encountered any notable positive outcomes other than the fact that they were reported to be relaxed and happy. Therefore, the purpose of the evaluative research was to discover how to improve ReacTickles Magic on the basis of observing the experiences of the young people when they were given time to engage on their own terms. Our approach was to remain mindful and to avoid target setting in this early phase. Importantly, we wanted to find out whether the pupils would be motivated enough to interact with ReacTickles Magic over a sustained period of time. Specifically, we were interested to find out whether they would become absorbed in the flow of the experience and evolve new actions, rather than repeat the same action. Csikszenmihalyi describes this as a form of autotelic play, whereby "people concentrate their attention on a limited stimulus field, forget personal problems, lose their sense of time and of themselves, feel competent and in control, and have a sense of harmony and union with their surroundings" (Csikszentmihalyi, 1978).

The boys took part in weekly sessions over a period of 6 weeks in the Magic Room. During the sessions the boys were allocated 20 min each to explore the interface. Either a classroom assistant or the class teacher was present together with the researcher and a research student. Each session was documented using field notes and video. At the end of the sessions, teachers were invited to review the video; the interview was also recorded. Although we were not able to gather the responses from staff after every session, we concluded that capturing the comments of teachers in the natural course of the conversation stream during the sessions provided a suitably rich description of each child's experience. In the next section, we provide a summary of the observations made during the 6 weeks of evaluation. We will refer to the experiences of three particular boys, Ben, Joseph and Ian, who showed the most notable interest in the system. Their names have been changed.

Ben

Ben is 15 years of age, has poor spatial awareness and shows no understanding of personal boundaries; he will quickly run and push his face very close to things, including other people, but makes little eye contact. He does not use speech but makes a few sounds; sometimes this seems to be for sensory stimulation as he presses his neck with his fingers during vocalisation. In the lab sessions, Ben could not tolerate being with the other boys; he knocked over the video camera and persistently tried to turn the light switches on and off. He wanted to stare at the projector light but showed little interest in the projected screen. Ben was often agitated when he came into the Magic Room and would circle repeatedly, jumping close to the corners or towards the researcher; he would then find a corner and rock for a while. We did not intervene until he appeared settled. Gradually his circling and erratic jumping reduced, and he no longer attempted to use the light switch. He was, however, attracted to light, and even though the room had been darkened for the sessions, he gravitated towards light sources. Each session began with the flocking circles application, *Trail*. Even though Ben did not show any obvious interest in *Trail*, it was important to maintain continuity and to give him time to absorb and process events occurring in the room. During the third session, as he was circling the room, he paused and watched the flocking circles of *Trail*. He then continued to circle but introduced a routine whereby he would stop at a certain point and watch while the circles appeared on his body. He remained calm and controlled in this routine for approximately 5 min. This bodily action enabled him to stimulate his interest in light patterns, and during the sessions that followed, we introduced *Cascade*. The graphics in *Cascade* were not as distinct as *Trail*, but the addition of sound input could accentuate the light and movement. While Ben did not pay much attention to this application, he was observed to find the light calming. We started to offer him physical objects that seemed to help him focus and he would go closer to the projections while holding an object. On one occasion he bounced and rocked on an exercise ball, moving it closer to the projected space. When using the ball, Ben took a lot more interest and controlled his rocking movements so that they went closer to the wall, beginning to introduce gentle rhythms. We used the ball in the next session and one of the adults joined in with Ben, rolling the ball back and forward towards the projected circles. He responded well to this and maintained his interest over a short period. Although Ben continued to circle the room in later sessions, the frequency of instances when he chose to move towards the projections and pause increased, and he gradually started to touch the circles; he was also observed to touch his neck and make vibrating sounds when he was happy. In the interview Ben's teacher reported that she felt he was making progress and that she had not seen him concentrate on any other activity for the amount of time he was spending of his own accord in the Magic Room.

Joseph

Joseph is 15 years of age. He is a very contented, placid pupil, eager to please and fascinated by other people. He makes regular eye contact, smiles a lot and likes to communicate by gently stroking the face, although he makes no sounds. A major problem for Joseph is his poor concentration. He really enjoys order and likes to put things away properly. During the lab Joseph was hard to engage. The design team had to leave the room as he was so interested in them that his attention could not be directed towards ReacTickles Magic projected onto the wall. Staff who remained with Joseph during the lab found it difficult to capture his interest apart from when he watched another pupil interacting and joined in. Although this only happened on one occasion, his teacher was surprised, reporting that she had never seen him intentionally join in an activity before. She went further to suggest that the two boys appeared to be collaborating using *Grid* by taking it in turns to change the square to a circle.

During the 6 weeks of regular activity, Joseph's interest increased as he began to engage with the applications that made a clear pattern. We started each session with his favourite application, *Grid*, and offered Joseph a drum and tambourine to help him use sound input. One problem, which we found with most of the group, was that as soon as he started to understand cause and effect, he wanted to touch the wall. As Kinect detects motion, the applications did not respond to touch, which meant that when he touched the circle, nothing would happen. In response to this, we set up the system so that if the sound of the wall being touched was loud enough, then the input would be picked up through the Kinect microphone and the shape would respond. Tentative touch was unlikely to elicit sufficient noise to trigger a change, so we used different props in the room to help Joseph to make a loud sound while touching the wall. By using some hard plastic cups against the wall, Joseph was able to make direct contact with the interface. He quickly gained confidence as each circle in the pattern reacted by changing to a square. This in itself was a serendipitous discovery. Joseph did not communicate by making sounds, so the sound clearly did not engage him, but the action of using the cups to control the pattern harnessed his desire for order. Of his own accord, he created a rhythmic game, and he would complete a row of circles and then hand over the cups to the researcher, as if to say, "your turn". The researcher followed this pattern by handing the cups back to Joseph on completion of the next line. This activity then became part of the weekly routine and we gradually introduced a new application, *Orbit*. *Orbit* offered a new challenge. Initially there is nothing visible apart from the black background, so there is no obvious shape to interact with. In order to trigger a response, the user needs to make a sound or touch. We demonstrated to Joseph that by tapping the cups together, not on the wall, he could create a pattern as each sound made a new small circle until a full clock-like *orbit* of circles completed the pattern and a new shape appeared in the centre. Joseph very quickly learnt to use *Orbit*, inventing a routine whereby whenever the clock completed, he would share the plastic cups before starting a new pattern. He also stopped touching the wall and was observed to pause before sharing the cups. He concentrated well and his enjoyment was obvious. Gradually we introduced Joseph to *Grid* and *Orbit* on the iPad. His initial interest in the device was only to close the magnetic cover and hand it to the researcher; his obsession with putting things away was more compelling than exploring the interface. When we removed the cover and showed Joseph how tapping on the surface could make a pattern, he started to take an interest. It appeared that directness of touch in relation to the patterns captured his attention. Since these sessions Joseph has been able to navigate the ReacTickles Magic interface and select different applications, although sometimes he needs some prompting.

Ian

Ian, aged 15, loves drumming and music. He is a sociable pupil, but has little awareness of personal boundaries, and he finds it difficult to regulate his need for proprioceptive stimulation; in relation to this, he is known to enjoy vigorous movements and deep pressure. He makes eye contact although he either stares at close proximity or looks away and puts his hand over his eyes. He laughs very loudly and often upsets the other children in his class. At the start of the study, Ian was beginning to use speech with prompts.

During the first days of the design lab, Ian demonstrated the most interest in the environment. He appeared to be highly aroused at being able to use sound and movement to create dynamic effects. He particularly enjoyed clapping as a mode of interaction and understood that he was causing the interface to change. He preferred clapping to using instruments, which suggested that the sensory feedback gained from hard clapping was more rewarding for him than playing music. Ian used the exercise ball to move forward and back in front of the projected area, causing shapes to cluster around him. He also used the ball rhythmically by drumming the sides to make the shapes change. This appeared to help him to manage his proprioceptive sensory regulation, and he gradually maintained concentration for longer periods.

We began each of the sessions with *Orbit*. This application had a clear structure as each sound contributed to a pattern, as described above. Ian enjoyed *Orbit* as he could interact by clapping, which at times became very loud. He gradually introduced new rhythms as the shapes changed and paused on completion of each clock pattern. In class he had started to learn shape names and following a prompt from his teacher, he verbalised each of the shape names. More significantly, he looked at the attending adults and pointed to the shape as he spoke, drawing attention to his actions. Over the following weeks, his teacher saw this as an opportunity to introduce the colour names, and he responded by pointing to the shape and saying the colour name. It became clear that Ian was responding well to the pleasure this gave his teacher, and he repeated this activity, verbalising the colour and shape name together. We used this as an opportunity to explore whether Ian could apply the colour and shape names to other ReacTickles Magic applications. He managed this easily and punctuated his hand clapping with pointing, looking to the adults in the room for recognition. While he was concentrating on these actions, his erratic, uncontrolled movements eased. Although his clapping was loud, when shown how to clap less violently, he responded well. In the last session, Ian and Joseph used *Grid* together – Ian said the shape names and Joseph interacted by touching the wall with the cups. When introduced to *Orbit* on the iPad, Ian tapped the screen gently to make the effects; he also smoothed the surface and explored the boundaries using *Trail*. Over time he has managed to sit quietly for long periods and concentrate, even when there are other pupils in the room; he has learnt how to select applications and change colours from a menu. He has also been able to share the device and take turns when required.

Summary of Evaluative Research

The responsive ideation and evaluation method enabled us to interpret the actions of children as abilities to be harnessed. When they felt relaxed and in control, their stereotypical, repetitive actions became more creative and experimental. Teachers were able to facilitate novel communicative exchanges with the children, and each child was able to interact according to emerging interests, rather than having to follow a routine set by others. For example, *Orbit* offered Joseph order and pattern and he initiated a turn-taking game; for Ian it provided a visual prompt for using speech and rhythm. *Ben* enjoyed light patterns and seeing the projection of *Trail* on his body, Ian used *Trail* to explore speed and enjoyed experimenting with the exercise ball to satisfy his need for more vigorous movement; he also enjoyed changing the shapes through sound. Although the visual design was informed by previous work and therefore not entirely novel, the opportunity to use the whole body as a means of control and expression allowed us to focus on the quality of interaction as a real-world experience rather than on judging whether or not an action was right or wrong or whether a skill had been learnt. A significant outcome of the process was that it led to the evolution of new research within the development cycle. From watching the children and listening to teachers, we were inspired to create an interface that actually mirrored the flow of movement rather than only cause and effect. These ideas became *soma-antics*, playful actions with the body.

Somantics Design Research

Somantics was motivated by the capacity of motion sensing and projection technology to convert gesture into visceral, real-world digital performances. Research in the ideation stage served to capture interest and generate responses from our young target group. Formative research in the prototyping stage sought to evaluate and improve prototypes in authentic user contexts. This stage was conducted over a period of 4 months during which we continued to refine prototypes to accommodate: (1) new ideas emerging, (2) usability issues, and (3) cross-platform appropriation.

Formative Research

Somantics began as a design lab with autistic children and students with a diagnosis of Asperger's syndrome, which was conducted within the art curriculum. We approached the school that had been involved in ReacTickles Magic as well as a residential college providing specialist education for students with ASD over the age of 16. Both parties were excited by the project and keen to use the technologies.

The Participants

At the suggestion of art teachers, we worked with young people with Asperger's syndrome. Asperger's is a form of autism characterised by highly aroused, restrictive interests and poor social imagination. The young people we worked with were all known to have difficulty with emotional regulation; they were prone to anxiety and meltdown, which was usually the result of frustration and feeling misunderstood. However, they had no problems in articulating their thoughts and, with the exception of one child, were generally sociable.

The first group we worked with were aged between 10 and 11 years. There were four in the group, three boys in full-time attendance and one girl who was attending the school in the mornings. The boys were good friends and enjoyed the art classes.

Typically, they enjoyed talking about their ideas but could respond negatively when questioned.

The second group comprised of six students aged between 19 and 22 years, four boys and two girls, in full-time residential care at a college of further education for students with ASD. They were verbally articulate; however, they had poor concentration when undertaking tasks that were not motivating for them.

Ideation

Knowing that the participants may find concentration difficult provided helpful constraints on the design process. We could not overwhelm with long explanations; we also wanted them to feel able to express their ideas without fear. We proposed to start the labs by showing some early abstract animation films. The idea being that the kinetic composition of flowing lines, colours and music may elicit emotional and rhythmic responses and help to generate ideas.

We began by showing three films as inspiration: *Colour Box* by Len Lye (1953), A*llegretto* by Oskar Fischinger (1936) and *La Merle* by Norman McLaren (1959). The first two films use shape and colour to create a visual syncopation with music that has strong percussive overtones; the third film was a depiction of a song, sung in French, using strong black lines and repetitive patterns. Another film, *Free Radicals* (Len Lye, 1958), was used for our first hands-on activity. We undertook the same activity in both settings. We introduced the films and talked about how the animators had created the movement by drawing or scratching directly onto thin strips of film. We projected the films and asked the groups to talk to each other briefly after each one. We then projected *Free Radicals* without the visuals so that they only heard the soundtrack, which was based on a traditional African drumbeat. We provided a variety of drawing materials and asked the participants to draw anything that came to mind while we played the soundtrack in the background. As soon as the music finished, we asked them in turn to talk about their drawings; we then projected the film again, this time with the visuals; and they compared their responses to those in the film. This was a relatively short activity; the films were no more than a few minutes in length. The children concentrated well and showed no signs of distraction; they seemed to enjoy the drawing activity and talked happily to us about their drawings. As we had consent to film all the activities, from parents and the children themselves, we captured the whole session on video and kept all their drawings for future reference.

Each drawing produced by the children was very different. While one child created a seemingly random series of yellow lines, another created an ordered pattern of different coloured circles with lines flowing around the edges of the paper. The girl designed a regular pattern of purple circles with lines flowing from each of them, joining the circles together. One of the boys created an abstract character and told a story of how the character was responding to objects in the scene.

The students at the college were more easily distracted; two of them paid little attention to watching the films. However, when they were invited to draw while listening to *Free Radicals*, each student worked well. We did not have consent to film the session, and the procedures for filming adults in residential care are far more complex than working with minors, so we documented the process by making comprehensive notes. We asked them to interview each other about their thoughts on the films and what their interpretations meant to them. We also asked them to imagine each of their drawings as something that other people could interact with. This line of enquiry produced the most imaginative responses and they all appeared to enjoy talking about how the artworks could respond to touch and movement.

The drawings were very carefully rendered and highly individual; ideas for interaction were plausible and clearly articulated. For example, one student created a triangle composed of coloured lines and talked about how it might feel to be inside the triangle, to be able to stretch his body and have the triangle behave as if it were made from elastic, stretching around the extremes of his body movement. Another student created the flow of pastel lines; she described how the colours could reflect mood and the lines could be an extension of the arms. She was a very musical student and performed the action as if conducting an orchestra. Another student made an intricate pattern of shapes that resembled a broken glass frame; she talked about being able to push the shapes out of the way and to make a new image appear. Another student talked about being able to see his own image inside a painting, and that as his reflection moved, so would the paint.

At the school we were sensitive to the fact that the children may become upset when questioned about their ideas and so we took a different approach to exploring how artworks may come to life when they have interactive properties. We took the children into the Magic Room and explained to them that we would be projecting some animation onto the wall. They were invited to imagine that they were inside the projections. The first film to be projected was Oskar Fischinger's silent black and white film, *Spirals* (1926). This was followed by *Motion Painting No. 1* (Fischinger, 1947), a colour film, accompanied by the music of Johann Sebastian Bach. Both films include patterns of circles, the latter introducing further flowing lines that appear to be hand drawn.

One of the children was having difficulty concentrating at the start of the session. The activity did not have an obvious structure and he did not cope well. We offered him a video camera and asked him to film the session. He responded well to this and not only captured the activity but also provided a spoken narrative from his point of view. While this had not been a planned activity, the resulting footage provided one of the most inspiring documents of the children's responses to the films. He moved in and out of the projected space and imagined that he was controlling the animation; he also turned the camera to focus on his friends as they performed within the environment. The other children moved in harmony with the animated lines. At times they put their hands on the wall as if directly drawing and at other times they moved away and performed in a synchronised manner using arms and feet, visibly changing the rhythm of their movement in response to the kinetics of the film.

In interpreting the ideas from the children and students, we cross-referenced both sets of drawings and created simple storyboards. We wanted to ensure that cause and effect was prioritised and that the flow of movement could be controlled and executed by knowing where the body existed within the projected image. In dance theory Laban refers to the fact that "form is produced by the limbs of the body and is governed by their anatomical structure which permits only certain movements to be made arising from the functions of stretching, twisting, and combinations of these" (Watts, 1977). In terms of our interpretation, this suggested that the range of bodily interaction could be restricted to particular actions rather than trying to translate every nuance into a matching graphical form.

Prototyping

The first prototypes were based on graphical lines that mapped three types of movement: *swaying*, *stretching* and *circling*. We created these initially for iPad with the intention of observing how the surface afforded movement and rhythm in relation to the graphics. The illustrations below (*Windmills*, *Tunnels* and *Kaleidescope*) show these graphics (Figs. 5.1, 5.2 and 5.3).

We gave these iPad prototypes to the participants. They enjoyed seeing the effects of movements mapped by the graphics. They concentrated well and were observed to squeeze, stretch and push the surface. They also responded well to multi-touch, at times experimenting in pairs as more fingers on the surface would change the image.

Over the following weeks, we created ten prototypes. The prototypes could use both iPad and Kinect inputs and could be disturbed, distorted or manipulated through body movement, leaving a visible trace of user interest. We also began to experiment with mirroring using camera inputs. Although our target group had not designed these, we attempted to recreate some of the ideas that emerged through conversation, such as ghosting, using the body to push paint, a human volcano, and making kaleidoscopic images.

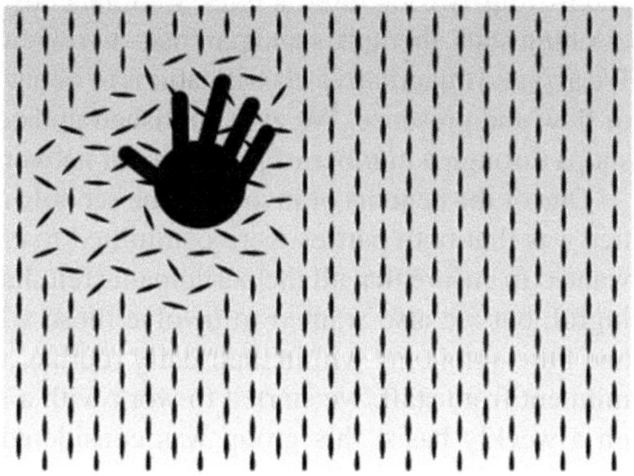

Fig. 5.1 *Windmills* – an orderly pattern of short lines can be disturbed by the finger

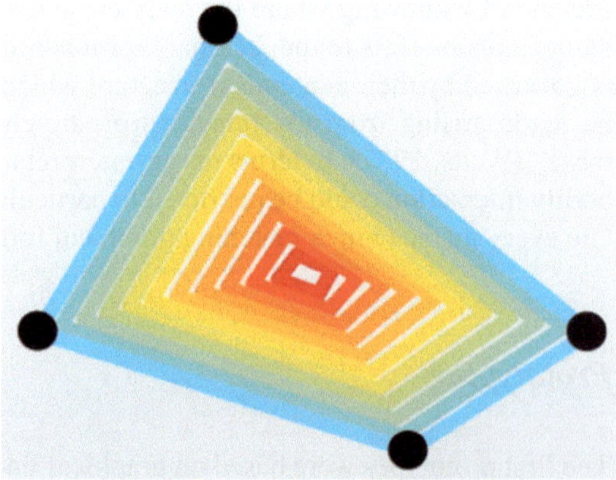

Fig. 5.2 Tunnels – lines form around points on the body, such as, head, arms and feet

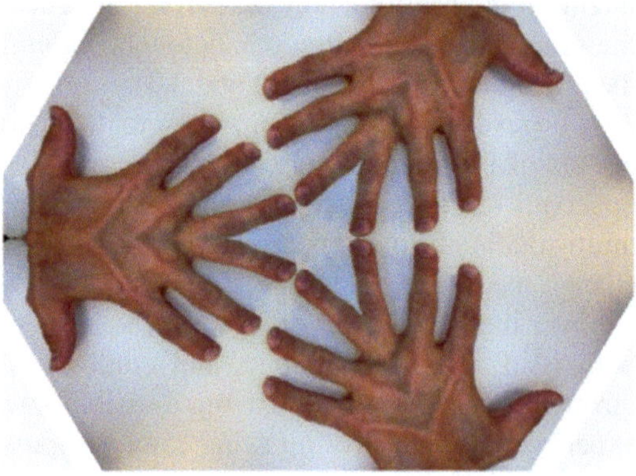

Fig. 5.3 Kaleidoscope creates an optical illusion of a slit screen mirror; a touch or sound can make the mirrors duplicate to form multiple kaleidoscopic images

Formative Evaluation

The evaluation was conducted through observation methods, with data captured using field notes, general observer feedback and inter-observer analysis of video taken from two or three angles simultaneously. We invited a range of experts – teaching staff, therapists and parents – to review and comment on the video footage. We avoided quantitative classifications of behaviour in favour of observing instances of flow and presence. We also published updates on the project blog and ran workshops through a number of professional networks.

One of the benefits of involving the school and college in the initial design activities was that both parties were committed to continuing to support the project. We wanted to ensure that all the participants felt that their contributions had been meaningful, but we also wanted to involve those with the most severe challenges, who had little autonomy within their daily routine. With consent from parents and commitment from staff, we started to work with a new group of students at the college on a weekly basis; this group was considered the hardest to engage and needed one-to-one support. We also met with our original co-design partners and offered them the opportunity to explore the interfaces we had created in response to their ideas.

At the school we introduced the prototypes to the group of boys who were regularly using ReacTickles Magic. By this time ReacTickles Magic was timetabled as a weekly activity and the boys were reported to be enjoying their sessions. The art teacher was confident with using the iPad and Kinect and had independently started to use Somantics with other groups of children. In the following sections, we describe the responses captured from these sessions.

Residential Further Education College

The first group we describe were our co-designers. We set up Somantics in a large activity room and projected the applications onto an interactive whiteboard. This was not ideal as the assumption was that the interface was controlled by touch; however, we were reliant on the existing technology set up for the projector.

Each of the students had very different personalities and interests, which were reflected in their reactions to the applications. Two were very good friends, but one was very reserved. The more confident student quickly involved the other and the two of them choreographed a number of different performances, taking time to observe how the interfaces were responding. They appeared to enjoy the application, *Painter*, in which the user can paint a large film of colour over a video image of themselves. The students remembered the ideas they had contributed towards *Painter*, which gave them a lot of satisfaction. In the lab the more reserved of the two had created a drawing of a triangle comprised of many coloured outlines and had talked about being able to stretch the triangle around his body. We translated this idea very closely and invited him to be the first to test the prototype, which we named *Tunnels*. His interest in *Tunnels* was palpable; he performed with confidence, as if testing the spatial parameters of the triangle. He moved closer and further away from the projection and from side to side. When he stretched his arm movements, the triangle stretched in harmony, causing him to move his arms up and add a leg movement. He was fully absorbed and occasionally looked for recognition from his friend. Other students watched the performance before trying out the different applications themselves. They generally began their explorations individually but very quickly interacted in pairs or as a group. While their attention was drawn towards watching their graphical body schema, they also made comments to one another and regulated their movements with respect to where in the real-world space each person was performing. They added shared rhythms, mirroring their gestures and giving one another verbal instructions. The students were also given Somantics on the iPad, which they also engaged with, but for a shorter period of time, as the temptation to use some of the games downloaded on the device was hard to resist. The musical student who had created a pastel drawing of flowing lines enjoyed *Windmills*, both with full-body input using Kinect and with touch on the iPad, stating that she found this very relaxing. While some of the other students were performing with the projected Somantics, she found the *GarageBand* application on the iPad and started to compose music to accompany the performances. She was having guitar lessons and transferred this knowledge easily to the iPad application. Her teacher informed us that to his knowledge she had not used the iPad before. When we asked her to compose music for her peers, she expressed delight and in the following weeks she took part in sessions with the less able students.

The second group from the college comprised of five students with low-functioning autism (LFA) aged 19–22 years. Their use of verbal language was confined to automatic, repetitive phrases – a condition known as echolalia – one of them also had unregulated body movements and was prone to running around and jumping.

When the students came into the room, the application *Sparkles* was set up. This application projects a monochromatic blue-grey mirror image from the camera, but movement produces a pattern of bright circles, which sparkle around the body. The brightness of the circles partly occludes the video image of the user; movement creates more sparkles, which follow the body, reinforcing the user's presence. Stillness causes the circles to fade and disappear. This idea came from the suggestion of a volcano erupting from the user as they move.

With some prompting, all the students concentrated on the projections, testing out their movements although they each had very different responses. The only female student in the group came into the session by approaching the researcher and repeating her favourite phrase. Her teacher encouraged her to try out *Sparkles*, which she grasped immediately and waved her arms energetically. She tried moving closer and further away from the projections, also standing still and moving different parts of the body. She gradually introduced dance moves. She did not repeat her favourite phase during the activity or while the other students were interacting. The student who liked to run around persistently moved into the projection space, occasionally pausing to look at his body. The teacher had to ask him to sit down, but he found this difficult. Later in the session, he explored *Sparkles* by holding hands with his teacher, keeping his feet still but moving his body slowly up and down.

Another student became a natural performer; he tested *Sparkles* with his favourite toy, using it as a prop to facilitate movement and maintaining a dialogue with the toy as he observed it projected on the screen. He held the toy on his head and began to exaggerate his own movements, letting go of the toy so that he could move his arms. Gradually he abandoned the toy and became immersed in his own performance. A student observing this performance in the background started to mimic the action. His teacher informed us that this student was very reserved and unlikely to join in, but as he was showing indications of wanting to move into the space, the researcher asked him if he wanted a turn. He moved enthusiastically into the area, remaining behind the student who he had been watching and continued to mimic his actions; however he was also able to divert his attention towards the projected images, and as a result, he began to introduce his own moves.

We introduced a new application called *Kaleidoscope*, which created an optical illusion of a slit screen mirror. As the body moves closer to the image, it is possible to make the body disappear. One touch or sound can make the mirrors duplicate to form multiple kaleidoscopic images.

All the students appeared to find this interesting. We felt this may have been due to the fact that using *Sparkles* had built up confidence and expectation that their movement could cause a reaction from the interface. What was of interest to the teachers was the degree of concentration and flow as the students experimented with using the body to effect a change in the patterns. They used their gesture as a form of control, as a form of expression and in harmony with each other. An example of this was when one student moved her arms as if they were wings, moving them far out and close in to see how *Kaleidoscope* responded; the other students copied her movements while watching the effects as they were projected. They tried standing in front of one another, appearing and disappearing. Their teachers and support staff spontaneously joined in by verbally describing what was happening. The patterns seemed to encourage natural rhythms and mimicry as the students were becoming more aware of the effects they were creating. This session was reported to be a success. All the students appeared to be very happy and as they were preparing to leave the staff quickly started to play in front of the screen.

Special School

The first group to try out the prototypes at the school was our co-design partners plus three extra peers, eight pupils in total. We set up Somantics in the Magic Room with a laptop, Kinect, projector and iPads. The room was arranged with one long bench positioned opposite the projection area and the laptop on a small table to the left. The bench became the audience area and the large space in front of the projector became the stage. We introduced Somantics as a turn-taking activity, allowing one student to choose from the desktop interface and then one student to perform. When the performer had explored and choreographed his movement, we invited another to join in. Those that weren't "*on stage*" could use the iPad or watch.

Pupils who had been using ReacTickles Magic were introduced to Somantics by including one new application within the ReacTickles routine. *Ian* made the biggest breakthrough, both in terms of his self-regulation and his verbalisation. When we showed him *Silhouette*, he recognised that his arm movements were causing the graphical triangle to become smaller and bigger and that it moved in response to the speed of his movement. He also noticed when it disappeared and he worked out the parameters of the "*stage*", intentionally moving in and out of the area. He pointed to the *Silhouette* shape and consistently looked at staff for recognition. After three sessions, when using *Tunnels*, he pointed to his graphical image as a series of coloured lines formed around his body and said "*look at that!*" His regular teacher was present and expressed complete surprise at this and repeated the phrase. She advised us that she had never before heard him use any such expression. He has since continued to use the phrase to draw attention to his action. When he was shown *Paths* and *Painter*, he spontaneously pointed to the colours, verbalising the names and changing them with his arms or body movement.

Ben was able to sit close to the wall and while rocking he watched his body creating *Sparkles*. The researcher experimented by moving behind him, making more sparkles and then moving to a different part of the space, taking the sparkles with her. He followed her movement and continued the interaction. We were advised that this level of interaction with another person was very rare.

Another pupil, who did not show much interest in ReacTickles Magic, became very engaged with his image in *Kaleidoscope*. This worked particularly well when he waved the researcher's bright pink scarf. The pink made a strong impression on the Kaleidoscope and he experimented with his movement. The most significant breakthrough for this pupil came when we showed him *Kaleidoscope* on the iPad. He had not used an iPad before; his teacher did not think that he would be able to use the device. Very quickly he moved the iPad screen in front of his face to make his projected image change. When he was shown how to manipulate this further through touch, he experimented with his fingers and concentrated while the image responded. Since this time his teacher has started to use the iPad on a regular basis.

In concluding this chapter, we describe an event for all the pupils at the school, called the Games Olympics. The event was held in a large hall and pupils took part at different intervals during over 1 day. The theme of games was explored in a number of activity bays, sectioned off in the hall. We rigged up a Somantics performance arena in one corner using a large white sheet as a projection screen. We positioned the projector behind the sheet and the Kinect camera on a bench in front.

In essence this inexpensive, easy set-up encapsulates the essence of the Somantics project. The environmental affordances facilitated phenomenological embodied interaction. The projected graphical output on the large sheet represented the body schema, and the temporality of the cause and effect reinforced the pupils' presence as they casually walked past the sheet, capturing their attention and the attention of others, which also prompted mirroring. Furthermore, the soft surface of the sheet appeared to reduce the temptation to touch the surface.

We documented the event using video captured from three angles: one camera pointing at the screen/sheet recording the graphical performance, one camera pointing at the live performance space and a wide angle from above showing the space in the context of the hall. This latter camera viewpoint enabled us to observe pupils before and after entering the space. We matched each of the three camera angles to create a composite video. We were also able to select different viewpoints and review these singly. We invited a number of teachers and the occupational therapist to review the footage and to pick out key moments. The process of capturing from multiple viewpoints and reviewing from a number of experts provided rich data for understanding autistic ability.

Although each of the pupils – ranging from 4 to 18 years – had very different interests, their sequence of actions followed a pattern:

1. Their attention was captured by seeing some form of graphical or video body schema moving in harmony with their movement.
2. Their interest was maintained as they sensed their control though cause and effect.
3. Their movements became increasingly imaginative and experimental.

4. They became immersed in the flow of movement and showed higher than expected levels of engagement.

What was even more surprising was how many pupils and staff on the periphery of the main action started to join in by mimicking the movements of the pupils interacting. On some occasions there were as many as five young people interacting with each other and the screen at the same time, with many others watching. There were some notable differences in interest when there was music playing in the background. The more confident pupils dominated the environment, clearly enjoying the performance. Their body movements corresponded to the rhythms and beats; sometimes they danced individually and at other times in pairs and small groups. When there was no music in the background, the less confident pupils were more active and were observed to maintain interest and interaction. Teaching staff were surprised at how motivated the students became, and they were able to make suggestions on how Somantics could be introduced to individuals and groups across the age and ability range. The occupational therapist pointed out that while pupils were watching themselves projected, their body movements were controlled and regulated.

Conclusion

This chapter has described how several young people on the autistic spectrum have engaged in bodily interaction with responsive, abstract interfaces. Experts have interpreted their interaction as creative and expressive – the participants have gained self-awareness and confidence during their explorations.

Our design methods have included young people on the autistic spectrum and those who support them in a series of ideation and prototyping activities, which have not only informed the technology development, but which have also demonstrated the abilities of the young people. These abilities emerged during the process of co-designing and became amplified through having access to prototypes in authentic settings.

From our observations, a pattern of interest has emerged, which will inform our future work in this area. This pattern can be summarised as:

1. The visual interface should capture attention through an iconic form that responds in harmony to bodily input.
2. Ensure that cause and effect is uncluttered and direct in order for control to be sensed.
3. Maintain interest by delicately adding new possibilities into this feedback loop, encouraging movement to become imaginative and experimental.
4. Enable the natural rhythms of bodily interaction to be the source of shared engagement by making the flow of interest visceral.

In developing ReacTickles and Somantics, we have come to realise that actions on the periphery of the main interface also contribute to the happiness and well-being of individuals. A particular benefit is the possibility of experiencing harmony and empathy with others, even when there may be difficulties with understanding other people's intentions. Many teachers, carers and peers have spontaneously joined in, either in close proximity and thus visible to the user and in the interface or in the background through mirroring and adding their own movements. The impact of this possibility for empathic co-experience is far reaching, but for the purposes of this work, it demonstrates that the greatest contribution these technologies can make to the well-being of individuals is to facilitate an environment for positive, rhythmic observation and exploration, effecting a change in approach from coping with disability to understanding ability.

Acknowledgements We all must thank the staff and children from Ashgrove Special School, Wales UK, particularly Ben Milne, Joy Price, Ruth Jenkins and Headteacher, Chris Britten; the staff and students from Beechwood College, Wales UK, particularly Robbie Gemmill, Jess Davies and Headteacher, Darren Jackson. Thanks also to Glynis Thomas and all the staff and children from the Hollies School, Wales, UK, for their trust and encouragement from the beginning.

ReacTickles was funded by the National Endowment for Science Technology and the Arts. ReacTickles Magic was funded by the Rayne Foundation. Somantics was funded by the Higher Education Academy, Technology Strategy Board and JISC/TechDis. All the projects have received additional funding from Cardiff Metropolitan University.

References

Baron-Cohen, S. (2001). Theory of mind and autism: A review. *International Review of Mental Retardation, 23*(169).

Binder, T., & Brandt, E. (2008). The design:Lab as platform in participatory design research. *CoDesign: International Journal of CoCreation in Design and the Arts, 4*(2), 115–129.

Bracken, C., & Lombard, M. (2004). Social presence and children: Praise, intrinsic motivation, and learning with computers. *Journal of Communication, 54*, 22–37.

Csikszentmihalyi, M. (1978). *Beyond boredom and anxiety: Experiencing flow in work and play*. Cambridge University Press.

Connolly, M. (2010). Constructing a curriculum of place: Embedding meaningful movement in mundane activities for children and youth with autism spectrum disorder (ASD). In L. Embree (Ed.), *Phenomenology 2010* (Vol. 5, pp. 107–134). Zeta Books.

Connolly, M., & Lathrop, A. (1997). Maurice Merleau-Ponty and Rudolf Laban – An interactive appropriation of parallels and resonances. *Human Studies, 20*, 27–45.

Desmet, P., & Jan Stappers, P. (2011). *CoDesign: International Journal of CoCreation in Design and the Arts* (Special Issue: Special Issue: Design and Emotion) (pp. 61–64). Taylor and Francis.

Dissanayake, E. (2000). *Art and intimacy: How the arts began*. University of Washington Press.

Dourish, P. (2001). *Where the action is: The foundations of embodied interaction*. MIT Press/ Bradford Books.

DSM 5, APA. (2011). http://www.dsm5.org/Pages/Default.aspx. Accessed March 2012.

Finlay, L. (2011). *Hermeneutic phenomenology, in phenomenology for therapists: Researching the lived world*. Wiley.

Foster, S. L. (2005). Choreographing empathy. *Topoi, 24*(1), 81–91.

Gallese, V. (2005). Embodied simulation: From neurons to phenomenal experience. *Phenomenology and the Cognitive Sciences, 4*, 23–48. Springer.

Gallese, V., & Goldman, A. (1998). Mirror neurons and the simulation theory of mind-reading. *Trends in Cognitive Sciences, 12*, 493–501.

Gibson, J. J. (1986). *The ecological approach to visual perception*. Lawrence Erlbaum.

Godoy, R. I., & Leman, M. (2010). *Musical gestures: Sound, movement, and meaning*. Routledge.

Goldin-Meadow, S. (2002). Constructing communication by hand. *Cognitive Development, 17*, 1385–1405.

Goldin-Meadow, S. (2003). *Hearing gesture: How our hands help us think*. Harvard University Press.

Gunnar, D., & Gapenne, O. (2009). Actuality and possibility: On the complementarity of two registers in the bodily constitution of experience. *Phenomenology and the Cognitive Sciences, 8*(3).

Head, H., & Holmes, G. (1911). Sensory disturbances from cerebral lesions. *Brain, 34*, 102–254.

Holmes, H. P., & Spence, C. (2004). The body schema and the multisensory representation(s) of peripersonal space. *Cogn Process. 2004 June, 5*(2), 94–105.

Held, R., & Durlach, N. (1993). Telepresence, time delay and adaptation. In S. R. Ellis, M. K. Kaiser, & A. C. Grunwald (Eds.), *Pictorial communication in virtual and real environments* (pp. 232–246). Taylor & Francis.

Jacklin, A., & Farr, W. (2005). The computer in the classroom: A medium for enhancing social interaction with young people with autistic spectrum disorders? *British Journal of Special Education, 32*(4), 202–210.

Jaffe, A. (1978). Symbolism in the visual arts, chapter. In C. Jung (Ed.), *Man and his symbols* (pp. 256–322). Picador.

Jolliffe, T., Lansdown, R., & Robinson, C. (1992). Autism: A personal account. *Communication, 26*, 12–19.

Keay-Bright, W. (2007). *Designing playful sensory experiences with interactive whiteboard technology: The implications for children on the autistic spectrum*. Dancing with Disorder: Design, Discourse and Disaster: 7th European Academy of Design Conference: Published conference proceedings.

Keay-Bright, W., & Lewis, J. G. (2011). *Co-Creating Tools for Touch: Applying an inspire-create-play-appropriate methodology for the ideation of therapeutic technologies, Include, 2011 proceedings*.

Kern, L., Koegel, R. L., & Dunlap, G. (1984). The influence of vigorous versus mild exercise on autistic stereotyped behaviors. *Journal of Autism and Developmental Disorders, 14*, 57–67.

Koegel, R. L., Koegel, L. K., & McNerney, E. (2001). Pivotal areas in intervention for autism. *Journal of Clinical Child and Adolescent Psychology, 30*(1).

Kruger, M. *Videoplace*. http://jtnimoy.net/itp/newmediahistory/videoplace/

Lawson, W. (2011). *The passionate mind: How people with autism learn*. Jesica Kingsley Publishsers.

Leekam, S. R., Prior, M. R., & Uljarevic, M. (2011). (2011) restricted and repetitive behaviors in autism spectrum disorders: A review of research in the last decade. *Psychological Bulletin, American Psychological Association, 137*(4), 562–593.

Marans, W. D., Rubin, E., & Laurent, A. (2005). Addressing social communication skills in individuals with high functioning autism and Asperger Syndrome; Critical priorities in educational programming. In F. R. Volkmar, A. Klin, & R. Paul (Eds.), *Handbook of autism and pervasive developmental disorders* (3rd ed.). John Wiley.

Martin, J. (1965) *The dance in theory*. Princeton Book Company Publishers. (Reprint 1989).

McNeill, W. H. (1995). *Keeping together in time: Dance and drill in human history*. Harvard University Press.

Merleau-Ponty, M. (1962). *Phenomenology of perception* trans. by Colin Smith, (New York: Humanities Press, 1962) and (London: Routledge & Kegan Paul, 1962) translation revised by Forrest Williams, 1981; reprinted, 2002).

Miranda, E. R., & Wanderley, M. M. (2006). *New digital musical instruments: Control and interaction beyond the keyboard* (A-R Editions). Spring.

Morris, R. R., Kirschbaum, C., & Picard, R. W. (2010). *Broadening accessibility through special interests: A new approach for software customization*. In *Proceedings of the 12th International ACM SIGACCESS Conference on Computers and Accessibility (ASSETS)*, Orlando, Florida, USA, October 25–27, 2010.

Mueller, F., Gibbs, M. R., & Frank, V. (2010). Towards understanding how to Design for Social Play in exertion games. *Journal of Personal and Ubiquitous Computing, 14*(5), 417–424. Springer.

Muller, P., & Warwick, A. (1993). Autistic children and music therapy: The effect of maternal involvement in therapy. In M. Heal & T. Wigram (Eds.), *Music therapy in health and education*. Jessica Kingsley.

Murray, D., & Aspinall, A. (2006). *Getting IT*. Jessica Kingsley Publishers.

Murray, D, & Lesser, M (1997). *Autism and computing*. Available URL: http://www.autismandcomputing.org.uk/. Accessed April 2012.

Murray, D. (1997). Autism and information technology: Therapy with computers. In S. Powell & R. Jordan (Eds.), *Autism and learning: A guide to good practice*. David Fulton Publishers.

Murray, D., Lesser, M., & Lawson, W. (2005). Attention, monotropism and the diagnostic criteria for autism. *Autism, 9*(2).

Murray, L., & Trevarthen, C. (1986). The infant's role in mother-infant communication. *Journal of Child Language, 13*, 15–29.

Nind, M., & Kellett, M. (2002). Responding to individuals with severe learning difficulties and stereotyped behaviour: Challenges for an inclusive era. *European Journal of Special Education, 17*(3), 265–282.

Norman, D. A. (1988). *The psychology of everyday things*. Basic Books.

Overbeeke, C. J., & Wensveen, S. A. G. (2003). Proceedings of the DPPI. In J. Forlizzi (Ed.), *From perception to experience, from affordances to irresistibles* (pp. 92–97). ACM Press.

Ozonoff, S., Strayer, D. L., McMahon, W. M., & Filloux, F. (1994). Executive function abilities in autism and Tourette syndrome: An information-processing approach. *Journal of Child Psychology and Psychiatry, 35*, 1015–1032.

Pavani, F., Spence, C., & Driver, J. (2000). Visual capture of touch: Out-of-the-body experiences with rubber gloves. *Psychological Science, 11*, 353–359.

Proffitt, D. R. (2006). Embodied perception and the economy of action. *Perspectives on Psychological Science, 1*(2), 110–122.

Proffitt, D. R., Stefanucci, J., Banton, T., & Epstein, W. (2003). The role of effort in perceiving distance. *Psychological Science, 14*, 106–113. https://doi.org/10.1111/1467-9280.t01-1-01427

Quek, F., McNeill, D., Bryll, R., Duncan, S., Ma, X.-F., Kirbas, C., McCullough, K. E., & Ansari, R. (2002). Multimodal human discourse: Gesture and speech. *ACM Transactions on Computer-Human Interaction, 9, 3*, 171–193.

Renner, P., Klinger, L. G., & Klinger, M. R. (2000). Implicit and explicit memory in autism: is autism an amnesic disorder? *Journal of Autism and Developmental Disorders Feb, 30*(1), 3–14.

Rizzolatti, G., Fogassi, L., & Gallese, V. (2006). Mirrors of the mind. *Scientific American, 295*, 54–61.

Seamon, D. (2012). Merleau-Ponty, perception, and environmental embodiment: Implications for architectural and environmental studies. In R. McCann & P. M. Locke (Eds.), *Carnal echoes: Merleau-Ponty and the flesh of architecture*. Routledge.

Sharp, L., & McGee, A. (2007). *The role of rhythm in the development, maintenance and management of stereotypic behaviours. A review of non-musical literature* (pp 23–27, Vol. 21 No 1 2007). British Association for Music Therapy.

Snibbe, S., & Raffle, H. (2009). *Proceedings of association of computer machinery computer-Human interface 2009* (ACM CHI 2009).

Steuer, J. Defining virtual reality: Dimensions determining telepresence. *Journal of Communication, 42*(4). (Autumn, 1992), 73–93. http://www.presence-research.org/papers/steuer92defining.pdf. Accessed April, 2012

Vischer, R., Mallgrave, H. F., & Ikonomou, E. (1994). *Empathy, form, and space: Problems in German aesthetics, 1873–1893*. Getty Center for the History of Art and the Humanities.

von Hippel, E. (1976). The dominant role of users in the scientific instrument innovation process. *Research Policy, 5*(3), 212–239. Accessed April 2012.

Watts, E. (1977). *Towards dance and art*. Lepus Books.

Wells, P. (2000). *Understanding animation*. Routledge.

Westerlund, B. (2007). A workshop method that involves users talking, doing and making. In *Human machine interaction conference, HuMaN'07*. Timimoun, Algerian Sahara.

Wetherby, A. (2006). In T. Charman & W. Stone (Eds.), *In social & communication development in autism spectrum disorders*. The Guilford Press.

Wimpory, D., Chadwick, P., & Nash, S. (1995). 'Musical interaction therapy for children with autism: An illustrative case study with two-year follow-up' (brief report). *Journal of Autism and Developmental Disorders, 25*(5), 541–552.

Witt, J. K., Proffitt, D. R., & Epstein, W. (2004). Perceiving distance: A role of effort and intent. *Perception, 33*, 577–590.

Wolf, M. M., Risley, T., Johnston, M., Harris, F., & Allen, E. (1967). Application of operant conditioning procedures to the behaviour problems of an autistic child: A follow up and extension. *Behaviour Research and Therapy, 5*, 103.

Wylie, M. (1996). A case study to promote hand use in children with Rett Syndrome. *Music Therapy Perspectives, 14*, 83–86.

Chapter 6
Investigating the Effectiveness of Paper-Based and Computer-Presented Social Stories for Children with Autism Spectrum Conditions in an Autism-Specific Special School

Clara Nevin and Nigel Newbutt

Introduction

Autism spectrum conditions (ASCs) are pervasive and enduring conditions, characterised by a qualitative impairment in social functioning and communication and restricted or stereotyped behaviours (Frith, 2003). It has been reported that the number of children in the Irish education system diagnosed with ASCs has increased from 1868 in the academic year 2006/2007 to 2741 in the academic year 2008/2009 (Parsons et al., 2009). This increase reflects the findings of prevalence-rate projects in the USA and UK (Centre for Disease Control and Prevention, 2009; Baron-Cohen et al., 2009). There is no equivalent study in Ireland. In light of the growing numbers of this community of children in schools, it is important that educational psychologists provide increased support in the form of effective interventions to alleviate difficulties and increase access to education. There has been a growing movement towards the concept of accountability in practice, resulting in an emphasis on evidence-based practice (EBP) and the evaluation of interventions (Dunsmuir et al., 2009; Frederickson, 2002).

C. Nevin (✉)
Educational Psychologist, Dublin, Ireland

N. Newbutt (✉)
School of Teaching and Learning, College of Education, University of Florida, Gainesville, FL, USA
e-mail: nigel.newbutt@coe.ufl.edu

E. Brooks, D. J. Brown (eds.), *Virtual Reality Games for Rehabilitation*, Virtual Reality Technologies for Health and Clinical Applications,
https://doi.org/10.1007/978-1-0716-3371-7_6

Social Stories

One intervention that is widely used and popular for the ASC community, but yet to be validated as an EBP, is that of Social Stories, short narratives that provide information about social situations in a clear, easily understandable way. Social Stories help to alleviate confusion, leading to improvements in social understanding and social functioning (Gray & Garand, 1993). In a 2009 survey, Reynhout and Carter (2007) found that, of teachers who worked with children with ASC, 100% had used Social Stories and 97% thought they were effective. In an American study, Day (2012) found that the majority of school psychologists surveyed recommended the use of Social Stories for children with ASC.

The use of Social Stories was developed by Carol Gray through direct work with children with ASC (Attwood, 2000), resulting in several published articles and books containing recommendations on their construction and implementation (e.g. Gray & Garand, 1993; Gray, 2004). Since the first description of Social Stories by Gray and Garand (1993), the concept has evolved, with updated instructions and criteria on how to construct and implement the stories. At their inception, the first set of criteria recommended the use of four different sentence types in story construction, namely, descriptive, perspective, directive and affirmative sentences (*see* Table 6.1). Two additional sentence types, control and cooperative sentences, were introduced in 2000 (Gray, 2000). The Social Story ratio – the ratio of the various categories of sentences that should be included – was established and included in publications following the initial introductory article (e.g. Gray, 2004). It is recommended that at least twice as many descriptive sentences as any other sentence type be included, to ensure the narrative focuses on describing events and explaining other people's behaviours (Gray, 2004).

Table 6.1 Social Story sentence types and their descriptions

Descriptive sentences	These are statements of fact, with no assumptions or opinions.
Perspective sentences	These describe, or refer to, the inner states of other people, including thoughts, beliefs, feelings, etc.
Cooperative sentences	These identify what other people will do to assist the child/young person.
Directive sentences	These identify responses, or a range of optional responses, to guide the child's/young person's behaviour.
Affirmative sentences	These enhance the meaning of surrounding statements, often expressing a widely held view or opinion in a given culture.
Control sentences	These are statements written by the child/young person themselves, identifying strategies that they will use to implement the Social Story.

Adapted from Gray (2004)

Evidence Base for Social Stories

In addition to their popularity, Social Stories have also been described as 'simple, acceptable, classroom friendly' (Chan et al., 2011). Despite the popularity and practical indications for the utility of Social Stories, along with their widespread use (Reynhout and Carter, 2006), their use has not yet been established as an evidence-based practice. Research into this form of intervention has produced variable results. The National Autism Centre (2009) lists story-based interventions amongst established practices in terms of interventions for people with ASCs. Other conclusions are more tentative, describing evidence as 'promising' while not yet established (Simpson, 2005). Early studies provided some positive results for the efficacy of Social Stories, both in reducing inappropriate behaviours and in increasing adaptive behaviours (Ali & Frederickson, 2006; Reynhout & Carter, 2006). On the other hand, the research base has been described as 'at best incomplete' (Sansosti et al., 2004).

A number of published reviews have highlighted methodological weaknesses inherent in much of the early research in the topic, which limits the extent to which results can support the efficacy of the intervention (Kuoch & Mirenda, 2003; Sansosti et al., 2004; Reynhout & Carter, 2006; Ali & Frederickson, 2006). Many studies have failed to isolate Social Stories as the sole variable, as they have included various other elements such as visual schedules, token economies and prompting and comic-strip conversations, making it difficult to ascertain which of the intervention agents were responsible for change. The use of experimental designs that can be described as pre-experimental, such as AB designs and case-study formats, was identified as a weakness in many cases. Failure to comply with the criteria and sentence ratios set out in the Social Story publications has also been highlighted as a weakness.

Some of the reviews identified a lack of data on a number of important aspects, including generalisation, maintenance, social validity, treatment integrity and lack of clear participant description (Ali & Frederickson, 2006; Reynhout & Carter, 2006). Reynhout and Carter provided the first review that examined outcome strength, reporting variable to weak effects for interventions. The variability in effect size across reviewed studies led the authors to suggest that there was particular intervention or participant characteristics that may have moderated the effects of the intervention.

More recently published studies in the area have demonstrated increased methodological rigour. This is evidenced in the increased use of study designs with greater internal validity, such as ABAB and multiple-baseline designs (Styles, 2011). However, reviews including more recently published and higher-quality research indicate that the results of studies remain highly variable, with some interventions assessed as highly effective and others as ineffective (Kokina & Kern, 2010; Test et al., 2011). In both meta-analyses and individually published studies, researchers have begun to investigate the causes of such variability, examining specific intervention and participant characteristics in relation to outcomes. In their meta-analysis, Kokina and Kern (2010) grouped studies according to various criteria and compared effect sizes between groups. Some interesting preliminary data is outlined, which suggests, for example, that brief interventions had higher effect sizes than longer ones; that interventions that targeted simple behaviours were more effective than those that targeted complex ones and that interventions with comprehension checks were more effective than those without.

Richmond Mancil et al. (2009) assessed the differential effects of paper- and computer-assisted Social Stories on inappropriate behaviour in children with autism. They found that the computer-based presentation was slightly more effective and was preferred by the children. In a study with three participants, Cummins (2010) found that the Social Story intervention was less effective for one child, who had lower IQ scores than the other participants. In a randomised control-group study, Quirmbach et al. (2009) found that the success of the Social Story for participants was predicted by their score on the Verbal Comprehension Index of the Wechsler Intelligence Scale for Children, Fourth Edition (WISC IV) (Wechsler, 2003). Specifically, children with scores within the borderline range or above made significant improvements, while those with lower scores did not make significant improvements.

There is a general trend for more recently published studies involving Social Stories to be of increasing quality. However, even the most recently published articles still fail to include important aspects of intervention analysis, such as data on generalisation, maintenance and peer comparison. Studies also include varying degrees of detail in participant description (Richmond Mancil et al., 2009; Schneider & Goldstein, 2010; Cummins, 2010; Chan et al., 2011). It has also been suggested that ecological validity has decreased with increased levels of methodological rigour (Styles, 2011). Two studies specifically discuss the possible confounding effects of researcher presence during data collection (Schneider & Goldstein, 2010; Cummins, 2010). Many studies also fail to conduct or report comprehension checks (Styles, 2011), despite evidence that increased comprehension can lead to increased effectiveness of the intervention (Reynhout & Carter, 2007) and of the study (Kokina & Kern, 2010).

There is a substantial body of research that points to the possible utility and effectiveness of computer-based interventions for individuals with ASC. Technology is desirable as an instructional tool, as it can replace costly personnel. Particular forms of technology, such as touchscreen tablet devices, can be used for multiple purposes. Reviews of studies utilising various types of computer technology indicate promising results for their use in improving social skills (DiGennaro Reed et al., 2011), communication skills (Ramdoss et al., 2011) and academic literacy (Pennington, 2010). It is suggested that computer-aided instruction may be particularly suited to individuals with ASCs and their unique pattern of difficulties – for example, for the teaching of social skills in rule-based format (Moore et al., 2000) and in compensating for difficulties in understanding naturally spoken language (Janzen et al., 2006). A review of studies into computer-aided social-skills interventions reveals that the majority of studies in the area used video/DVD technology (58.6%), followed by audio script (17.2%) and computer programmes (13.8%).

None of the studies utilised the relatively new smart technology available in handheld devices or tablet computers.

One early study (Hagiwara & Smith-Myles, 1999) and some recent studies (Richmond Mancil et al., 2009; Chan et al., 2011) have begun to inform us about the impact of different modes of presentation on outcome data, employing the use of technology to present stories. Howley and Arnold (2005) highlight the importance of the mode of presentation. They suggest that technology may be used to enhance stories, as it allows for a visual mode of presentation, a mode of learning often preferred by individuals with ASC. The use of technology represents an efficient, cost-effective and flexible method for creating Social Stories. Richmond Mancil et al. (2009) also provide data to suggest that children may have a preference for this type of story. However, none of the studies that presented Social Stories using technology employed the use of the increasingly popular range of devices with touch technology, such as the Apple iPad. Children with ASC, their parents and even therapists are beginning to use iPads and apps as tools for education and augmentative communication, as well as for leisure (Davis, 2011). The current study will investigate the use of this technology in creating and presenting Social Stories.

Echoing calls from numerous researchers and reviewers, it is suggested that more methodologically sound research, with clear participant description and addressing the effects of moderator variables, should be conducted. The current study will attempt to extend the literature further by addressing some of these flaws and by investigating particular intervention characteristics. The particular research questions addressed in the current study were:

- Can Social Stories presented in paper-based and computer-based formats increase adaptive social behaviours in children with ASC in an autism-specific school setting?
- Are there characteristics of the participants, the intervention or the social and environmental context that can be used to predict the effectiveness of the intervention?

Methodology

Participants

An autism-specific special school in the Dublin area of Ireland was selected to take part in this research. For inclusion in the study, children had to have (a) a current diagnosis of ASC, (b) at least some basic skills in oral communication and reading, and (c) a skill area, not currently targeted by another intervention, that was identified by teachers and parents as an area in need of improvement. Teachers in the school were first consulted to identify whether there were children who matched these criteria, and two children were identified. Information letters and consent forms were then sent to the parents of these children, both of which were returned with consent given. Prior to the intervention, the participants were assessed using the Social Responsiveness Scale (SRS) (Constantino & Gruber, 2005) and the Diagnostic Reading Analysis (DRA) (Crumpler & McCarthy, 2008).

Names of participants have been changed to protect anonymity.

Christopher

Christopher was aged 15 years and 3 months at the time of the current study. Christopher received a diagnosis of autistic disorder and general developmental delay in 2002 (CA: 5:8). The diagnostic instrument used in the assessment was not specified in the report. In a psychological report dated 4 February 2010 (CA: 13:4), Christopher obtained a score that was reported to be within the range of 42–50, consistent with a profile of Moderate Intellectual Disability. His performance on the DRA reading test indicated a reading age of 8 years and 3 months, with a comprehension standard score of <69 – in the 'very weak' category. The teacher report questionnaire of the SRS resulted in a 't' score of 62 – in the 'mild to moderate' range. Christopher had been exposed to Social Stories, both in school and at home, prior to the current study.

David

David was aged 9 years and 3 months at the time of the current study. David received a diagnosis of Pervasive Developmental Disorder Not Otherwise Specified (PDDNOS) in 2007 (CA: 4:6). The instruments used to make this diagnosis were the Childhood Autism Rating Scales and the Autism Diagnostic Observational Schedule. In a psychological assessment dated 18 January 2008, David obtained a score on the Wechsler Preschool and Primary Scale of Intelligence Third Edition (WPPSI III) in the range of 56–66, consistent with a profile of Mild Intellectual Disability. His performance on the DRA reading test indicated a reading age of 7 years and 0 months, with a comprehension standard score of <69 – in the 'very weak' category. The teacher report questionnaire of the SRS resulted in a 't' score of 65 – in the 'mild to moderate' range. David had been exposed to Social Stories at home to alleviate anxiety about novel events, but not in school, prior to the current study.

Target Behaviours

Behaviours were selected in consultation with parents and teachers using interview and observation data. For both children, the target behaviour was to begin a conversation by getting a person's attention. The behaviour was specifically defined as gaining a person's attention before initiating a conversation, either (a) physically, e.g. by tapping the person on the shoulder, or (b) verbally, e.g. by saying 'excuse me' or the person's name at a volume level audible over the typical classroom noise level.

Social Stories

Through random assignment, Christopher was assigned to the computer-based Social Story, while David was assigned to the paper-based version. A story was written for each child according to Gray's (2004) criteria, including descriptive, perspective and directive sentences and adhering to the Social Story ratio. The stories contained information on when the behaviour might occur and described some options for obtaining attention and what the result might be.

The computer-based story was created and presented on an Apple iPad using the *Stories2Learn* application. Photographs of Christopher himself in the school setting were used to illustrate the story (see Fig. 6.1). The story was presented in the default font and settings of the application. The paper-based story was printed on white paper in 16-point comic sans font, laminated and spiral bound and included colour photographs of David to illustrate the story (see Fig. 6.2).

Design

A single-subject AB multiple-baseline-across-participants design was employed, whereby there was an initial baseline phase, followed by the intervention phase. The multiple-baseline design is a widely used experimental design that allows researchers to evaluate the effects of an independent variable across different behaviours,

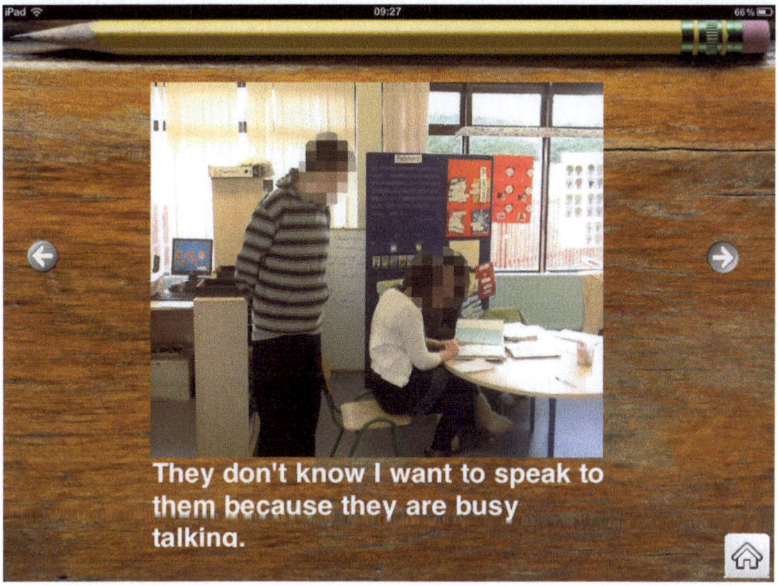

Fig. 6.1 Sample page layout for computer-based Social Story

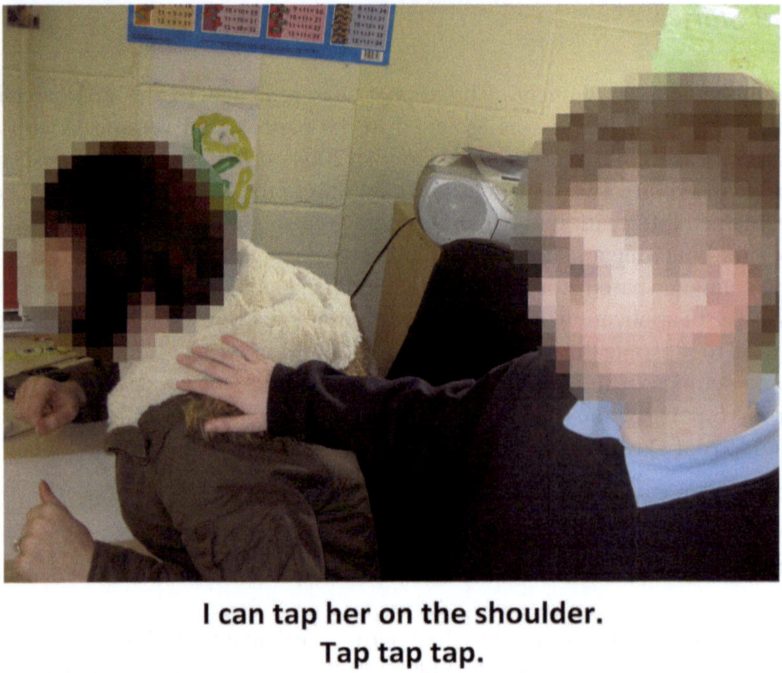

Fig. 6.2 Sample page layout for paper-based Social Story

settings or participants (Cooper et al., 2007). Using this design, baseline measures were initiated for both participants, but intervention was initiated with the first participant, while the second remained under the baseline conditions. When the first participant demonstrated maximal response, intervention began with the second participant.

Procedure

Data collection took place in the participants' respective classrooms in the morning, between the beginning of the school day and the first break at eleven o'clock. Two special needs assistants (SNAs), who were typically involved in the children's school day, were trained by the researcher to record the behaviours. Participants were currently receiving individual instruction in communication tasks as part of their Individual Education Plans. This was part of their normal school day and involved tasks requiring them to speak with other members of the school staff, e.g. to make requests and ask questions. The SNAs recorded whether or not the target behaviour occurred during these interactions. If it did occur, a '+' was recorded on a pre-designed recording sheet; if it did not occur, a '–' was recorded.

The baseline phase lasted for five sessions for Christopher, and nine sessions for David, after which the intervention phase began. The Social Story was read to the children once by the SNA on the first day it was introduced, following which the children read the story themselves, both in the initial session and on subsequent days in the intervention phase. Comprehension was checked following story reading by asking three questions from a selection of five comprehension questions that were predetermined and written on a separate sheet.

As the intervention did not produce the same gains for David as it did for Christopher, a third phase was introduced. This involved adding role play, a model prompt and verbal praise as reinforcement in order to ascertain whether the skill could be learned by augmenting the Social Story with additional strategies.

Inter-observer Agreement (IOA)

The current study utilised trial-by-trial IOA, involving dividing the total number of trials by the number of trials for which the observers agreed and multiplying this figure by 100. The minimum number of recommended trials for which IOA should be calculated is 20%, with preferable levels of 25–33% (Cooper et al., 2007). The current study calculated IOA for 33% of trials for Christopher and 30% of trials for David, by comparing the observations of trained staff and the researcher. Inter-observer agreement was 100% for Christopher and 96% for David.

Treatment Integrity

The terms 'treatment integrity' and 'procedural fidelity' refer to the extent to which the independent variable is applied consistently (Cooper et al., 2007). In order to assess treatment integrity in the current study, a checklist was provided to teachers on which to record the completion of the different steps of the procedure during the intervention phase. Treatment integrity for each step (story reading and asking of comprehension questions) was calculated by dividing the number of times the step was completed by the number of days of the intervention and multiplying by 100. Treatment integrity was 100% for both participants.

Treatment Acceptability

The Intervention Rating Profile (IRP 15) is a measure of treatment acceptability (Martens et al., 1985). Items are rated on a six-point Likert scale, ranging from 'strongly disagree' to 'strongly agree', with higher scores indicating greater acceptability. The IRP-15 has high internal consistency (Cronbach's a = 0.98) and high validity coefficients with related measures (r = 0.86). The participants' two class teachers completed the questionnaires and both returned a score of 85 out a maximum of 90, indicating high treatment acceptability. They also reported in interviews that they would use the intervention again. They thought that it was easy to implement and that it fitted in well with the daily running of the classroom.

Data Analysis

Each participant's behaviour was graphed on a line graph, as a percentage of expressions of the target behaviour per opportunity during their communication tasks. Data points in the baseline and intervention conditions were analysed visually for variability of performance, level of performance, direction and degree of trends in the data.

Maintenance and Generalisation

Maintenance was assessed for Christopher at 1 week and 2 weeks after finishing the Social Story intervention phase, after which the Social Story was no longer available. The communication task was repeated without the reading of the Social Story, as it had been in the baseline phase. Generalisation was assessed for Christopher by prompting him to speak with another person outside of the context in which the skill was taught, e.g. in another classroom while he was on a break. It was also assessed qualitatively through teacher observations, which were relayed through interview to the researcher. For Christopher, the effects of the Social Story maintained within the communication task that it was taught in at the 1- and 2-week follow-up stages. In terms of generalisation, Christopher demonstrated the target skill in areas of the school other than the classroom he learned it in. Qualitative reports suggest that he initiated conversations appropriately in different contexts only some of the time and not often at home. Some generalisation was seen for David, as he was observed by the researcher to initiate conversations appropriately. David was reported by the teachers to do this some of the time, but not all of the time, in school.

Results

Data Analysis

The children's performance in the baseline and intervention phases were recorded daily, and results were plotted on a line graph (Fig. 6.3). Christopher demonstrated a significant increase in the target behaviour during the initial intervention phase, while David did not.

Christopher

During the baseline phase, Christopher's target behaviour was completely absent. On the sixth day, when the Social Story was introduced, an immediate increase in the target behaviour was observed. The target behaviour increased throughout sessions, reaching the maximum level of 100% by day 8. It dropped back to 80% on day 9, before becoming stable at 100% on day 10 and remaining at this level until the end of the intervention phase. During the intervention phase, the percentage of interactions with the target behaviour ranged from 40% to 100% (M = 87%). During his communication tasks in the baseline phase, Christopher approached people who were speaking to other people and interrupted without any initiation or spoke to people who were not listening as he had not gained their attention. During the

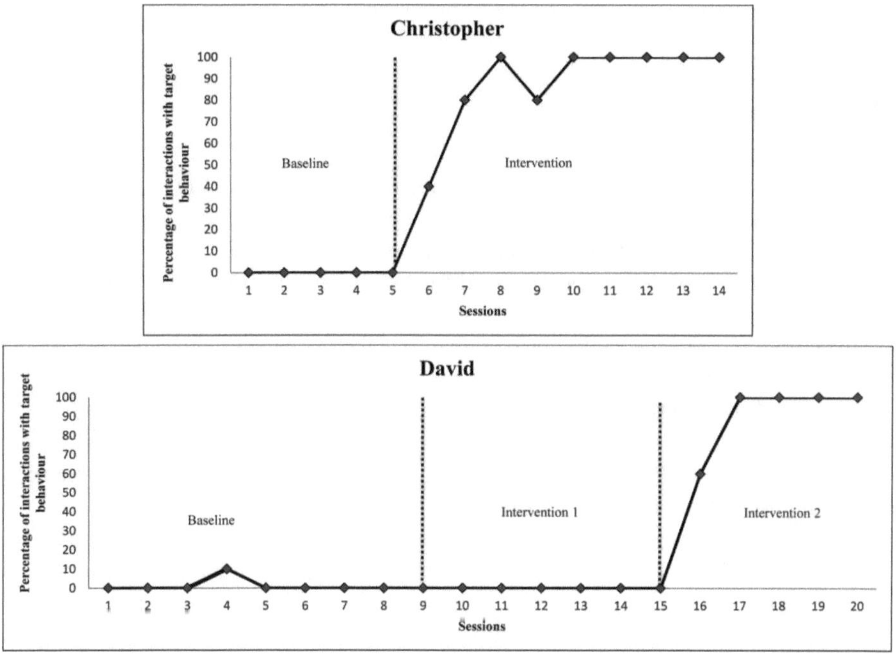

Fig. 6.3 Percentage of interactions within communication task in which target behaviour was observed

intervention phase, Christopher was observed to say 'Excuse me', followed by the person's name, in order to gain someone's attention. Christopher's number of correct responses to the comprehension questions correlated positively with the level of the target behaviour. On the first 2 days of the intervention phase, he got a number of the comprehension questions incorrect, but by the third day, he was responding correctly to all of the questions.

David

During the baseline phase, the target behaviour was completely absent for David, except for one occurrence on day 4 in which he gained the attention of a listener by saying 'Excuse me'. Teacher reports suggested that this anomaly was due to inadvertent verbal prompting by a staff member. During baseline, David approached people during his communication tasks but spoke in a quiet voice, standing far away from the listener and without any formal initiation to the conversation. The Social Story was introduced on day 10, as Christopher's level of response was reaching its maximum level. The target behaviour remained absent during this phase, and similar behaviours were observed during the communication tasks as in the baseline phase. After 2 days David was responding correctly to all comprehension questions. A second intervention phase was introduced on day 16, involving significant amounts of additional teaching including role play, model prompting and verbal praise as reinforcement. The level of interactions with the target behaviour increased with this level of additional support and reached the maximum of 100%. Maintenance was not assessed for David, due to time restrictions.

Discussion

This study evaluated the effects of two Social Story formats on the level of socially appropriate behaviour of two children in an autism-specific school setting. The frequency of the target behaviour – appropriate conversation initiations – increased for the first child, using the computer-based format, but not for the second child, using the paper-based story. The introduction of role play, model prompting and verbal praise led to an increase in the target behaviour for the second child. Such variable results for different participants within studies have been demonstrated previously in the research (Sansosti & Powell-Smith, 2006; Cummins, 2010; Schneider & Goldstein, 2010). Evidence of short-term maintenance for one participant and some generalisation of skills for both participants were found. Treatment acceptability was found to be high for both participants.

For Christopher, the level of the target behaviour increased from 0% in the baseline condition to 87% in the intervention phase. These results are consistent with recently published, methodologically rigorous studies investigating the effects of Social Stories as the sole intervention variable and demonstrating increases in socially appropriate behaviour in participants (Schneider & Goldstein, 2010; Chan et al., 2011). This is despite some indications that Social Stories may be more effective in decreasing inappropriate behaviours than increasing appropriate behaviours in research that predates these publications (Kokina & Kern, 2010). Young people of Christopher's age group have been relatively neglected in Social Story research. Kokina and Kern (2010), in their review of single-case research in the area, report that only 19% of studies included participants of age 12 or above. This study suggests that children of secondary school age may benefit from the intervention.

The results for the second participant, David, were quite different, reflecting the variation in the success of Social Stories, both within studies (Sansosti & Powell-Smith, 2006; Cummins, 2010; Schneider & Goldstein, 2010) and between studies, as highlighted in reviews (Reynhout & Carter, 2006; Kokina & Kern, 2010). A variety of participant and intervention characteristics have been proposed as differently moderating the effects of Social Stories by the authors of previous studies and reviews, including the type of behaviour targeted (Schneider & Goldstein, 2010), the IQ level of the participants (Cummins, 2010; Kokina and Kern, 2010), the level of communication deficits (Cummins, 2010; Kokina & Kern, 2010) and the level of treatment integrity and quality of the Social Story (Sansosti & Powell-Smith, 2006). In the current study, the Social Story was successful with the child within the Moderate Intellectual Disability range of intelligence, but not for the child within the Mild Intellectual Disability range. This is the converse to previous research, in which children with higher IQ levels demonstrated greater gains (Cummins, 2010; Kokina & Kern, 2010). IQ level is unlikely therefore to be a moderating variable in this study.

There may be aspects of the social and environmental context that contributed to the lack of success of the intervention for David. Reports from teachers and parents indicated that Christopher was more likely to readily approach people than David. The results of the SRS also indicated that Christopher's score on the Social Motivation scale (58) was lower than David's (76), indicating that David had greater difficulties in this area. As it appeared that David understood the story, evidenced through his correct responses to the comprehension questions, it is possible that a lack of motivation prevented him from initiating conversations successfully as outlined in the story. Crozier and Tincani (2007) discuss the possibility that a participant in their study may not have demonstrated gains after a Social Story intervention due to a similar lack of motivation. The participants' Social Communication score on the SRS differed to a smaller degree. Christopher's score was seven points lower than David's, indicating fewer difficulties. Differences in communication may also therefore have moderated the intervention effects.

Prior exposure to Social Stories for skills learning may have influenced the outcome of the intervention – Christopher had been exposed to Social Stories in school, but David had not. David's educational history involved the use of the Applied Behaviour Analysis model for teaching. This involves prompting, modelling and reinforcement, amongst other things, but not teaching through narratives. In the second intervention phase, familiar teaching strategies were added to the Social Story, and these resulted in success. The teaching methods added in this phase with David are similar to those used in a Social Stories intervention package reported by

Chan and O'Reilly (2008), in which Social Stories combined with role play and verbal prompts were successful in increasing appropriate social behaviour and decreasing inappropriate behaviour. This also suggests that for some children, Social Stories alone may not be enough to acquire skills.

The results of the maintenance probes for Christopher indicated that, at 1-week and 2-week follow-up stages, the treatment gains were maintained. It is noted in several reviews that early studies in the Social Story literature often neglect to report maintenance effects (Sansosti et al., 2004; Reynhout & Carter, 2006; Ali & Frederickson, 2006). More recently, maintenance effects have been more routinely reported by researchers but with variable results (e.g. Sansosti & Powell-Smith, 2006; Richmond Mancil et al., 2009). Some generalisation of skills was seen for both participants in the current study. This is similar to the results of a study by Delano and Snell (2006), which noted generalisation from a play area setting to a classroom setting for two out of three of the participants.

Measures of treatment acceptability – quantitative data (IRP-15) and qualitative data in the form of teacher and parent interviews – indicate that the intervention was highly acceptable to both teachers and parents, who rated it as effective. It should be noted that the addition of other teaching strategies in the second intervention phase for David meant that his teacher's ratings probably did not reflect her opinion of the Social-Story-alone phase. Teachers and parents stated that they would use the intervention in the future, reporting that they found it easy to use and a good fit for the environment they were working in. This adds to the findings of previous studies, which suggest that this intervention is very acceptable and classroom-friendly (Chan et al., 2011; Cummins, 2010; Reynhout & Carter, 2009).

This study indicates that the *Stories2Learn* app on an iPad is an effective mode of presentation of Social Stories, which also has high social validity in terms of acceptability as well as practicality. The use of such technology is flexible and cost-effective. Machines such as iPads can be used for several different purposes, such as augmentative and alternative communication, as well as for generating and presenting Social Stories. The Social Story presented on an iPad was seen as easier to construct, better presented and possibly more attractive to children. Richmond Mancil et al. (2009) also found that computer-based stories were preferred by children in their study. In a book endorsed by Carol Gray, Howley and Arnold (2005) highlight the importance of the mode of presentation used for Social Stories. They suggest that technology may be used to enhance stories, as it allows for a visual mode of presentation, a mode of learning often preferred by individuals with ASC.

This study adds to the literature in a number of ways. Firstly, the study demonstrates increased methodological rigour over much of the previously published research, by including a number of indicators of quality research. Secondly, ecological validity was maintained: using school staff to implement the Social Stories and collect data provides ecological validity and reduces the confounding effect of researcher presence discussed in previous studies (Schneider & Goldstein, 2010; Cummins, 2010). Finally, the study also extends the literature by investigating a previously unexamined mode of presentation, in the form of iPad technology. This, along with clear participant descriptions, allowed for the consideration of the results in the light of potential participant and intervention moderating variables. Moreover, the study triangulated results by adding qualitative data from interviews and observations to the quantitative data gathered. Purely positivist paradigms are predominantly employed in many Social Story studies. Such studies could be enhanced with more interpretivist approaches, which would allow for an analysis of additional within-subject factors as well as social and environmental variables that may moderate intervention effects (Styles, 2011).

Limitations

Although the study addresses some of the flaws inherent in previous research, a number of limitations remain. Peer comparison data was not collected, as there were no typical peers available in the autism-specific setting. This type of data is gathered in order to ensure that skills being taught and acquired are valid in terms of what would be expected for a typical peer (Cooper et al., 2007). Using the design in the current study, it was not possible to experimentally compare the effects of using the two different formats of the Social Story, the computer-based and paper-based formats. Previous studies have used designs that would allow for such a comparison, such as the ABABABCBC multicomponent reversal design used by Richmond Mancil et al. (2009). This study includes data on the children's preference for computer- or paper-based stories. This was not possible in the current study – the participants used only one format each, so they could not choose a preference.

Conclusions and Future Directions

The current study confirms previous findings that Social Stories as a sole intervention variable presented in computer format can be effective for increasing socially appropriate behaviour in some children with ASC within particular settings. It also demonstrates that the intervention has variable effects and may not be effective as a sole intervention variable for all children with ASC. The study provides preliminary evidence for the efficacy of presentation of Social Stories via tablet computer and smart technology, as well as the acceptability and practicality of this mode of presentation. Some of the possible participant, intervention and environmental characteristics that may moderate the effects were discussed, such as the moderating effect of social motivation, the level of communication deficits and prior exposure to Social Stories. Despite a plethora of individual studies, as well as reviews into Social Stories, there are few that use Social Stories as the sole intervention agent and are experimentally rigorous, with even the most recent studies neglecting to report important information such as generalisation and maintenance data. Future research should continue to isolate Social Stories as the sole intervention agent and employ rigorous experimental designs incorporating quality research practices.

Moreover, consideration should be given to ensuring that qualitative data is included and used to provide a reliable and valid context in which the quantitative data can sit. Further work might also consider larger sample sizes across a variety of settings and compare the use of Social Stories on touchscreen devices to paper-based stories. Future studies should provide clear and detailed participant information and attempt to experimentally manipulate moderator variables, in order to generate profiles of responders and non-responders to the intervention.

References

Ali, S., & Frederickson, N. (2006). Investigating the evidence base of Social Stories. *Educational Psychology in Practice, 22*, 355–377.

Attwood, T. (2000). Strategies for improving the social integration of children with Asperger's Syndrome. *Autism, 4*, 85–100.

Baron-Cohen, S., Williams, J., Bolton, P., Matthew, F., & Brayne, C. (2009). Prevalence of autism-spectrum conditions: UK school-based population study. *British Journal of Psychiatry, 194*, 500–509.

Centres for Disease Control and Prevention. (2009). *Autism and developmental disabilities monitoring network*. Retrieved November 27, 2011, from http://www.cdc.gov/mmwr/preview/mmwrhtml/ss5810a1.htm

Chan, J. M., & O'Reilly, M. F. (2008). A Social Stories™ intervention package for students with autism in inclusive classroom settings. *Journal of Applied Behavior Analysis, 41*(3), 405–409.

Chan, J. M., O'Reilly, M. F., Lang, R. B., Boutot, A., White, P. J., Pierce, N., & Baker, S. (2011). Evaluation of a Social Stories intervention implemented by pre-service teachers for students with autism in general education settings. *Research in Autism Spectrum Conditions, 5*, 715–721.

Constantino, J. N., & Gruber, C. P. (2005). *Social responsiveness scale*. WPS.

Cooper, J., Heron, T., & Heward, W. (2007). *Applied behavior analysis* (2nd ed.). Merrill Prentice Hall.

Crozier, S., & Tincani, M. (2007). Effects of social stories on prosocial behavior of preschool children with autism spectrum disorders. *Journal of Autism and Developmental Disorders, 37*(9), 1803.

Crumpler, & McCarthy. (2008). *Diagnostic reading analysis* (2nd ed.). Hodder Education.

Cummins, S. (2010). *An investigation into the effectiveness of Social Stories for children with Autistic Spectrum Disorders*. Unpublished master's thesis, University College Dublin.

Davis, M. R. (2011). *Virtual ed. targets rise of autism.* Retrieved October 2, 2011, from http://www.edweek.org/ew/articles/2011/08/24/01edtech-autism.h31.html?qs=apps+autism

Day, A. S. (2012). Social skills intervention for students with autism spectrum disorders: A survey of school psychologists. *Dissertation Abstracts International Section A: Humanities and Social Sciences, 2365*. Retrieved January 15, from http://search.proquest.com/docview/964202861?accountid=14507

Delano, M., & Snell, M. E. (2006). The effects of social stories on the social engagement of children with autism. *Journal of Positive Behavior Interventions, 8*(1), 29–42.

DiGennaro Reed, F. D., Hyman, S. R., & Hirst, J. M. (2011). Applications of technology to teach social skills to children with autism. *Research in Autism Spectrum Disorders, 5*(3).

Dunsmuir, S., Brown, E., Iyadurai, S., & Monsen, J. (2009). Evidence-based practice and evaluation: From insight to impact. *Educational Psychology in Practice, 25*, 53–70.

Frederickson, N. (2002). Evidence-based practice and educational psychology. *Educational and Child Psychology, 19*, 96–111.

Frith, U. (2003). *Autism: Explaining the Enigma*. Blackwell Publishing.

Gray, C. (2000). *Writing Social Stories with Carol Gray*. Future Horizons.

Gray, C. (2004). Social Stories 10.0: The new defining criteria and guidelines. *Jenison Autism Journal, 15*, 2–21.

Gray, C., & Garand, J. D. (1993). Social stories: Improving responses of students with autism with accurate social information. *Focus on Autistic Behavior, 8*, 1–10.

Hagiwara, T., & Smith Myles, B. (1999). A Multimedia social story intervention: Teaching skills to children with autism. *Focus on Autism and Other Developmental Disabilities, 14*(2), 82–95.

Howley, M., & Arnold, E. (2005). *Revealing the hidden social code: Social stories for people with autistic spectrum disorders*. Jessica Kingsley Publishers.

Janzen, J. E., Baron, M. G., & Groden, J. (2006). Understanding the role of stress in autism: The key to teaching for independence, Chapter 12. In *Stress and coping in autism* (pp. 324–350).

Kokina, A., & Kern, L. (2010). Social Story interventions for students with autism spectrum disorders. *Journal of Autism and Other Developmental Disabilities, 40*, 812–826.

Kuoch, H., & Mirenda, P. (2003). Social Story interventions for young children with autism spectrum disorders. *Focus on Autism and Other Developmental Disabilities, 18*, 219–227.

Martens, B. K., Witt, J. C., Elliot, S. N., & Darveaux, D. (1985). Teacher judgements concerning the acceptability of school based interventions. *Professional Psychology: Research and Practice, 16*(2), 191–198.

Moore, D., McGrath, P., & Thorpe, J. (2000). Computer-aided learning for people with autism: A framework for research and development. *Innovations in Education and Training International, 37*, 218–228.

National Autism Centre. (2009). *National standards report: Addressing the need for evidence-based practice guidelines for autism spectrum disorders*. Retrieved November 25, 2011. from http://www.cdc.gov/mmwr/preview/mmwrhtml/ss5810a1.htm

Parsons, S., Guldberg, K., MacLeod, A., Jones, G., Prunty, A., & Balfe, T. (2009). *International review of the literature of best practice provision in the education of persons with autism spectrum disorders*. Retrieved September 12, 2011, from the National Council for Special Educational Needs website http://www.ncse.ie/uploads/1/Autism_Report.pdf

Pennington, R. C. (2010). Computer-assisted instruction for teaching academic skills to students with autism spectrum disorders: A review of literature. *Focus on Autism and Other Developmental Disabilities, 25*(4), 239.

Quirmbach, L. M., Lincoln, A. J., Feinberg-Gizzo, M., Ingersoll, B. R., & Andrews, S. M. (2009). Social stories: Mechanisms of effectiveness in increasing game play skills in children diagnosed with autism spectrum disorder using a pretest posttest repeated measures randomized control group design. *Journal of Autism and Developmental Disorders, 39*(2), 299–321.

Ramdoss, S., Lang, R., Mulloy, A., Franco, J., O'Reilly, M., Didden, R., & Lancioni, G. (2011). Use of computer-based interventions to teach communication skills to children with autism spectrum disorders: A systematic review. *Journal of Behavioral Education, 20*(1).

Reynhout, G., & Carter, M. (2006). Social Stories for children with disabilities. *Journal of Autism and Developmental Disorders, 36*, 445–469.

Reynhout, G., & Carter, M. (2007). Social Story™ efficacy with a child with autism spectrum disorder and moderate intellectual disability. *Focus on Autism and Other Developmental Disabilities, 22*(3), 173–181.

Reynhout, G., & Carter, M. (2009). The use of social stories by teachers and their perceived efficacy. *Research in Autism Spectrum Disorders, 3*(1).

Richmond Mancil, G., Haydon, T., & Whitby, P. (2009). Differentiated effects of paper and computer-assisted social stories on inappropriate behaviour in children with autism. *Focus on Autism and Other Developmental Disabilities, 24*, 205–215.

Sansosti, F. J., & Powell-Smith, K. A. (2006). Using social stories to improve the social behavior of children with asperger syndrome. *Journal of Positive Behavior Interventions, 8*(1), 43–57.

Sansosti, F. J., Powell-Smith, K. A., & Kincaid, D. (2004). A research synthesis of social story interventions for children with autism spectrum disorders. *Focus on Autism and Other Development Disabilities, 19*(4), 194–204.

Schneider, N., & Goldstein, H. (2010). Using Social Stories and visual schedules to improve socially appropriate behaviors in children with autism. *Journal of Positive Behavior Interventions, 12*(3), 149–160.

Simpson, R. L. (2005). Children and youth with autism spectrum disorders: The search for effective methods. *Focus on Exceptional Children, 20*, 140–149.

Styles, A. (2011). Social Stories: Does the research evidence support the popularity? *Educational Psychology in Practice, 27*(4), 415–436.

Test, D. W., Richter, S., Knight, V., & Spooner, F. (2011). A comprehensive review and meta-analysis of the Social Stories literature. *Focus on Autism and Other Developmental Disabilities, 26*, 49–62.

Wechsler, D. (2003). Wechsler Intelligence Scale for Children, Fourth Edition (WISC-IV).

Chapter 7
A Colour-Coded Analysis of Movement Dynamics Associated to Potentials of Motion-Based Commercial Games to Supplement Training of Patients Diagnosed with Fibromyalgia Syndrome

Anthony Lewis Brooks and Eva Brooks

Introduction

Fibromyalgia syndrome (FMS) is considered a condition that impacts one's sensing of their body that results in a long-term experience often reflected upon as a holistic wide-bodily form of pain that to an extent is as unexplainable as it is unspecific. Additionally, this condition, as a result of the pain, commonly affects patients' well-being by them also experiencing fatigue, limb stiffness, headaches, sleep deprivation, numbness, mood swings, impairment to cognitive performance, irritable bowel movements and other life-impacting states related to anxiety and depression. Both male and female can be affected; however, statistically, increased diagnosed reports are of the condition impacting females (Boissevain & McCain, 1991; Clauw, 1995; Henriksson et al., 1992; Olsen et al., 2013; Sørensen et al., 2019; Waylonis & Heck, 1992; Wolfe et al., 2010).

The research studies originated as a result of discussions between a specialist rheumatologist (who was also an adjunct professor at Aalborg University Esbjerg campus) and the authors who are both senior researchers exploring technologies for inclusive wellbeing and empowering behavioural approaches relating to play and creativity. A typical general advice from the specialist rheumatologist to his patients was for them to 'stay as physically active as possible'. This is in line with related literature stating that exercise therapy is an established treatment for fibromyalgia,

A. L. Brooks (✉)
Department of Architecture, Design and Media Technology, Aalborg University, Aalborg, Denmark
e-mail: tb@create.aau.dk

E. Brooks
Department of Culture and Learning, Aalborg University, Aalborg, Denmark
e-mail: eb@ikl.aau.dk

E. Brooks, D. J. Brown (eds.), *Virtual Reality Games for Rehabilitation*, Virtual Reality Technologies for Health and Clinical Applications,
https://doi.org/10.1007/978-1-0716-3371-7_7

with efficacy studies in adults documenting significant improvements in patient's physical fitness, pain threshold and intensity and sleep (McCain et al., 1988; Busch et al., 2008a; Gowans et al., 1999, 2001; McCain, 1986).

In these two studies, as reported previously in this thread (Brooks & Petersson-Brooks, 2012; Mortensen et al., 2015), participants were patients diagnosed by their various doctors as having fibromyalgia syndrome (FMS). These patients had been subsequently assessed by the specialist rheumatologist at his local private treatment clinic who confirmed their condition and offered participation in the studies. As well as FMS, the clinic treated conditions such as rheumatoid arthritis and related other associated connective tissue diseases.

A posited initial hypothesis was on the potentials of such patients' self-training to exercise towards alleviating their movement pain(s) associated with FMS through gameplay. Inclusion conditions were women of age 18 or above diagnosed with FMS according to the commonly used American College of Rheumatology (ACR) criteria (1). Exclusion criteria were patients diagnosed with other diagnosed rheumatic diseases or conditions as determined by the specialist rheumatologist.

Both research studies were conducted in a large room with space for free and dynamic gameplay movements at the SensoramaLab – a human-centred behavioural laboratory complex exploring primarily virtual reality, interactivity, games, motivation and empowerment via adaptable interfaces and systems, alongside creative expression through motion performance. The SensoramaLab was situated at Aalborg University Esbjerg city campus on the west coast of Denmark.

The first intervention acted as a primary proof-of-concept and feasibility pre-study where three patients participated. Fifteen patients participated in the second study with seven completing sessions. The first study was where a single commercial game platform was used with interactive content responding to physical motion activities to substantiate a hypothesis on the potentials of patients' self-training to exercise.

Three game platforms were used in the second study. An outcome reflection relates to the history of the field whereby typical has been where a solitary game experience is used. This can lead to boredom and posited is how a narrative that consists of tasks/challenges along a journey or adventure may more fully engage a patient over a treatment period.

In both studies where the focus was on fibromyalgia, senior students conducted sessions with supervision led by the authors as senior researchers. A focus was on studying interactive gameplay content that responded to physical motion activities. The students who conducted the tests were considered competent at using the game controllers and the selected game platforms. They were also native Danish speakers, which enabled easier communication when interfacing with the participants.

In the established scenarios, the participants could select a preferred game aligned to how they believed it could best help their situation whilst stimulating motivation to play. The gameplay motion data was generated using selected devices that used either handheld or camera-based controllers. A primary goal was to motivate patients' compliance in their home-based exercise regime as a part of their activities in daily living (ADL). Results indicated positive potentials from the gameplaying, however, a negative was the high dropout/noncompliance from the original batch of proposed participants/patients.

Methodology

In the second study, a qualitative description approach was used supported by quantitative observation measures in the description of the primary outcome: participants' experience with the selected MCVGs. Quantitative measures were used in description of the secondary outcome consisting of indicators of pain and fatigue symptom severity and performance of ADL. All data were treated confidentially, and to assure anonymity, pseudonyms were used in all cases. As reported in (Mortensen et al., 2015), Test of Playfulness (ToP) was used as an observational tool for assessment of play experience. This tool considers aspects of (1) intrinsic motivation, (2) internal control, (3) suspensions of reality and (4) framing, with each aspect consisting of a number of items, e.g. actively engaged and acts self-direct, which separately have three subcategories: extent, intensity and skilfulness. The ToP tool is considered as reliable and valid in observation of both children and adults.

The Importance of Game Knowledge and Competence by Instructors

It was clear from the baseline that the participants had little or no experience of gameplay with such game platforms. Thus, the importance of the students' knowledge and capacity to instruct was of great importance to support and assist the experience towards a positive reflection.

In these studies the students' profiles were of (study 1) a single male Medialogy Msc student (Medialogy is an education based upon creativity and technology where typically projects are game-based with a focus upon human performance and gameplay) and (study 2) two Msc occupational therapy students.

Theoretical Method of Analysis Posited from Prior Research

In the authors' 2005 publication titled 'Play Therapy Utilizing the Sony EyeToy®' (Brooks & Petersson, 2005), two hospitals, one in Denmark and one in Sweden, collaborated where rehabilitation medical staff, doctors and play therapists supervised children patients playing the affordable, popular and commercially available Sony Playstation 2 EyeToy®. This was to investigate potentials of games utilising mirrored user embodiment in therapy.

The published work from this investigation is the first part of our resourced prior work that is built upon for this reflection on fibromyalgia method of analysis. In this prior work it states how aesthetic resonance (AR) was targeted in the study. Aesthetic resonance (AR) is when the response to intent is so immediate and aesthetically pleasing as to make one forget the physical movement (and often effort) involved in the conveying of the intention. This mind-body relation is posited as relating to the authors' approach to fibromyalgia alongside and integral to how an immersed 'play' mindset rather than a 'therapy' mindset is targeted which our prior research has shown as optimal. The set-up in this study utilised the same data used as control data to the interactive feedback content (gameplay) parallel to that used for monitoring simultaneous performance progress by the player/patient.

System set-up tailoring to each individual's preferences was adaptable towards optimising gameplay performance. In this prior paper (Brooks & Petersson, 2005), the often-used all-encompassing term of presence was challenged with a positing of aesthetic resonant state of the user being beyond 'a feeling of being there' as is typically interpreted in defining presence (Brooks, 2003).

In this prior work, systems such as the EyeToy®, that focus on the body as the interface, was posited as being an under resourced opportunity for therapists to include into training as, unlike traditional biofeedback systems, specific licensing is not required as there are no attachments to the patient. In the paper this was related to Flow (Csikszentmihalyi & Csikzentmihaly, 1990). We hypothesised in that study on how tools such as the EyeToy® have potentials to decrease the physical and cognitive load in a daily physical training regime, and this we stated as being central to our concept.

This thread continues by the first author's most recent research presentations on 'cognitive decoupling' associated to his SoundScapes concept as presented in five keynotes around the world in the fall/winter of 2021 (Brooks, 2021a, b, c, d, e). Herein, by bringing together the prior and recent research, we posit how cognitive decoupling can be achieved via digital gameplaying where body tracking interacting with the game content control may assist fibromyalgia patients in distancing (decoupling) from the pain associated with the disease: related can be the use of VR in pain decoupling in line with Hoffman's work as an example – see, e.g. https://depts.washington.edu/hplab/research/virtual-reality/. This directly associates to our statement in the prior paper (Brooks & Petersson, 2005) where we state how gameplaying actions do not need to be conscious, as at a certain level they can be unconscious skills, which, supported by playful aspects of the game, proactively push the participant's limits towards new levels of movements (p. 304). This claim substantiated from prior field research interventions.

We further stated in the prior paper (Brooks & Petersson, 2005) how we attempted to understand movements according to a semiotic interplay between participants' inner and outer world via elaborating with our theoretical framing citing related literature.

In the prior studies with the two hospitals, the planned method incorporated triangulated methodologies of video observations, interviews, questionnaires and diaries/field notes.

The video recordings underwent numerous temporospatial analyses by two independent coders where the units of analysis were the qualitatively different expressions of movement.

This methodology is detailed in the publication (Brooks & Petersson, 2005) with text and figures illustrating technique, approach and outcomes. Included in the analysis/coding was observed expressive gesture, action and pause periodic segmentations and performances. Alongside was compared temporal specific aspects concerning rhythm as a periodic repetition, dynamic kinetic changes and structural patterns of gameplay.

Detailed spatial analysis was also correlated with foci on specifics of range and intentionality of movements alongside facial expressions and utterances of participants.

Cumulatively, we referred to this as our manual multimodal analysis method. Alongside this manual method we conducted an automated computer analysis using the software EyesWeb by the University of Genoa and specifically from the 'EyesWeb Gesture Processing Library' (see Figs. 2 and 3 herein associating to Figs. 4 and 5 in (Brooks & Petersson, 2005)). These figures correspond to the appendixes in (Brooks & Petersson, 2005) where generated graphs and tables from these analyses are exemplified as well as detailing the created algorithms. For example, Fig. 4 in the paper details the quantity and segmentation of movement with threshold/buffer/motion phase indicators – buffer image, pause and motion phase durations. Further, Fig. 5 in (Brooks & Petersson, 2005) (Fig. 3 herein) illustrates the Contraction Index (CI) analysis via silhouette bounding rectangle initially set on buffer image. Finally, Table 3 in (Brooks & Petersson, 2005) informed on temporospatial analysis of one annotated session video file from the archive. This is not replicated herein as our focus is on colour coding of motion but may be of interest for readers to cross-reference our temporospatial analysis approach. A Silhouette Motion Image (SMI) algorithm was used that is capable of detection of overall quantity, velocity and force of movement.

The extracted measures related to the 'temporal dynamics of movement' were computed, and an adjustable threshold value slider was changed according to each participants' functional ability so that he or she was considered to be moving if the area of the motion image was greater than the related (threshold) percentage of the total area (Figs. 7.1, 7.2 and 7.3).

Building on (1) above, we similarly resource from our previous work where a focus was on empowering a participant to be able to digitally paint based upon dynamics of motion. This we determine as (2) where a focused selection is from the research in Portugal that led to a paper titled *Ao Alcance de Todos*. *Ao Alcance de Todos* is Portuguese for 'Within Everyone's Reach' in English and was realised as a 2-week workshop festival that was hosted at Casa da Música, Porto, Portugal in April 2008 (Brooks, 2008). This included a collection of the first author's works combined as an interactive installation in a space 14 m by 18 m, built as the national orchestra rehearsal room with a suspended/sprung wooden floor.

Extracted from this body of work are the algorithms used in the body painting section of the installation. This was where participants could move in front of a

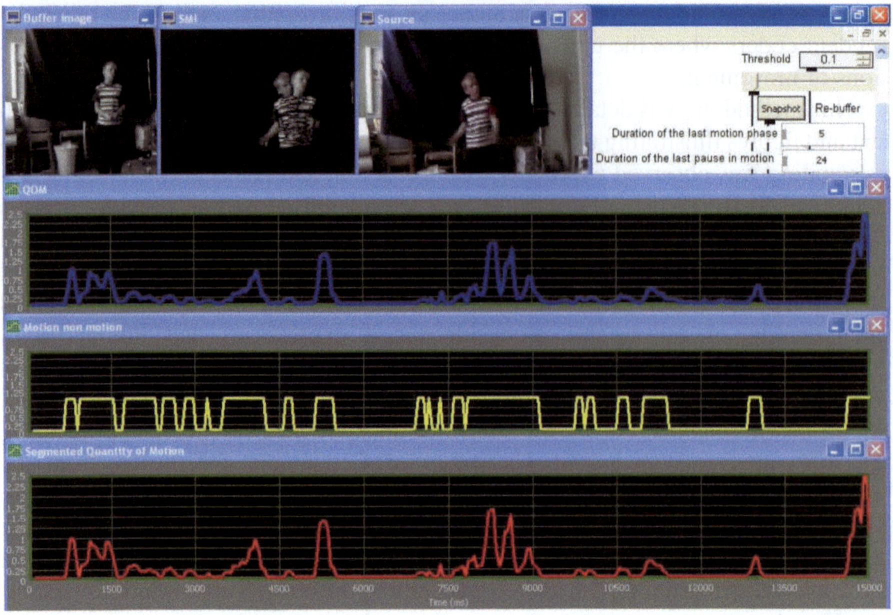

Fig. 7.1 Quantity and segmentation of movement. Threshold/buffer/motion phase indicators (upper right). Buffer image, Silhouette Motion Image (SMI) and source windows (upper left) – see also Fig. 4 in (Brooks & Petersson, 2005)

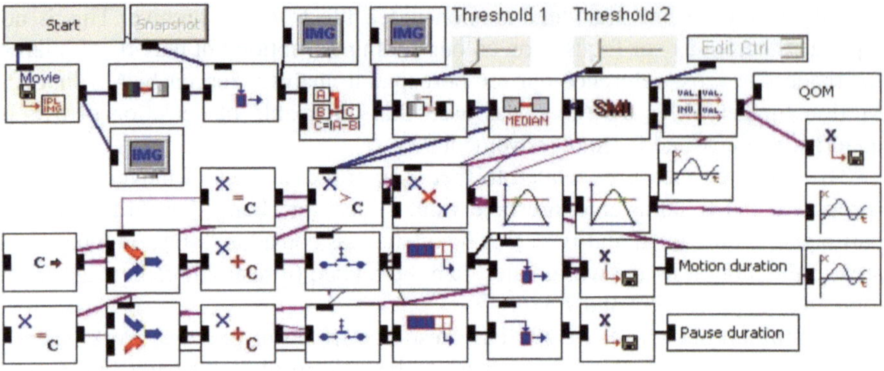

Fig. 7.2 EyesWeb algorithm for processes illustrated in Fig. 7.1 above: see also Fig. 4 (Brooks & Petersson, 2005)

camera and play music and simultaneously digitally paint and generate A3 size paintings of their creations. The algorithms originated from the first author's role in leading a European project based upon his research within the field of handicapped, elderly and (re)habilitation (Brooks & Hasselblad, 2004). Figure 9 in the original paper illustrates the exhibition of paintings and a group of attendees with special

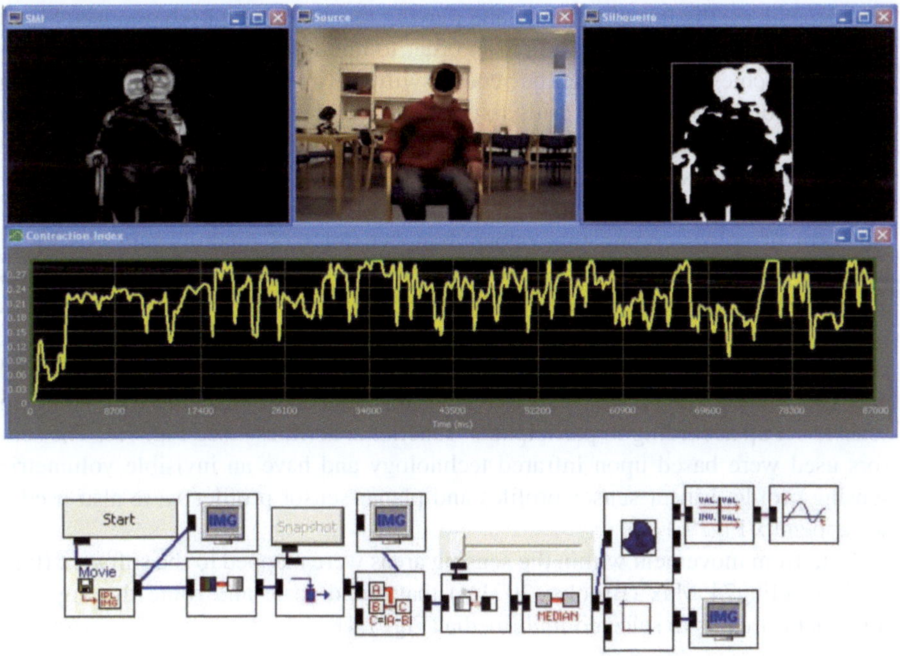

Fig. 7.3 Upper = Contraction Index (CI) analysis of motion. Upper right shows silhouette bounding rectangle initially set on buffer image. Lower = EyesWeb algorithm for CI analysis process as illustrated (Fig. 5 in (Brooks & Petersson, 2005))

needs who were painting (details of the participants is in the original paper). The second author was involved in interviewing and questioning on the participants' experiences in the workshops.

The EyesWeb algorithm for body painting was programmable to match individual nuances of control – across dysfunctionality – via a threshold control. Input motions are qualified and input to a threshold value to enable control of the process of stepping through a colour selector. As a participant's motion diminishes below the threshold, the algorithm stops painting, and when the dynamics of motion are once again above the threshold, the painting restarts but at the next step of the selector processing, i.e. the next designated colour in the selected paint chart (according to participant function versus threshold sensitivity control).

By combining from studies (1) and (2), it is posited how a manual annotation of fibromyalgia participants, such as conducted in our works, can be supplemented by an automated process that determines a colour coding schematic to identify dynamics of motion. Albeit a low-level indication of motion dynamics, this is speculated as being a significant addition to real-time analysis of such motion performance.

The feedback painting and/or gameplay is hypothesised as approaching a 'cognitive decoupling' such that the pain for the fibromyalgia patients is more bearable due to the motivation and enjoyment of playing the game alongside (simultaneously or independent) the fun of painting and playing music through body motion. Slight adjustments are foreseen as required in order to fine-tune the analysis method posited, but if achievable, then a colour-coded swift analysis of motions above a certain threshold for each individual with associated pains that typically prevent reaching such dynamics would be a contribution to this field for others to also explore and improve and is thus speculated to contribute to advance the study of fibromyalgia.

A further and earlier study (Brooks et al., 2002) by the authors includes a different form of colour-coding that rather than dynamics of quantity and quality of movement, it focused upon range and area of motions where the colouring of shapes alongside generated sounds was the multimedia feedback for participants. A focus was on achieving closure of the afferent/efferent loop to empower the participants who were from a school for children and adolescents with special and profound needs in Sweden. This was achieved using three (or more) specific data sourcing sensors set up according to participants' functional abilities – see Fig. 7.4. The sensors used were based upon infrared technology and have an invisible volumetric sensing profile. Linear sensor profiles and planar sensor profiles were also used – see appendix Fig. 7.11.

Data from movement within the sensing areas were mapped to the software (typically Cycling74 Max (Brooks, 2021a)) that could scale and route the big- and thick-data streams to selected multimedia (Fig. 7.4).

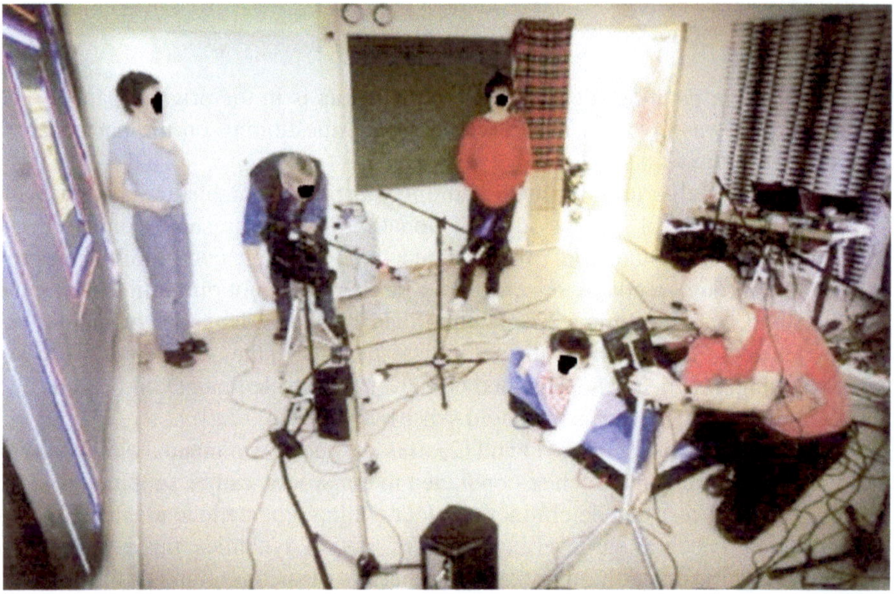

Fig. 7.4 A three-sensor set-up using infrared sensing with volumetric profiles with participant on vibroacoustic chamber generating motion data that results in sounds and coloured images on a large projection screen in front of her

The selection of the multimedia (visuals, sounds, robotics, games, etc.) could be according to each participant's preferences, but herein the focus is on the interactive visuals in the form of colour that result from the set-up (Figs. 7.4, 7.5 and 7.6). This earlier study gives a more digital representation of the motion as the generated data in each invisible sensing zone is representational of a proportional addition of colour. In other words, in each sensing zone (of three in this case) where motion is detected, a proportional saturation of the selected hue relates to the distance/range of motion and is not dependent on the dynamic of the motion.

In the case of the later research (Brooks & Petersson, 2005), the dynamic motion is represented by a duration of colouring, whilst the dynamic data is above a programmed threshold of motion according to the programming of the selected colour (Figs. 7.7, 7.8 and 7.9).

The colours are not mixed and projected in the later studies as one sensor is used (camera with planar profile) versus in the early research where three sensors were used, such that three colours could be mixed. The different colouring in the figures are time-based projections of each threshold change stepping through the selected colour chart in the algorithm.

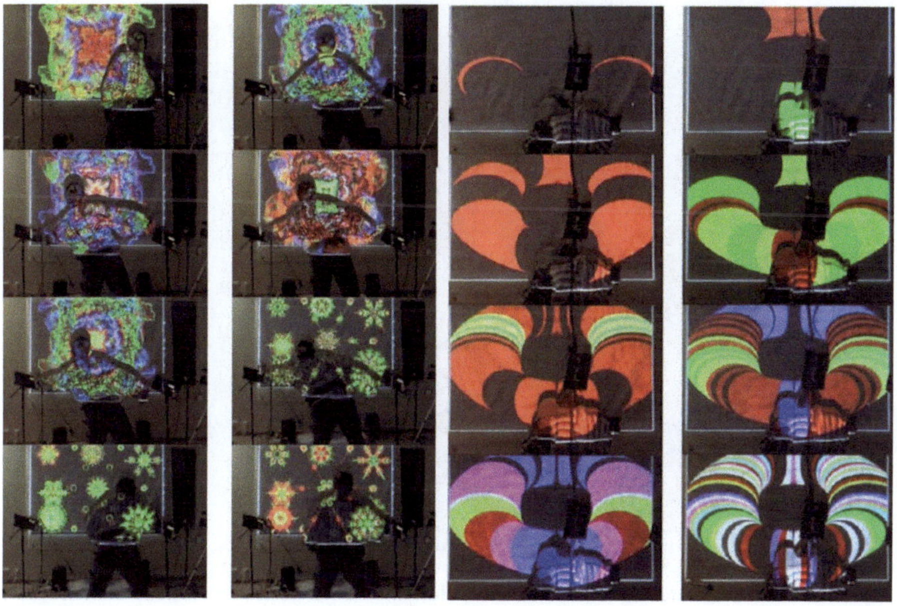

Fig. 7.5 A three-sensor set-up using infrared sensing with volumetric profiles with two different participants illustrating how different selected images are coloured versus the cited later studies where colouring was determined by the actual body movement silhouette

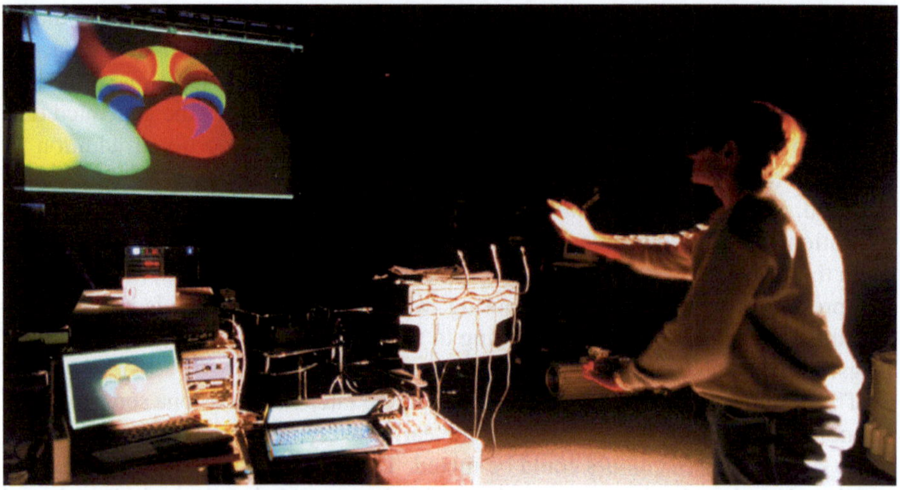

Fig. 7.6 The author's three-sensor set-up using infrared sensing with volumetric profiles mapped to red, green and blue colouring, with a participant illustrating how a selected image (doughnut shape on screen) is coloured as well as control of corresponding robotic moving head lighting colouring (in the figure the coloured lighting circles over and to left of the multicoloured doughnut shape – the computer screen lower left shows without lighting overlay)

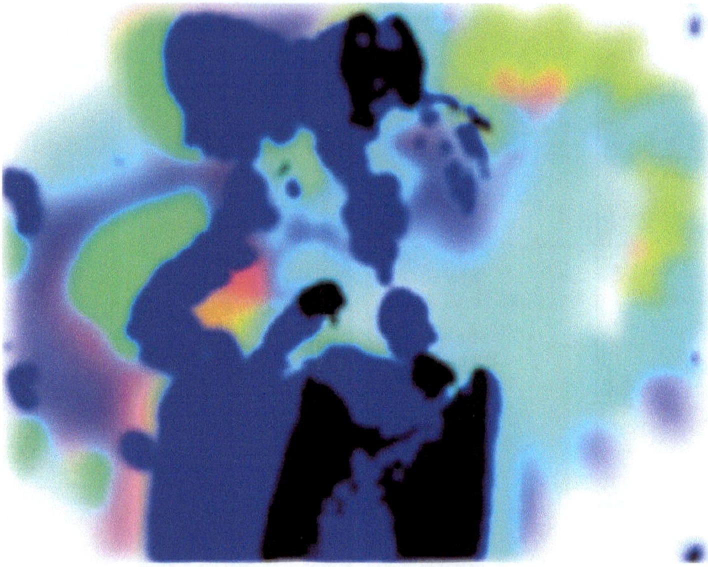

Fig. 7.7 A single camera sensor set-up where colouring was determined by the actual whole body movement silhouette (black areas in figure = head, two hands and two upper thighs) according to a programmable threshold of activity that steps through a selected colour chart

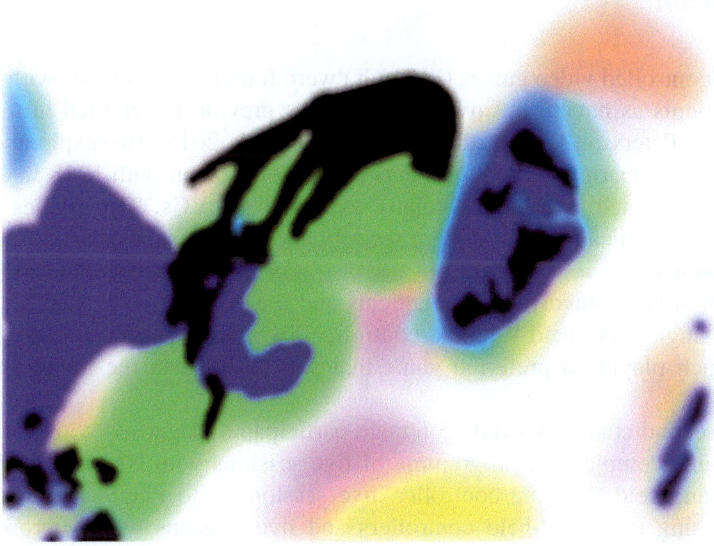

Fig. 7.8 A single camera sensor set-up where colouring was determined by the actual hands and head of a participant's movement silhouette (black-filled shapes) according to a programmable threshold of motion activity that steps through a predetermined colour chart

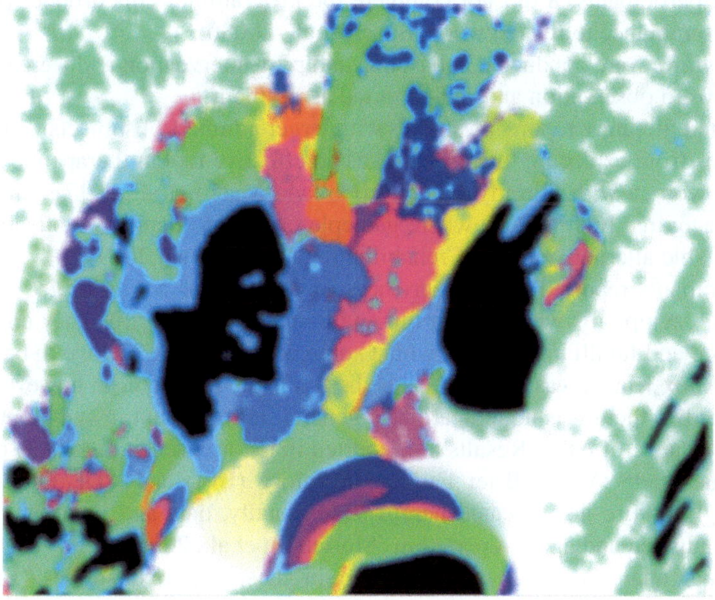

Fig. 7.9 A single camera sensor set-up as Figs. 7.7 and 7.8, where colouring was determined by the participant's and therapist's head movement silhouette (black-filled shapes)

Discussion

Motion-controlled video games (MCVGs) were found in our studies with fibromyalgia patients as having positive potentials. As previously reported in this thread (Brooks & Petersson-Brooks, 2012; Mortensen et al., 2015), two explorations were undertaken to learn and study the experiences of women with FMS in exploring through motivated play commercially available MCVGs. The studies included investigating indicators of symptom severity and performance of activities of daily living (ADL).

The first study involved three patients and the Nintendo Wii gaming platform using a single hand-held Wiimote controller. Two participants completed ten sessions, each playing a preferred game that was selected in the initial instruction session.

The second study involved 15 female participants diagnosed with FMS. Seven participants completed a programme of five sessions with Nintendo Wii using a single hand-held Wiimote controller, five sessions with PlayStation Move (PS3 Move) using two hand-held controllers and five sessions with Microsoft Xbox Kinect – a hands-free camera-based interface.

The sessions in the second study were planned to be conducted over a period of around 7 weeks, which, on reflection, may have influenced adherence as (Mortensen et al., 2015) shows the actual period was 9–17 weeks duration. Of the 15 originally selected participants, 8 did not complete the programme. This dropout percentile bears resemblance to related work (Busch et al., 2008b).

Interviews were conducted at baseline and post-intervention and were supported by data from observation and self-reported assessment.

Related literature reports on studies with larger numbers of subjects with positive outcomes from exploring 'exergaming' as an effective tool in therapeutic intervention for women with fibromyalgia, e.g (Collado-Mateo et al., 2017)., and beyond (e.g. in acquired brain injury) where gameplay was considered as motivational and an enjoyable alternative form of rehabilitation (Burke et al., 2009).

Participants reported their experiences of MCVGs as a way to get distraction from pain symptoms whilst doing fun and manageable exercise. They enjoyed the slow pace and familiarity of Wii, whilst some considered PS3 Move to be too fast-paced. Xbox Kinect was reported as the best console for exercise; however, overall in the studies there was no indication of general improvement in symptom severity or performance of ADL. Results are reported in (Mortensen et al., 2015) on Visual Analogue Scale (VAS), Brief Fatigue Inventory (BFI) and ADL Questionnaire (ADL-Q) and are not repeated herein. Additionally, data and interview analyses were conducted and again reported in (Mortensen et al., 2015).

Manual analysis only was conducted in these reported studies (Brooks & Petersson-Brooks, 2012; Mortensen et al., 2015). Herein, based upon the authors' prior researches and ongoing work in progress, a means to automate low-level analysis of body motions that can be associated to fibromyalgia pain-restricted movement via colour-coding is posited. The data that achieves the colour-coding can also be analysed in line with the authors' 2005 methodology where quantity and quality of movement was determined. These approaches offer opportunities for next-generation researchers to explore such analysis of the big and thick data at different levels according to desired outcomes. Our subsequent hypothesis from this work related to how artificial intelligence (explainable AI and/or deep learning) can add to this analysis set-up to inform (e.g. Brooks, 2021e).

In this body of work, it has been demonstrated how MCVG can act as an effective healthcare intervention for persons with FMS associated to temporary pain relief (to be discussed further relating to cognitive decoupling) and enjoyable low-impact exercise such as resulting from gameplay and or digitally creating music and/or painting. The literature indicates how rehabilitation exercise is recommended in the management of fibromyalgia syndrome (FMS). People with FMS often find it counterintuitive to exercise because of pain exacerbation, which may influence adherence to an exercise programme. In general it would seem that motion-controlled video games may offer temporary pain relief and fun as a low-impact exercise for women with FMS.

An illustration of the overview of the first author's SoundScapes concept (a 'Communication method and apparatus' – see patent number US6893407B1) of invisible sensing of dynamic movement mapped to multimedia feedback in (re) habilitation (Fig. 7.10) and the three sensing technology and differing profiles typically used in SoundScapes (Fig. 7.11) are illustrated in the Appendix. The term 'Communication' in this context and with upper case refers to the SoundScapes' modular and flexible feed-forward and feedback loop that affects achieving of afferent-efferent neural feedback loop closure that is reflected as motivational for participants whilst communicating causality of their own sensed motion dynamics. Correspondingly, the set-up 'Communicates' data to the system that is informing, logged and archivable for post-session analysis. It also 'Communicates' to the facilitator or therapist if the system is optimally matched to the patient/participant.

In this paper a colour-coding of motion dynamics is posited that gives a real-time opportunity for analysis and thus corresponding system parameter change in order to fine-tune the system to each individual patient/participant. Thus, a reflection on the methodology was that a previously used motion-based body-painting algorithm could be tested to determine dynamic changes of body movements during gameplay. This would generate a colour-coded result to indicate (as in further 'Communicate') within or between adjacent or initial and final sessions any potential benefits that were otherwise unseen. Whilst this could potentially advance the field of evaluating in a quantitative manner, it is only speculated at this time without testing.

Summary of Related Studies on Fibromyalgia/Pain and Digital Technologies

Summarising related studies on fibromyalgia/pain and digital media technologies (here we focus on sensors, virtual reality environments and games) that associate to the approach taken by the reported studies herein notable is an article by (Wiederhold et al., 2014) that approximately a decade ago stated how:

> Recent studies indicate that computer-generated graphic environments—virtual reality (VR)—can offer effective cognitive distractions for individuals suffering from pain arising from a variety of physical and psychological illnesses. Studies also indicate the effectiveness of VR for both chronic and acute pain conditions. Future possibilities for VR to address pain-related concerns include such diverse groups as military personnel, space exploration teams, the general labor force, and our ever increasing elderly population. VR also shows promise to help in such areas as drug abuse, at-home treatments, and athletic injuries.

More recently, aligned with technological advances and gaming industry pervasiveness, VR is commonly associated to gaming whereby head-mounted displays (HMDs) have become affordable alongside stand-alone platforms or personal computers with online access to VR games (and other) content. Educations have been initiated around the world on gaming due to market size and potentials across disciplines, and the authors were founder leaders of such an education from 2002 in Denmark titled 'Medialogy' (Medialogy, 2002).

Previous to those studies reflected in this text, the authors were awarded with a best paper award at the International Conference on Disability, Virtual Reality and Associated Technologies (ICDVRAT 2012), Laval, France, with their contribution titled 'Perceptual Game Controllers and Fibromyalgia studies' (Brooks & Petersson, 2012). This 2010–2011 investigation was of gesture-based control of video games to promote and motivate self-driven home-based aerobic exercise (AE) training regimes to improve pain threshold associated to fibromyalgia. Forty-nine patients with fibromyalgia in total participated within two studies where control was other registered patients with the involved Norwegian medical doctor (expert in fibromyalgia) who had a local practice conducting assessments. Pre- and post-interviews, tests and VAS registrations of pain, disturbed sleep, lack of energy and depression were supplemented by patient-reported global subjective improvement or otherwise – conducted by the patients' doctors. Multiple angle (3) video cameras synchronised to the gameplay for correlation analysis. Outcome measures were at baseline and completion. Three game platforms were studied: the MS Kinect, Sony MOVE and Nintendo Wii, with the first study with 10 sessions of 1 h each per patient and second study with 5 game sessions of 1 h being played by each patient on each platform (15 sessions in total each). Positive outcomes with completion involved patients reporting purchasing their own game platform for self-driven home training.

Building on the positive finding from our initial studies that ongoingly involved expert fibromyalgia medical professionals, subsequent investigations involved therapist students alongside the experts, as reported online (Mortensen et al., 2015)

(Epub 2013 Sep 12) in the *Journal for Disability Rehabilitation Assistive Technology*, which fed into another study as reported in 2014 under the title '*Engagement in Game-Based Rehabilitation for Women with Fibromyalgia Syndrome*' (Brooks & Brooks, 2014).

Around the same time, (Botella et al., 2013) reported on the effectiveness of VR as an adjunct to cognitive behavioural therapy (CBT) in the treatment of fibromyalgia (FM) with a small sample of six patients. Reported results '*showed the long-term benefits of significantly reduced pain and depression and an increased positive affect and use of healthy coping strategies.*'

In (Villafaina et al., 2019) a single-blinded randomised controlled trial was conducted with fifty-five women with fibromyalgia in a university setting investigating '*the effects of a 24-week exergame-based intervention on health-related quality of life (HRQoL) and pain in patients with fibromyalgia as well as to analyze the effectiveness of the intervention in subgroups of patients with different pain intensity levels.*' Conclusions indicate how the results point to how exergames '*could be a useful tool to improve perceived health status and pain intensity level in women with fibromyalgia with a reduced health-related quality of life.*'

More directly associated to the reported studies conducted by our team, (De Carvalho et al., 2020) reported on a randomised control study where thirty-five women, divided into two groups (control group where $n = 19$, performing stretching exercises; and a Wii exergame group, $n = 16$) where assessments were using the fibromyalgia impact questionnaire (FIQ), algometry, step tests, cardiopulmonary parameters, and fatigue in the lower limbs. Treatments lasted for 7 weeks with 3 1-h sessions weekly with re-evaluations after the tenth and the 20th sessions. Results indicated how (De Carvalho et al., 2020):

> The exergames group showed significant reduction of their fibromyalgia symptoms, as demonstrated by lower FIQ scores in the key domains on questions regarding missed work, pain, fatigue, problems resting, stiffness, anxiety, and depression. Significant improvements were observed in mean algometric values in the cervical region, the second chondrocostal junction, the lateral epicondyle, left medial knee border, left occipital region, trapezius, supraspinatus, gluteal muscles, and the greater trochanter. Improved cardiovascular adaptation was reflected by decreased systolic blood pressure, reduction in fatigue of the lower limbs assessed by the CR10 Borg scale, and improved exercise capacity assessed by a step test.

Conclusions being that '*Exergames have the potential to increase exercise capacity, decrease the impact of fibromyalgia, promote cardiovascular adaptation, reduce fatigue of lower limbs, and improve the pain threshold in women with fibromyalgia.*' (De Carvalho et al., 2020).

In a subsequent report (de Carvalho et al., 2021) is more specific on analysing the effect of exergaming on muscular activity at rest and on maximum voluntary isometric contraction which was conducted by the same team with the same participants/groupings/sessions/design. This time evaluations involved EMG, dynamometry by load cell, baropodometry and algometry before interventions with reassessments after the tenth and 20th sessions. Again reported results were positive with conclusions that the exergaming showed potentials to increase the peak torque for dorsiflexion and plantar flexion movement for the participants by also producing a decrease in tender point count equal to that with flexibility exercises and does not produce changes in the static balance.

In the same year, (Polat et al., 2021) investigated motion-controlled video games and their effect on women ($n = 40$, split into control [VR] and conventional training groups) with fibromyalgia on their pain, functionality, cardiopulmonary capacity and quality of life. MS XBox Kinect was used with the VR group lab, and home exercising was scheduled with all patients evaluated at baseline and 4th and 8th weeks. '*Primary outcome measure was Fibromyalgia Impact Questionnaire. Visual Analogue Scale (VAS), Hospital Anxiety and Depression Scale, Fatigue Severity Scale (FSS), Symptom Severity Scale, EuroQol-Five Dimensions Index Scale/Visual Analogue Scale (EQ-5D-index/VAS) and Six Minute Walk Test (6MWT) were used as secondary outcome measures*'. Outcomes indicated how VR '*game exercises along with aerobic exercise increased cardiopulmonary capacity and quality of life in fibromyalgia syndrome. In addition, they increase patient satisfaction and may improve patient compliance to exercise*'.

More recently, (Gava et al., 2022) reviewed the effects of gaming on pain-related fear, pain catastrophising, anxiety and depression in patients with chronic musculoskeletal pain. Findings were based on very low- or low-quality evidence. In a conclusion, the review showed how gaming modalities may have positive effects on some mental health outcomes, but there were conflicting results with low-quality evidence, which indicates that more high-quality randomised controlled trials are needed.

Conclusive Comments

From our individual and combined positions, we have explored interactive sensor-based activities including virtual reality environments/virtual interactive space (VIS)/human performance/entertainment, etc. for many years since the early 1990s. The first author's investigations of sensor interfaces mapped to different multimedia interactive digital content in the form of auditory/musical, visual/effect and robotic content as direct feedback to a participant; and the second author's mature body of research investigating play associated to formal/informal and non-formal learning. The combination of the two bodies of research gave credence to the researchers' concept on how games (exergaming) could be used in therapeutic environments where entertainment, enjoyment and simple fun led to new advancements in wellbeing and (re)habilitation. Different participants with different profile of age/condition have volunteered over the years, and many of the corresponding studies were undertaken with healthcare experts externally (hospitals, treatment clinics, etc.) or located at the SensoramaLab that was founded by the researchers in 2004 at Aalborg University Esbjerg campus in Denmark. Games and virtual reality related to human behaviour were the core foci at the lab complex.

Following their initial studies in the field, their findings align with others who have reported that the effects of exergaming on fibromyalgia can result in additional benefits for patients such as improvements in lower-body strength, cardiorespiratory fitness autonomic control, exercise capacity, cardiovascular adaptation and pain threshold and also decreases the impact of fibromyalgia reducing fatigue – especially of the lower limbs.

Positive results in favour of aerobic exercises, flexibility exercises, strength training, stretching and body awareness therapies for fibromyalgia treatment have also been reported. The conclusions (Botella et al., 2013; Brooks & Brooks, 2014; Brooks & Petersson, 2012; De Carvalho et al., 2020, 2021; Gava et al., 2022; Herrero et al., 2014; Medialogy, 2002; Mortensen et al., 2015; Polat et al., 2021; Villafaina et al., 2019; Wiederhold et al., 2014) as reported in this text of expert teams in their respective field reflect our findings (as non-experts in pain/fibromyalgia conditions but who research with such experts). Further, (Brooks, 1999) reported on a system along with data regarding the acceptability, satisfaction and preliminary efficacy of a virtual reality (VR) environment for the promotion of positive emotions where results showed significant increases in general mood state, positive emotions, motivation and self-efficacy. These preliminary findings show the potential of VR as an adjunct to the psychological treatment of such an important health problem as chronic pain and align with such applications of technology in healthcare (Brooks, 1999, 2011).

These related findings support our addendum in recommending that further studies should be undertaken investigating additional games and interfaces that, through adaptability to achieve optimisation and personalisation, may advance coping with fibromyalgia as well as increasing compliance through their adaptability to a given physical condition and (thus) limitation. Aligned from this text and our posit of means to support interventions and treatment design, we also believe the investigation of means for subject/participant and intervention therapist to (in real time) identify through colour-coding (or other) feedback methodology is fruitful as a support for the therapists and individuals in their self-driven home sessions to improve their own life quality. To end, however, it must be stated that from the concluded studies it is unclear from those volunteers who completed the research sessions and continued to play such games at their home. This has no follow-up re-testing to conclude from in this work as following 2015 that which was scheduled was cancelled due to management closure of the SensoramaLab where the studies took place in Aalborg University Esbjerg, Denmark, soon after the fibromyalgia investigations that were located therein. However, the authors are positive to their contribution to this field and welcome correspondences as appropriate.

Acknowledgements The authors wish to thank all of the participants for their time and efforts across all cited studies. Special thanks in the cited (1) and (2) studies go to the senior Medialogy student and Occupational Therapy students, rheumatologist Hans-Jacob Haga for recruiting participants and gathering data on pain and fatigue and also Eva Ejlersen Wæhrens for allowing use of the ADL-Q. The other cited works acknowledge the patients/participants, doctors, play therapists from the research partner hospitals and staff at the special school in Landskrona, Sweden.

Appendix

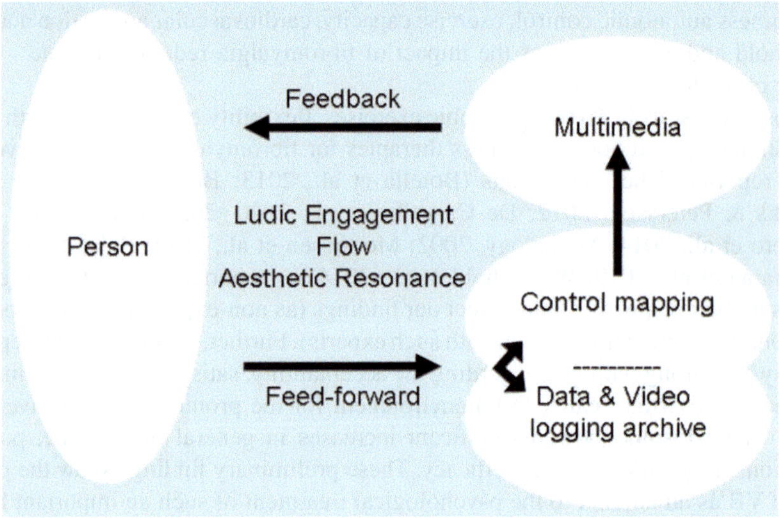

Fig. 7.10 Overview of the signal flow where movements result in data generation (feed-forward) that is processed and routed in software to affect multimedia software (or, e.g. robotic lighting hardware) that generated multimedia content that is sensed by the participant. The thick data is archived with video recording for post-session correlation analysis. The generated multimedia content is representational of the movement dynamics and/or range of motion whereby the quality and quantity of the movement is within the thick data

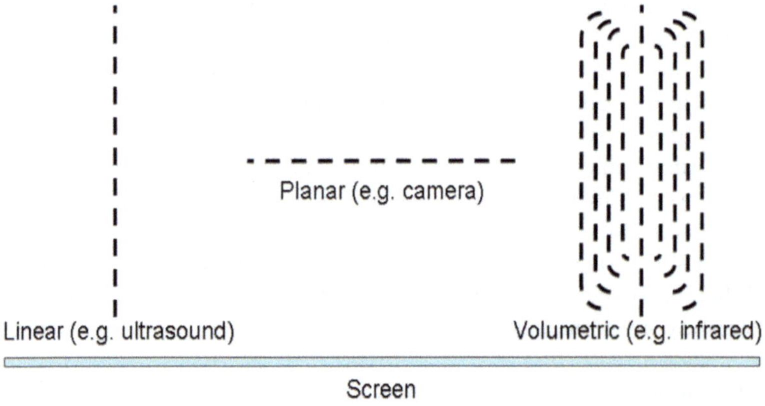

Fig. 7.11 The three sensing profiles and technology typically used in this research being linear (ultrasound), planar (camera) and volumetric (infrared) relational to a screen where the colouring of the image is viewed by participants. Dotted lines indicate data profile regions

References

McCain, G. A., Bell, D. A., Mai, F. M., & Halliday, P. D. (1988). A controlled study of the effects of a supervised cardiovascular fitness training program on the manifestations of primary fibromyalgia. *Arthritis and Rheumatism, 31*, 1135–1141.

Boissevain, M. D., & McCain, G. A. (1991). Toward an integrated understanding of fibromyalgia syndrome. Psychological and phenomenological aspects. *Pain, 45*(239), 48.

Botella, C., Garcia-Palacios, A., Vizcaíno, Y., Herrero, R., Baños, R. M., & Belmonte, M. A. (2013). Virtual reality in the treatment of fibromyalgia: A pilot study. *Cyberpsychology, Behavior and Social Networking, 16*(3), 215–223. https://doi.org/10.1089/cyber.2012.1572

Brooks, A. L. (1999). *Virtual interactive space (V.I.S.) as a movement capture interface tool giving multimedia feedback for treatment and analysis WCPT*. Science Links Japan. https://www.researchgate.net/publication/257536704

Brooks, A. L. (2003). SoundScapes – A concept and methodology of "being there". In *Proceedings 6th annual international workshop on presence*.

Brooks, A. L. (2008). Towards a platform of alternative and adaptive interactive systems for idiosyncratic special needs. In *Proceedings of the 7th ICDVRAT with ArtAbilitation, Maia, Portugal*. ICDVRAT/University of Reading. ISBN 07 049 15 00 6.

Brooks, A. L. (2011). *SoundScapes: The evolution of a concept, apparatus, and method where ludic engagement in virtual interactive space is a supplemental tool for therapeutic motivation*. (PhD dissertation) https://vbn.aau.dk/ws/portalfiles/portal/55871718/PhD.pdf

Brooks, A. L. (2021a). *Keynote speech presentation at the 13th international conference On disability, virtual reality & associated technologies (ICDVRAT2021)*, Serpa, Portugal. http://icdvrat2020.ulusofona.pt

Brooks, A. L. (2021b). *Keynote speech 24th rehabilitation international world congress*, Aarhus, Denmark. https://www.riworldcongress2021.com

Brooks, A. L. (2021c). *Keynote speech 15th international conference on information technology and applications (ICITA)*, Dubai UAE https://www.icita.world

Brooks, A. L. (2021d). *Keynote speech 14th world down syndrome congress (WDSC) 2021*, Dubai UAE. https://wdsc2021.org.ae

Brooks, A. L. (2021e). *Keynote speech 11th international conference on internet technologies & society*, Sydney, Australia, https://its-conf.org

Brooks, E., & Brooks, A. L. (2014). Engagement in game-based rehabilitation for women with fibromyalgia syndrome. In C. Stephanidis & M. Antona (Eds.), *Universal access in human-computer interaction. Aging and assistive environments. UAHCI 2014* (Lecture notes in computer science) (Vol. 8515, pp. 359–367). Springer. https://doi.org/10.1007/978-3-319-07446-7_35

Brooks, A. L., & Hasselblad, S. (2004). CAREHERE – Creating aesthetically resonant environments for the handicapped, elderly and rehabilitation: Sweden. In P. Sharkey, R. McCrindle, & D. Brown (Eds.), *5th international conference on disability, virtual reality, and associated technologies*.

Brooks, A. L., & Petersson, E. (2005). Play therapy utilizing the Sony EyeToy. In *Proceedings of the presence 2005*. http://matthewlombard.com/ISPR/Proceedings/2005/Brooks%20and%20Petersson.pdf

Brooks, A. L., & Petersson, E. I. (2012). Perceptual game controllers and fibromyalgia studies. In *Proceedings international conference on disability, virtual reality & associated technologies (ICDVRAT 2012)*, Laval, France (Best paper award) https://isvr.org/ICDArchive2021/2012/P/2012_SP06_Brooks_Petersson_Brooks.pdf

Brooks, A. L., & Petersson-Brooks, E. (2012). Perceptual game controllers and fibromyalgia studies. In *Proceedings of the 9th international conference on disability, virtual reality and associated technologies (ICDVRAT)* (pp. 439–442).

Brooks, A. L., Hasselblad, S., Camurri, A., & Canagarajah, N. (2002). Interaction with shapes and sounds as a therapy for special needs and rehabilitation. In P. Sharkey (Ed.), *6th international conference on disability, virtual reality, and associated technologies*.

Burke, J. W., McNeill, M. D. J., Charles, D. K., Morrow, P. J., Crosbie, J. H., & McDonough, S. M. (2009). Optimising engagement for stroke rehabilitation using serious games. *The Visual Computer, 25*, 1085–1099.

Busch, A., Schachter, C., Overend, T., Peloso, P., & Barber, K. A. R. (2008a). Exercise for fibromyalgia: A systematic review. *Medicine The Journal of Rheumatology, 35*(6), 1130–1144.

Busch, A. J., Schachter, C. L., Overend, T. J., et al. (2008b). Exercise for fibromyalgia: A systematic review. *The Journal of Rheumatology, 35*, 1130–1144.

Clauw, D. J. (1995). The pathogenesis of chronic pain and fatigue syndromes, with special reference to fibromyalgia. *Medical Hypotheses, 44*(369), 78.

Collado-Mateo, D., Domínguez-Muñoz, F. J., Adsuar, J., Merellano-Navarro, E., & Gusi, N. (2017). Exergames for women with fibromyalgia: A randomised controlled trial to evaluate the effects on mobility skills, balance and fear of falling. *Medicine: PeerJ, 5*, e3211.

Csikszentmihalyi, M., & Csikzentmihaly, M. (1990). *Flow: The psychology of optimal experience*. Harper & Row.

De Carvalho, M. S., Carvalho, L. C., da Silva Menezes, F., Frazin, A., da Costa Gomes, E., Lunes, H., & D. (2020). Effects of Exergames in women with fibromyalgia: A randomized controlled study. *Games for Health Journal, 9*(5), 358–367. https://doi.org/10.1089/g4h.2019.0108

de Carvalho, M. S., Carvalho, L. C., da Silva Menezes, F., Frazin, A., da Costa Gomes, E., Lunes, H., & D. (2021). Analysis of the muscular activity, peak torque in the lower limbs, and static balance after virtual rehabilitation in women with fibromyalgia: A randomized controlled study. *Games for Health Journal, 10*(3), 190–197. https://doi.org/10.1089/g4h.2020.0206

Gava, V., Fialho, H. R. F., Calixtre, L. B., Barbosa, G. M., & Kamonseki, D. H. (2022). Effects of gaming on pain-related fear, pain catastrophizing, anxiety, and depression in patients with chronic musculoskeletal pain: A systematic review and meta-analysis. *Games for Health Journal – Online Ahead of Print*. https://doi.org/10.1089/g4h.2021.0232

Gowans, S. E., deHueck, A., Voss, S., & Richardson, M. (1999). A randomized, controlled trial of exercise and education for individuals with fibromyalgia. *Arthritis Care and Research, 12*, 120–128.

Gowans, S., deHueck, A., Voss, S., Silaj, A., Abbey, S., & Reynolds, W. (2001). Effect of a randomized, controlled trial of exercise on mood and physical function in individuals with fibromyalgia. *Arthritis and Rheumatism, 45*, 519–529.

Henriksson, C., Gundmark, I., & Bengtsson, A. (1992). Living with fibromyalgia: Consequences for everyday life. *Medicine: The Clinical Journal of Pain, 8*(2), 138–144.

Herrero, R., García-Palacios, A., Castilla, D., Molinari, G., & Botella, C. (2014). Virtual reality for the induction of positive emotions in the treatment of fibromyalgia: A pilot study over acceptability, satisfaction, and the effect of virtual reality on mood. *Cyberpsychology, Behavior and Social Networking, 17*(6), 379–384. https://doi.org/10.1089/cyber.2014.0052

McCain, G. A. (1986). Role of physical fitness training in the fibrositis/fibromyalgia syndrome. *The American Journal of Medicine, 81*, 73–77.

Medialogy. (2002). Msc = https://www.en.aau.dk/education/master/medialogy and Bsc = https://www.en.cph.aau.dk/degree-programmes/bachelor-programmes/medialogy/

Mortensen, J., Kristensen, L. Q., Brooks, E. P., & Brooks, A. L. (2015). Women with fibromyalgia's experience with three motion-controlled video game consoles and indicators of symptom severity and performance of activities of daily living. *Disability and Rehabilitation: Assistive Technology, 10*(1), 61–66. https://doi.org/10.3109/17483107.2013.836687. with Epub 2013, Sep 12.

Olsen, M. N., Sherry, D. D., Boyne, K., McCue, R., Gallagher, P. R., & Brooks, L. J. (2013). Relationship between sleep and pain in adolescents with juvenile primary fibromyalgia syndrome. *Sleep, 36*(4), 509–516.

Polat, M., Kahveci, A., Muci, B., Günendi, Z., & Kaymak Karataş, G. (2021). The effect of virtual reality exercises on pain, functionality, cardiopulmonary capacity, and quality of life in fibromyalgia syndrome: A randomized controlled study. *Games for Health Journal, 10*(3), 165–173. https://doi.org/10.1089/g4h.2020.0162

Sørensen, L., Jensen, M. S. A., Rathleff, M. S., & Holden, S. (2019). Comorbid insomnia, psychological symptoms and widespread pain among patients suffering from musculoskeletal pain in general practice: A cross-sectional study. *BMJ Open, 9*(6), e031971.

Villafaina, S., Collado-Mateo, D., Domínguez-Muñoz, F. J., Fuentes-García, J. P., & Gusi, N. (2019). Benefits of 24-week Exergame intervention on health-related quality of life and pain in women with fibromyalgia: A single-blind, randomized controlled trial. *Games for Health Journal, 8*(6), 380–386. https://doi.org/10.1089/g4h.2019.0023

Waylonis, G. W., & Heck, W. (1992). Fibromyalgia syndrome. New associations. *American Journal of Physical Medicine & Rehabilitation, 71*, 343–348.

Wiederhold, B. K., Soomro, A., Riva, G., & Wiederhold, M. D. (2014). Future directions: Advances and implications of virtual environments designed for pain management. *Cyberpsychology, Behavior and Social Networking, 17*(6), 414–422. https://doi.org/10.1089/cyber.2014.0197

Wolfe, F., Clauw, D. J., Fitzcharles, M. A., Goldenberg, D. L., Katz, R. S., Mease, P., Russell, A. S., Russell, I. J., Winfield, J. B., & Yunus, M. B. (2010). The American College of Rheumatology preliminary diagnostic criteria for fibromyalgia and measurement of symptom severity. *Arthritis Care & Research (Hoboken), 62*, 600–610.

Chapter 8
The Design, Development, and Evaluation of an Accessible Serious Gaming System for Children with Cerebral Palsy

David A. Hobbs, Brett G. Wilkinson, Max B. Hughes, Alexander (Sandy) W. Walker, Remo (Ray) N. Russo, Susan L. Hillier, and Karen J. Reynolds

Introduction

Cerebral palsy (CP) is a permanent condition and the most common cause of physical disability in childhood (Reddihough, 2011; Herbert et al., 2016). The term comes from two words used to define the condition – *cerebral* relating to or of the brain – and *palsy* referring to involuntary muscle tremors. Affecting between 1.4 and 2.1 per 1000 live births in Australia (ACPR, 2016) and 17 million people

D. A. Hobbs (✉)
Medical Device Research Institute, College of Science and Engineering, Flinders University, Adelaide, Australia

Allied Health and Human Performance, University of South Australia, Adelaide, Australia
e-mail: david.hobbs@flinders.edu.au

B. G. Wilkinson · K. J. Reynolds
Medical Device Research Institute, College of Science and Engineering, Flinders University, Adelaide, Australia
e-mail: brett.wilkinson@flinders.edu.au; karen.reynolds@flinders.edu.au

M. B. Hughes · A. W. Walker
Medical Device Research Institute, College of Science and Engineering, Flinders University, Adelaide, Australia

UniSA Creative, University of South Australia, Adelaide, Australia
e-mail: sandy.walker@flinders.edu.au

R. N. Russo
Women's and Children's Hospital Network, Adelaide, Australia

College of Medicine and Public Health, Flinders University, Adelaide, Australia
e-mail: ray.russo@sa.gov.au

S. L. Hillier
Allied Health and Human Performance, University of South Australia, Adelaide, Australia
e-mail: Susan.Hillier@unisa.edu.au

E. Brooks, D. J. Brown (eds.), *Virtual Reality Games for Rehabilitation*, Virtual Reality Technologies for Health and Clinical Applications,
https://doi.org/10.1007/978-1-0716-3371-7_8

worldwide (Impact for CP, 2021), the consensus definition defines CP as 'a group of permanent disorders of the development of movement and posture, causing activity limitation, that are attributed to non-progressive disturbances that occurred in the developing fetal or infant brain. The motor disorders of cerebral palsy are often accompanied by disturbances of sensation, perception, cognition, communication, and behaviour, by epilepsy, and by secondary musculoskeletal problems' (Rosenbaum et al., 2007, pg. 9).

Engaging children with CP in meaningful therapy or exercise can be difficult, despite the merits of the intervention, the potential therapeutic benefits that accompany compliance, and the best intentions of family and rehabilitation specialists to motivate and encourage the child. Using computer games for physical therapy in the treatment of children with CP began in 1998 (Bonnechère et al., 2014, pg. 1905) due to the games' ability to promote a willingness to participate and engage compared with traditional therapy approaches. In this context the games are known as 'serious games' (SG); however, different terms have been used to describe games used for a health or rehabilitation context. Such terms include health gaming, interactive computer play (Sandlund et al., 2009), 'Exer-gaming' ('Exer' from the word 'exercise'), rehab gaming, active video gaming, 'Wiihabilitation' (specifically when the *Nintendo Wii* system is used), and aspects of virtual or augmented reality, depending on the application.

By their very nature, the participatory aspect of computer gaming allows the child to be both engaged and distracted by the game as they become immersed in the challenge of the game activity. Moreover, SGs create 'fun and engaging environments that motivate the child to exercise' (Sandlund et al., 2009, pg. 173). Dunne et al. highlighted the need for engaging children with CP in an immersive and engaging environment, noting that '…a large challenge in administering therapy, however, is to maintain the child's interest and enthusiasm during these exercises' (Dunne et al., 2010, pg. 1751). Consequently, the aim of most SG interventions is to utilise technology to improve attention, engagement, and motivation, which most therapists acknowledge is a challenge when it comes to a rehabilitation programme.

Rehabilitation practitioners began taking an interest in SG technology when it was recognised that gaming actions could be used to substitute the boredom often associated with exercises including stretching, strengthening or mobilisation (Sharan et al., 2012), and skill acquisition (Annema et al., 2010) and that it could also act as a distraction from pain (Pearson & Bailey, 2007; Annema et al., 2010). Sandlund et al. (2012) described the range of interactive technologies as potentially being 'excellent tools to increase motivation for practice in rehabilitation' (pg. 926). Staiano and Flynn (2014) concluded that this combination of entertainment and distraction could '…be just as useful to completing therapy and restoring positive mood as the actual physical improvements attained' (pg. 361), while Sandlund et al. (2009) noted the role SGs can play in delivering home-based rehabilitation and reducing travel time and hospital or clinic costs. Deutsch and colleagues critically analysed the literature within a rehabilitation setting for evidence of SG being able to increase energy expenditure and exercise intensity, identifying preliminary evidence of moderate energy expenditure for children with CP with mild deficits

(Deutsch et al., 2015). Moreover, Bonnechère and colleagues' review concluded that 'SG shows enough evidence to be included within conventional treatment of CP children since it proved to be efficient for increasing patients' motivation' (Bonnechère et al., 2014, pg. 1910).

'Custom built' or 'specially developed' games developed for therapeutic purposes, however, are typically limited in their engagement and participatory content. To engage users actively in the game experience, appropriate interactive elements and a rewarding story progression are required. Sweetser and Wyeth introduced the idea of game enjoyment in greater detail outlining the *GameFlow* model (Sweetser & Wyeth, 2005) and its eight core elements: concentration, challenge, skills, control, clear goals, feedback, immersion, and social interaction. Aspects of this game theory are seen in the development of traditional entertainment applications and research continues to look at the psychology behind game design and the user's continuing buy-in to the game experience. All these aspects are part of the design methodologies behind computer game development for traditional entertainment purposes.

To maintain interest, enthusiasm, and motivation in a computer game therapy session, the games on offer need to be appealing and captivating, promoting repeated, continual, and enjoyable play. This research utilised proven design strategies seen in commercial products to develop an accessible SG system – hardware and software – as an alternative therapeutic intervention for children with CP. The target group was children aged between 5 and 15 years, with a confirmed diagnosis of CP. While most therapy attention focusses on the motor impairment associated with CP, the literature reports that somatosensory impairments of the upper limbs (i.e. impaired sensation, including touch, related to the hands) is common amongst children with CP, as first reported by Tizard and Crothers more than 70 years ago (Tizard & Crothers, 1952).

Where this study differs from all other applications of SG for this population is that the therapeutic application is *not* targeting motor rehabilitation. The research focus was investigating the therapeutic effect of providing targeted afferent vibration feedback to the hands of children with CP to complement their gameplay experience. Rather than focusing on movement and motor rehabilitation, this research examined if contextually relevant and appropriate mechanical stimuli that reinforce gameplay can aid in improving tactile sense in the hands of children with CP with a known sensory loss. Our hypothesis, that upper limb somatosensation could be improved through the use of an accessible, integrated SG system, was to be tested through a home-based randomised controlled trial.

To undertake the project, we employed a multidisciplinary team (Hobbs et al., 2015) to develop an accessible SG system that featured an integrated catalogue with multiple custom-made 2D and 3D computer games, with full data logging capability, in conjunction with a novel, accessible gaming controller. The games were developed with an emphasis on cognitive engagement (ensuring player buy in) and system longevity to encourage long-term and repeat play. Industrial design expertise was used to ideate, conceptualise, design, prototype, test, and fabricate the accessible controller, where the focus was on form and intuitive use. A patent has been filed for the overall gaming system, recognising the design novelty and application. This chapter will discuss the design philosophy and evaluation process of the overall system in readiness for the home-based trial.

Background

There are four types of CP, with the most common type being called spastic CP. Spastic CP accurately describes the nature of the stiff or tight muscle tone present and affects approximately 80% of all people with CP (CDC, 2021). The remaining types are known as dyskinetic CP, ataxic CP, and mixed CP (CDC, 2021). CP can be heterogeneous in nature and presentation, and there is currently no cure for the condition. The most significant risk factors for CP are low birth weight, intrauterine infections, and multiple gestation (Odding et al., 2006).

Included in the consensus definition of CP (Rosenbaum et al., 2007) is the specific mention of 'disturbances of sensation'. This was a neglected area of clinical investigation and understanding for this population until J.P.M. Tizard and Bronson Crothers published their landmark paper in 1952 (Tizard & Crothers, 1952) and subsequent follow-up paper two years later (Tizard et al., 1954). Identifying somatosensory impairments in the hands of children with CP is important. Tactile sensory inputs are invaluable as they provide important cues for cutaneous and proprioceptive information, and intact sensory hand function is essential for the initiation and execution of refined hand, grasp, and finger movements. Sensory input is an essential component of motor function and motor control, and sensory deficits may constitute limits on the functional outcome of children with CP (Cooper et al., 1995).

If a child with CP has a sensory loss in their hand(s), the most commonly reported impaired modalities are stereognosis or haptic perception (with vision occluded, the ability to identify an object placed in the hand through form only), two-point discrimination (the ability to identify that two nearby objects touching the skin are two distinct points and not one), and proprioception (in this circumstance, the ability to identify the position of the thumb or finger in space). Studies have consistently highlighted that sensory deficits are not just restricted to the impaired or hemiplegic side – they are also present in the 'unaffected' or 'dominant' hand (such as Monfraix et al., 1961; Cooper et al., 1995; Arnould et al., 2007; Wingert et al., 2008; Auld et al., 2012; Hobbs et al., 2014). Prevalence rates on the affected side vary from 42% (Tachdjian & Minear, 1958) to 97% (Van Heest et al., 1993) and depend on the type of CP (Wigfield, 1966). However, the studies are difficult to group for a number of reasons, including the lack of a definition as to what constitutes an impaired sense, poor methodological quality, the lack of a standardised testing suite, and unclear details of the testing protocols that were used.

Computer or video games are pervasive and a part of everyday life. With the advent of laptops, tablets, and smartphones, a player doesn't have to be at home in front of their console to be 'gaming' anymore – able-bodied gamers can 'game' in transit on public transport or in the park during a lunch break. Despite their popularity, and the profile of groups such as Game-Accessibility (http://gameaccessibility.com) and the philosophy of Universal Design (Story, 1998), off-the-shelf or commercial games generally remain inaccessible for people with a disability – meaning they are socially excluded from participating in such activities and often isolated from peer conversations involving games as they cannot contribute their first-hand experience. Consequently, this project aimed to develop a home-based accessible SG system that children with CP could independently play and engage with. This meant addressing both software and hardware accessibility issues simultaneously – developing a suite of accessible games as well as an accessible controller. A design emphasis for the system as a whole was the incorporation of sensory (haptic) feedback into both the games and the controller to augment the potential therapeutic effects of play.

System Design and Development

The Software – Game Development

Many computer games built for the traditional commercial market take full advantage of the complex game control systems available and assume the player has the dextrous ability to manipulate those controls rapidly and with precision. Children with CP typically struggle with button size, location, and the speed with which a button is required to be pressed due to their impaired hand function, as highlighted in the literature (Bierre et al., 2005). An additional challenge is that while some buttons might be accessible (such as the four coloured buttons, A, B, X, and Y, on a *Microsoft Xbox* controller), most commercial games utilise all available inputs and functionality of the controller, meaning that access to the full range of input options and not a subset is required to successfully play a given game.

Our approach and philosophy for developing a suite of accessible games was to develop games that relied on joystick control only and avoided all in-game button activity (Henschke et al., 2012). When coupled with the system controller, this paradigm encouraged sustained, bimanual (two-handed) use that didn't require coordinated, controlled, and precise digit movements. Significant effort went into the design, conceptualisation, and development of the games to ensure features such as game appeal, re-playability, player interest, and intuitive gameplay were part of the gaming experience despite the modified control system adopted.

Consequently, every game was required to conform to the specific design requirements of:

- Utilising only four control options for in-game movement and control – forward, backward, left, and right
- Providing an engaging experience, where each relevant game action (such as collecting a reward, achieving a milestone, or bumping into an object) produced a

corresponding haptic event that was felt via the controller, thereby reinforcing the game action (Geerdink et al., 2004)

- Ensuring haptic events were (a) often, specified as enabling the player to experience a haptic event at least once every 10 s of gameplay and (b) tailored to the particular game event, providing an opportunity for the player to experience a range of vibration intensities and durations while playing and not a single, repetitive burst of vibration each time;
- Increasing game difficulty at a slower rate compared to commercial games, but still providing a degree of challenge and sense of progression and achievement within the game
- Integrating with the central gaming system catalogue so that (a) all data logging and game statistics could be recorded in a common format and (b) the central in-game pop-up menu could work across all games, ensuring the player could pause and exit their game when the single out-of-game button was pressed

The most significant design challenges during game development were the restrictive control mechanic that was adopted and the requirement for frequent haptic feedback during gameplay. The first challenge was addressed, usually in team meetings, by brainstorming a game concept and possible storyline and identifying an intuitive control mechanic. Once the framework for a given game was drafted, opportunities for providing haptic feedback were identified, and possible levels of intensity (on a 0.1–1.0 full scale) and duration (typically from 0.5 s to approximately 3.0 s) were assigned to relevant game events. Both aspects (vibration intensity and duration) were tested using both a standard *Microsoft Xbox 360* game controller and the prototype controller that was developed at the time, to ensure the vibration assigned accurately represented the game event. Values were subjectively adjusted where a 'vibration-game event' mismatch was identified, and a uniform approach to providing haptic feedback across all games was implemented (i.e. picking up a collectable in all games provided a vibration of the same intensity and duration). The suite of games, and a short overview of each game, is presented in Table 8.1.

System Features

All games were programmed using the *Microsoft* XNA 4.0 framework, and the chosen platform was an off-the-shelf *HP ProBook 4730 s* laptop (Intel Core i5 (2nd Gen) 2450 M/2.5 GHz, AMD Radeon HD 6490 M, 1GB GDDR5 SDRAM graphics card, 17.3″ display). XNA was chosen for its flexibility and the fact that it is the language that students at Flinders University learn during the topic 'Computer Game Development'. From a system performance perspective, the laptop was specified to run the complete XNA environment, all the games and associated 2D and 3D assets, and the required data logging of player performance. On-board data logging removed the need for families to keep a journal of system use during the home trial, which requires diligent record keeping and can be burdensome for families

Table 8.1 An overview of the custom games developed for the project

Game name	Brief game overview
A Bridge Too Far	Similar to '*Temple Run*', the main character has to navigate an endless pathway, jumping gaps and collecting gems and coins
Alex Adventure	A side-scroller game where the main character, Alex, explores themed landscapes while collecting carrots and avoiding obstacles
Alien Attack	Similar to '*Space Invaders*', the player must cleanse each planet of alien spaceships while moving through the solar system and an asteroid field
BiPlane 1922	A 3D flight simulator that has the player fly over the English countryside, avoiding obstacles while navigating through farm barns. Levels are presented from different perspectives, such as the cockpit and chase-cam
DragonFly Dodge	A side-scroller game that has the main character, a dragonfly, fly over a stream and collect coins while avoiding frogs, reeds, birds, and rocks
Driving Maniac	A vertical-scroller game that has players avoid obstacles and challenges on the road, such as other cars, road works, and lane changes
Marine Life	An underwater swimming game that has players attempt to move up the food chain by eating other underwater creatures while avoiding predators
Move Gravity	A puzzle-based game that requires players to combine multiple asteroid masses in space into a single mass, taking into account gravitational forces and black holes
Planet Fall	An action game where players control a laser and rocket-shooting moon lander, trying to stop meteorites from reaching the ground
Snake	Similar to the '*Snake*' game on Nokia™ mobile phones, players guide a moving snake around the screen, trying to eat as many objects as possible while avoiding running into themselves and the edge of the screen
Space Stuntz	A 3D spaceship simulator where players fly through an endless tunnel of rings to score points while avoiding asteroids and other objects
Squirrel	An endless running game that has players control a squirrel as it climbs a giant tree, collecting coins and avoiding tree knots and branches
Sunday Driver	A 3D exploratory driving game that has players search for hidden objects and avoid enemies, before progressing to the next world
Swimma	A side-scroller game that requires players to control a snorkeler, collecting as many gems and air bubbles as possible while avoiding predators
The Fancy World	A dress-up game that challenges players to suitably dress their character for a given event, such as going to the movies or the beach

(Preston et al., 2016). A 17.3-inch screen was chosen to maximise player immersion in the game and hence player buy-in. The games and overall software system design, development, evaluation, testing, and commissioning process took 2 and a half years from start to finish, through a combination of final year Engineering, Digital Media, and Information Technology student projects to seed the study. Grant funding secured for the project enabled a graduate computer scientist/game developer to be employed as a Research Assistant to act as a central coordinator to ensure consistency and to fine tune the work.

The games catalogue and menu system manage all 15 games, collate and present high scores for each game, and manage system functions (such as the sound level, the profile of the player, the colour of the game menu background, the vibration

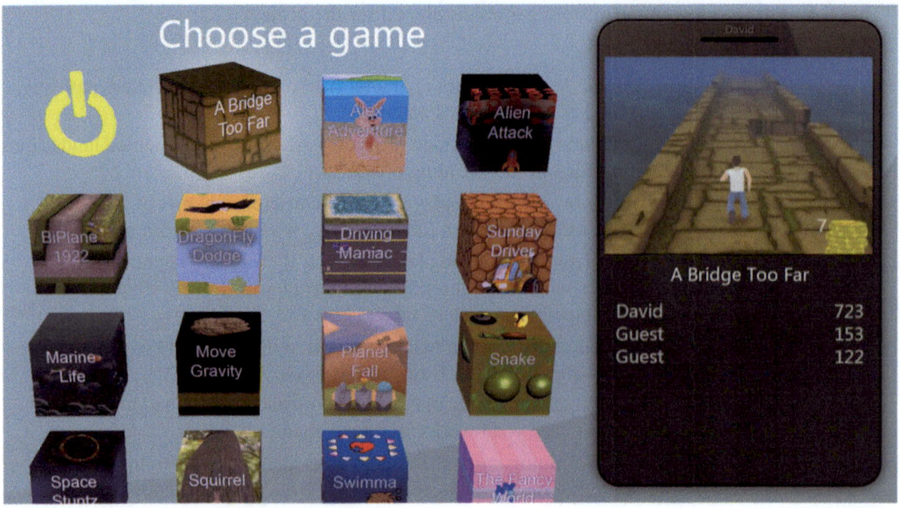

Fig. 8.1 The tablet-style main menu screen for the gaming system, where game selection is made. In this instance, the game *A Bridge Too Far* has been selected. Players can preview any game by selecting the relevant game 'cube' and watching a short video of the game on the smartphone on the right-hand side

profile, and the system credits). The main menu went through a number of iterations and designs before arriving at the final design (see Fig. 8.1). Fourteen of the 15 games were coded using procedural generation, meaning the games generated random events each and every time the game was played. For example, in *Sunday Driver* (a 3D driving game that encourages players to explore different worlds as they search for hidden objects and try to progress to the next world), the location and reward for collectables, the location of obstacles to avoid, and the progression portal between levels change every time the game is played. The games were designed this way to reduce boredom and game fatigue, meaning players couldn't memorise where certain items or enemies were within games and levels, as the scenario changed each time. Offering multiple games was a specific strategy to appeal to a broad audience and to reduce game boredom and fatigue, which had been reported by other studies (Li et al., 2009; Preston et al., 2016).

The final design of the main menu (Fig. 8.1) adopts a contemporary tablet-style look and presents the player with a single view of all 15 games in a 4 by 4 grid layout. The universal computer symbol for 'on/off' is depicted as a bright yellow icon in the top left-hand corner position, and each of the 15 games is represented by a cube that has the name of the game in white text on the front face, and the cube itself is wrapped in artwork from the game. To the right of the game grid layout is a 'smartphone' that is integrated within the system and provides additional information to the player.

The player must log in to the system before they can play any of the games. The login screen always presents two options – the default profile, which is the name of the child who is participating in the trial on the left-hand side, and a 'guest' login on the right-hand side. The guest login is for players other than the child who is part of the trial, meaning trial participants can share their gaming system with siblings and friends if they wish and potentially enjoy some of the socially binding and competitive experiences that gaming can bring in a multi-player environment. When a game finishes the player is returned to the login screen, meaning they must consciously choose their name every time they wish to play a game.

When the player logs in by choosing the appropriate profile, the main menu is loaded and the default starting position is the computer 'on/off' icon. In this grid position, the smartphone screen shows the player the system time, day and date, and the battery charge level. To move within the grid, the player simply moves the controller in the desired direction – 'right' to move to the cube immediately right of their current position, 'down' to move to the cube immediately beneath their current position, and so on. When moving within the game menu the player receives haptic vibration via the controller, to reinforce the on-screen action of moving between game cubes. They also receive a small vibration when they push the out-of-game button to choose the game they wish to play.

When a particular game cube is selected, it moves forward from its static position within the grid, adopts a glow around its edges, and starts to rotate to signify it is the currently chosen game (seen in Fig. 8.1 for the game '*A Bridge Too Far*'). At the same time, the smartphone shows a video preview of the game on the right-hand side of the screen, and if the game has been played previously, the area beneath the video screen shows recent high scores for that game, including who achieved the score. Players can personalise their system by changing the background colour of the game menu as well as adjust the system volume level, which is done by selecting the relevant options within the yellow 'on/off' icon area.

If the player removes their hands from the controller during gameplay and presses the large red out-of-game button on the front of the controller, a universal pop-up menu is presented that pauses the game. The player can then choose to resume their game, change the volume level of the current game they are playing, or exit the game and return to the login screen. If they choose 'resume', the player is counted back into the game using an animated '3-2-1' countdown sequence to enable the player time to prepare for the next game action without being suddenly thrust back into gameplay.

User Evaluation of the Custom Games

Game development was supervised and tracked weekly (by Hobbs and Wilkinson) and progress was monitored in line with academic milestones throughout the development phase. The team used Scrum-based agile software engineering practices to rapidly prototype each game. An important aspect was to seek external opinion and feedback on the quality and appeal of the games being developed – particularly considering the restrictive control mechanic adopted across all games and what this meant for game enjoyment and playability. However, given children with CP typically find commercial gaming systems inaccessible, meaning they have little or no prior experience to draw on and hence may lack knowledge of commercial game expectation and quality, an experienced and knowledgeable typically developing cohort was sought. This decision was driven by the fact that the accessible controller development lagged game development and hence wasn't ready to be trialled. It also meant the games would be critiqued by a knowledgeable group that is used to having all available inputs (all buttons, thumb sticks, and thumb pads) available to them for gameplay, meaning they could make an informed comparison with respect to the games and the gameplay experience.

Two local schools were approached for the evaluation. The first round of testing involved 31 primary school students aged 4–13 years (15 females), and the second round of testing, conducted a year later, involved 17 high school students aged 14–16 years (8 females). Information packs about the study were provided to all families, and consent to participate was provided by the child's main parent/caregiver. Children could assent to the study if they were old enough to read and understand the 'plain English child's version' of the study information sheet. Permission to conduct the user evaluations was provided by Flinders University's Social and Behavioural Research Ethics Committee and the Government of South Australia's Department for Education and Child Development Research Unit.

An unused classroom was utilised for both evaluation sessions. This provided enough room for up to ten laptops to be set up while still being able to access mains power and suitable desk space. Each participant was assigned a unique two-digit ID, which the researchers used to log participants in with. This number also formed the filename for the log files that the system generated for each participant. Participants were assigned a laptop each and asked to play as many games as they liked in the time allowed.

It was a conscious decision not to segregate participants during the evaluation as the games for the main intervention trial were intended to be played within the family home. When the games were eventually deployed, it was expected that the trial participants would discuss the games with their family, peers, and siblings to engender a sense of ownership, competition, and buy-in to the games. Allowing the game evaluation participants to play the games within the one room meant that a sense of competition and comparison was evident. During both evaluations the participants would often call out to their friends asking if they had completed a particular stage or how many points they had scored in a particular game, or compete side by side in the same game.

Each round of game testing provided an opportunity to also test the performance and stability of the laptops chosen for the trial (the *HP* laptops referred to earlier), the stability of the current game catalogue (at that point in time), the performance and accuracy of the data logging system, and the stability of the games themselves when running for up to 5 h continuously. Each laptop was set up with identical software and a *Microsoft Xbox 360* controller for *Windows* was used to control the games. All joystick control was routed through the left thumb stick and the green 'A' button represented the out-of-game button.

Beside each laptop was a set of instructions for all games. The instructions were simple one-page documents that briefly identified the theme of the game and the controls required to play it. They were prepared for the average-aged student playing the game; however, some of the younger children required additional support to understand some of the game requirements (i.e. the instructions were read or more fully explained to the younger children), but images for the control systems helped most children understand what was required. The primary school cohort tested and evaluated the first six games developed for the project (Wilkinson & Hobbs, 2015), whereas the high school cohort tested and evaluated eight games – six new games and two from the earlier evaluation.

Participants were allowed 1 h to play the games. For the primary school cohort, this was a continuous hour of play, but for the high school cohort the hour was divided into two half-hour sessions with an alternate paper-based activity being conducted in a separate room. The paper-based activity was an exercise in creative game development, where the students were asked to brainstorm and develop their own game, from any genre, that used the same game controls and no in-game button activity. They were asked to write and/or draw a 'storyboard' for their game idea.

At the beginning of each evaluation a brief introduction was given to provide background to the study, the simple instructions, and the expectations of the session. A summary of the games was provided for the primary school cohort to provide participants with a context for the games they were to play. Participants were allowed to select the order of play that suited their game interests; however, they were encouraged to play every game and were able to go back to previous games they enjoyed toward the end of the session. The individual game designers and developers were not present during either evaluation session.

Prior to each session starting, participants were asked a series of background questions addressing their age, gender, the frequency of their computer gameplay, the devices they used, the genre of games they enjoyed, and the reason for their preference of their favoured system. For the primary school cohort, while playing the games the researchers circulated throughout the room asking the participants about their impressions of the games via set questions. The questions sought to address a range of game evaluation aspects, including whether the participants enjoyed the games, if they needed to read the instructions to be able to play the game, their opinion on specific aspects of the game, their level of interest in the game, if they would buy the game if it were in a store, if they felt there were aspects missing from the game, what didn't work within the game, the level of difficulty, if they had played similar games, whether the scoring made sense, and if they would be willing to replay the game to beat their previous score. Due to time restrictions, each primary school participant's response was recorded for at least two of the six possible games they played. For the high school cohort, each participant was asked to record their own responses to the above questions on the sheets provided, and they were encouraged to do this after they had played a given game enough times to be able to critique it.

While the games were being played, player activity was logged by the system and stored locally. The information collected included the length of time the game was played, the X and Y locations of the thumb stick, the duration of vibration events, and the intensity of each vibration. The system created an individual log file for each game played. A post-evaluation analysis of the log files indicated that the primary school cohort played a total of 362 individual games (average number of games per student, 11.7; range, 4–21 games played per student), while the high school cohort played a total of 246 games (average number of games per student, 14.5; range, 6–28 games played per student).

The participants provided a wealth of qualitative feedback and information on all the games, including comments on the graphics and artwork quality, the sounds used, the game storyline, opportunities for improvements such as power-ups or extra lives, and what aspects of a particular game they liked or didn't like. Responses to questions that produced a 'yes' or 'no' answer were collated and presented as a percentage that agreed with the question being asked, and participants were asked to rate their interest in the particular game they were playing (out of ten). Across both evaluations, the integration and use of haptic vibration feedback to complement gameplay was described as being 'good' by most participants (where 'good' was the highest ranked response). All feedback was passed on to the individual game designer/developer for consideration and was incorporated into future game development.

From the values shown in Table 8.2, it can be seen that both cohorts enjoyed playing the games during the evaluation, with most games showing high replay value (85% for the primary school cohort compared to 77% for the high school cohort). The largest discrepancy between the two cohorts was in response to the 'would you buy this game if it were available in a store?' question. Nearly three-quarters of the younger cohort said they would buy the game, compared to 38% of the older cohort. This discrepancy can be explained by the simple fact that most of the older cohort were game-savvy enough to know that our games took inspiration from popular existing games currently on the market, and that most of these were able to be downloaded as an app or game to their phone. As one participant said: 'I like the game a lot, but why would I buy it when I can download it for free?', indicating their straightforward, pragmatic approach to games and today's technology.

At two different time points during the game development process, two teenage children with CP (1 female, average age 13.5 years) volunteered to test and evaluate the games in a more extended, home-based trial, lasting 2 and 3 weeks, respectively.

Table 8.2 Summary of responses to sample questions asked during the game evaluation

Question ('yes' response only)[a]	Primary school cohort ($n = 31$)	High school cohort ($n = 17$)
Enjoyed playing the game?	88%	88%
Would play the same game again?	85%	77%
Would buy the game?	74%	38%
Average interest in the game (/10) (range)	7.3 (5.9–8.7)	7.0 (4.5–8.2)

[a]Percentages are for 'yes' responses only. If a response was not a 'yes' or 'no' (i.e. unsure) or was left blank, it was not included in the above calculations

Again, this was an opportunity to test the games, the laptops, and the robustness and stability of the system and its logging capability in an unsupported environment. As the controller was still in development, both children were set up with a traditional *Microsoft Xbox 360* controller with all joystick control routed through the left thumb stick and the green 'A' button, identical to the school trials. One of the teenagers had a right-side involvement, meaning their left hand was unimpaired, and the other had a mild left-side impairment, meaning they could use a traditional *Xbox* controller without duress or discomfort. Neither child reported a problem with using the traditional *Xbox* controller during their trial.

The system was in the early stages of development during the first trial and the data logging system wasn't functioning correctly – consequently inaccurate results were recorded. The second trial occurred later in the development phase, when the data logging system was fully functional. An analysis of the results indicated that this participant played with the gaming system sporadically, playing 78 games on 3 separate days over a 3-week period. The total amount of time spent using the system was 76 min and 23 s, which comprised 67 min and 28 s of gameplay and 8 min and 55 s spent in the system menu. The longest time spent playing one game was 7 min, 53 s (for one game of *BiPlane 1922*) and *Snake* was the game that was played the most number of times. The total amount of vibration that was delivered was 15 min, 45 s, of which 49 s was delivered when navigating the menu system and 14 min, 56 s was delivered during gameplay.

A written assessment and detailed feedback was received from only one participant, who rated the system highly. They reported the games as being 'exciting', 'fun' and 'mostly creative' and described the game vibration events as 'very creative and easily felt'. The participant concluded that 'I had the best 2 weeks of my life playing the games, from early morning to afternoon'. The participant's mother reported anecdotally that their child preferentially chose to play games on the system during their trial instead of their normal favourite past-time, which was competitive swimming. Following a podium presentation on the games developed to date for SG system at the biennial *Australian Rehabilitation and Assistive Technology Association* (ARATA) National Conference, the authors were awarded first Prize in the *Soft Technology Awards*, for 'developments, improvements and innovations in service delivery to Assistive Technology users' (Hobbs et al., 2012).

The Hardware – Controller Development

The controller was developed with a primary focus on form, to maximise physical accessibility and to facilitate intuitive use given the restrictive game control mechanic. The seven *Principles of Universal Design* were used as a framework for accessible design (Story, 1998). Based on a *Microsoft Xbox 360* technical package, the controller was required to promote and intuit bimanual (two-handed) use, interface with the existing XNA-based gaming system, have no in-game buttons but one large and easily accessible out-of-game button for menu selection, self-centre, and be robust enough to withstand 'above average' wear and tear due to the possibility of the end user having uncontrollable arm and/or hand spasms that may twist or knock the controller during use. Additionally, the controller was required to have a high degree of aesthetic and visual appeal so children would want to use it and have it in their homes.

An iterative Industrial Design approach was utilised for the ideation, conceptualisation, design, and prototyping of the controller, where the requirements and function were tightly specified but the form was not. An initial 4-month project with four postgraduate Industrial Design students seeded the project, with each student taking on the task of designing and developing a unique, working prototype controller. Four working, diverse prototypes that all met the design brief were produced and two were selected to proceed to the second phase of the design process, which involved further refinement, ideation, and prototyping, but over a longer 12-month period to complete a master's level project. A structured, stage gate process was used to guide the design process (Walker & Hobbs, 2014).

The first prototype design, Design A (Fig. 8.2), took inspiration from a trackball and used a sphere or dome to control joystick movement. When assessed by the design team, the control was thought to be very intuitive – tilting the sphere forward moved the player's character forward, tilting it back moved the character back, etc. The motion was smooth and logical. Different colour oval pads were recessed slightly into the top portions of the sphere to act as a guide as to where the player should place their hands. To use the controller, the player simply rested their hands on the oval pads of the sphere, which placed their wrists, hands, and fingers in a neutral position (meaning the wrists and fingers were neither flexed nor extended). The out-of-game button was located centrally on the front of the controller. The form of this controller removed the need to be able to grip a joystick handle. Due to the variability of the condition that is CP, provision for a strap that could hold the

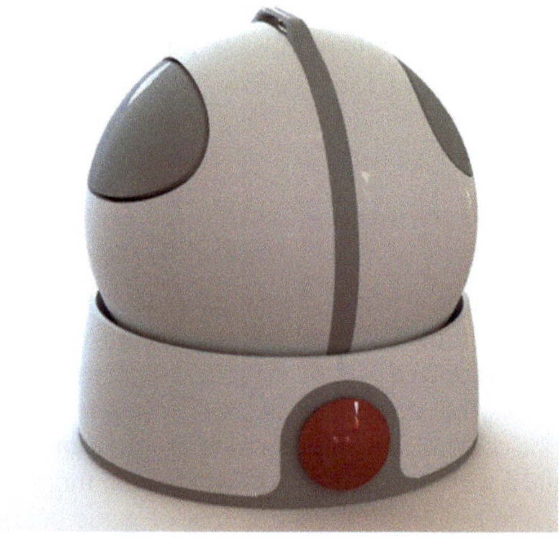

Fig. 8.2 CAD model of Design A, which utilised rotation of a sphere or dome for game control

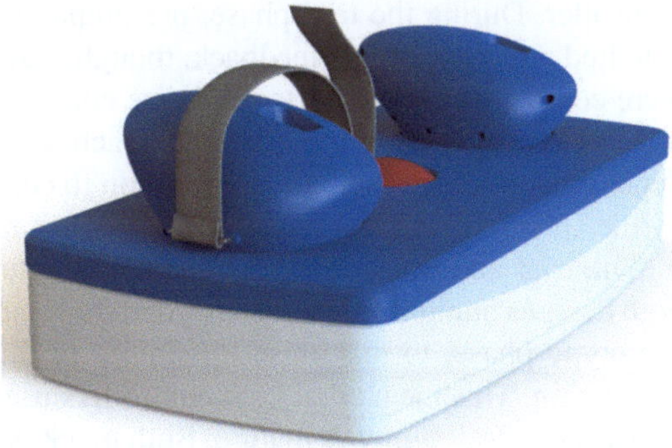

Fig. 8.3 CAD model of Design B, which utilised horizontal planar movement for game control, with a single hand strap shown

hand in place, over the oval pad, was incorporated into the design, should the player require additional hand support.

The second prototype design, Design B (Fig. 8.3), took inspiration from a combination of the form of a computer mouse combined with that of an indoor rock climbing handhold. Two handholds were fixed to a horizontal top plate that provided planar (X-Y) movement relative to a fixed base to control the on-screen character. Control was achieved through a planar sliding motion instead of rotation. From the central neutral position, sliding the top plate forward produced forward or up movement, sliding it back produced backward or down movement, etc. The motion was smooth and the handholds were comfortable, although they did require a hand that could grip slightly more than what was required for Design A. The out-of-game button was located midway between the handholds, in an easily accessible location, and provision for a strap was included (shown in Fig. 8.3).

Both prototype controller designs were routinely reviewed, assessed, and critiqued by the main supervisory team (Walker, an Industrial Designer, and Hobbs, a Biomedical/Rehabilitation Engineer) throughout the process, and at key milestones broader feedback was solicited from other professionals within the team, including a Biomedical Engineer (Reynolds), Computer Scientist/Game Developer (Wilkinson), Paediatric Rehabilitation Consultant (Russo), Physiotherapist (Hillier), and other allied health professionals associated with the project. Approximately two-thirds of the way through the process, both controllers were trialled and evaluated by two teenagers with CP who volunteered to be a part of a focus group session that involved using the controllers to play and interact with the gaming system software.

User Evaluation of the Prototype Controller Designs

The user evaluation was conducted with two teenage children with CP (1 female, average age 14.5 years), who both had commercial game experience. The sessions began with an introduction to the project, a brief presentation by the designers of the two different controllers using CAD models, and an opportunity to trial each controller. During the trial phase, pre-prepared questions about the controller that solicited the participant's feedback, thoughts, and feelings were asked. The sessions were conducted separately to minimise comments or observations from one volunteer biasing or leading the other, and each session lasted between 30 and 45 min, depending on the participant. Permission to conduct the user evaluations was given by the University of South Australia's Human Research Ethics Committee.

The trial and evaluation session was scheduled at a point in the project where both designs could be presented beyond the conceptualisation phase and at the early prototype phase, to maximise the ability to incorporate feedback from the target population. This meant that both controllers used 'mock prototypes' for the evaluation as neither design was mature. Both mock prototypes functioned as intended but differed in look and feel compared to what the final prototype design would eventually be (see Figs. 8.4 and 8.5). This was communicated to the participants by drawing their attention to the CAD models of the current design (shown on a large projector screen, as shown in Figs. 8.2 and 8.3) during each trial. They were asked to provide comment on the use of the controllers while playing with them, but on the aesthetic and visual appeal by studying the CAD models.

Upon studying the CAD images and the mock prototype in front of them, both participants thought the controllers looked simple and easy to use, using words such as 'novel', 'different', 'creative', 'new', and 'great' to describe both controllers. Both participants wanted to buy one, with their parents commenting that if it was robust and performed as desired, they would spend 'around AUD$100 or more' if they thought it would help their child play computer games. Colour, durability, and a compact design were highlighted as important features, which they felt were

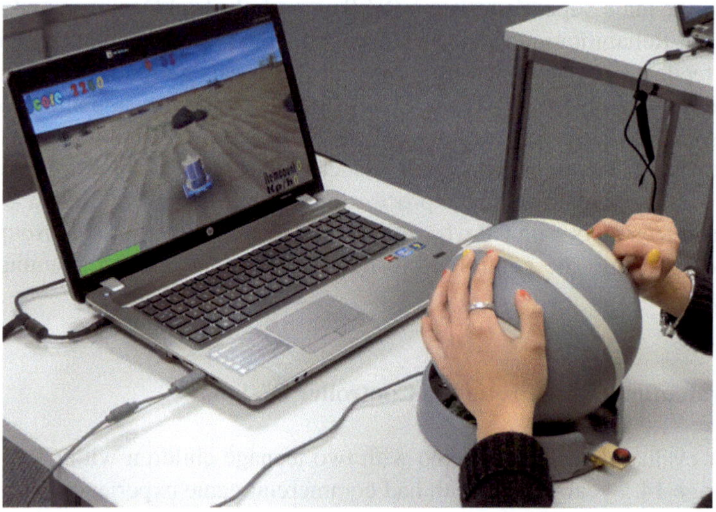

Fig. 8.4 A participant trialling a 'mock prototype' of controller Design A during the user evaluation

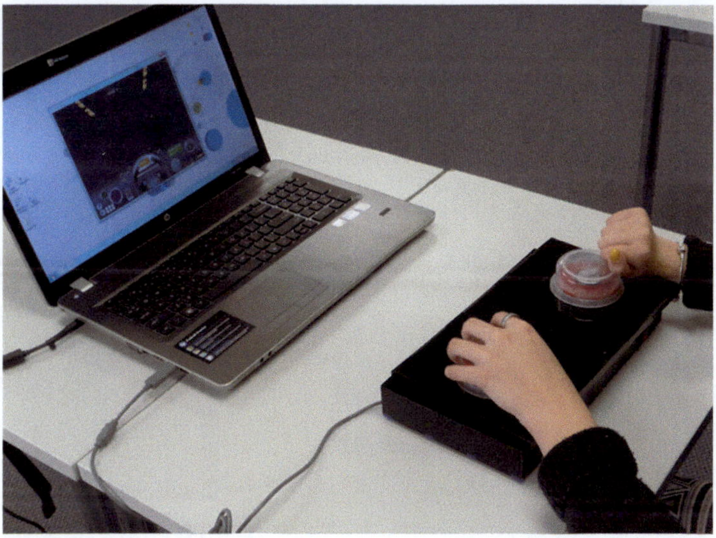

Fig. 8.5 A participant trialling a 'mock prototype' of controller Design B during the user evaluation

strong features of both designs. Design A was identified as being more 'instantly natural' and intuitive, implying the player knew how to use it just by looking at it and putting their hands on it.

During the user trial the research team noticed that both participants were able to play and perform well with both controllers when playing 2D games – as well as the typically developing participants that had previously evaluated the games. However, there was a stark difference in performance and gameplay when 3D games where played, due to the perception of depth created by the game. The sphere-shaped controller (Design A) was found to be much more intuitive, natural, and easier to use within a 3D environment. When using the horizontal plate controller (Design B) to play 3D games, both participants tried to twist or rotate (instead of sliding left or right) or lift the top plate from the base (instead of sliding forward) when attempting to control their game character. There were no such control incompatibility issues with Design A.

Both participants were able to interact with the controller, the games, and the game menu screen as well as anticipated. Design A received more favourable and positive comments than Design B and performed better in terms of providing a more natural control interface. Consequently, Design A was chosen as the preferred design for the eventual trial. At the conclusion of the academic year, and following further iterative design changes based on the feedback received, both controller designs won individual awards at the University of South Australia's end of year design exhibition.

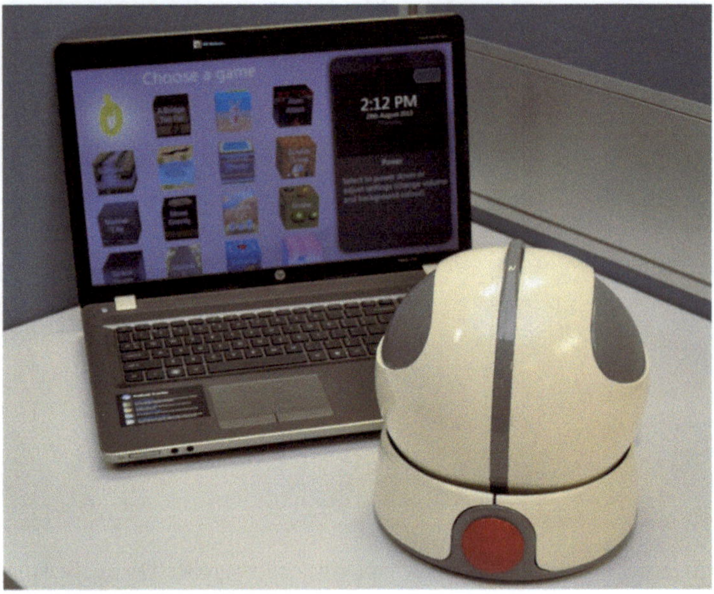

Fig. 8.6 The final prototype game controller (foreground) with the final version of the gaming system (background)

Future Work

The final prototype SG system was the product of a series of software and hardware design iterations and is shown in Fig. 8.6. Future work includes improving the vibration feedback that is delivered to players during gameplay through the controller, and the implementation of sensors into the oval pads of the controller for hand detection purposes, to ensure two hands are always used during gameplay. A desirable system feature, reported during one of the evaluations, is the ability to incorporate multi-player remote gaming into the system so children with CP can compete against each other from the comfort of their homes. This is being investigated.

Conclusion

This chapter describes the process of design, development, testing, and user evaluation for a custom-made haptic SG system for children with CP, aimed at providing an immersive, engaging, and interactive therapeutic experience. End user evaluation of both the games and the controller were positive, with most participants excited and interested to know more about the final version of the system.

The present software system comprises a comprehensive and integrated menu system that contains fifteen 2D and 3D haptic games, with full game logging capability, and an integrated accessible controller for menu navigation and gameplay. School and extended multi-week home-based trials, as well as multiple demonstrations at different university campuses on multiple occasions, have demonstrated that the system is stable and robust.

Both prototype game controllers (hardware) won individual awards at the University of South Australia's end of year design exhibition, and the game catalogue (software) was awarded first prize in the ARATA *Soft Technology Awards*. A patent has been filed for the overall SG system.

The chosen prototype controller design is currently undergoing further design iteration and revision prior to the overall SG system being deployed into family homes for a 6-week randomised controlled trial.

References

ACPR. (2016). *Report of the Australian Cerebral Palsy Register, birth years 1993–2009*. Available via https://cpregister.com/wp-content/uploads/2018/05/ACPR-Report_Web_2016.pdf. Accessed 28 Jan 2021.

Annema, J-. H., Verstraete, M., Abeele, V. V., Desmet, S., & Geerts, D. (2010, September). *Videogames in therapy: A therapist's perspective*. Paper presented the 3rd International Conference on Fun and Games, Leuven, Belgium. https://doi.org/10.1145/1823818.1823828

Arnould, C., Penta, M., & Thonnard, J.-L. (2007). Hand impairments and their relationship with manual ability in children with cerebral palsy. *Journal of Rehabilitation Medicine, 39*, 708–714.

Auld, M. L., Boyd, R., Moseley, G. L., Ware, R., & Johnston, L. M. (2012). Tactile function in children with unilateral cerebral palsy compared to typically developing children. *Disability and Rehabilitation, 34*(17), 1488–1494.

Bierre, K., Chetwynd, J., Ellis, B., Hinn, D. M., Ludi, S., & Westin, T. (2005). *Game not over: Accessibility issues in video games*. HCI International.

Bonnechère, B., Jansen, B., Omelina, L., Degelaen, M., Wermenbol, V., Rooze, M., & Van Sint, J. S. (2014). Can serious games be incorporated with conventional treatment of children with cerebral palsy? A review. *Research in Developmental Disabilities, 35*(8), 1899–1913.

CDC. (2021). *What is cerebral palsy?* https://www.cdc.gov/ncbddd/cp/facts.html. Accessed 28 Jan 2021.

Cooper, J., Majnemer, A., Rosenblatt, B., & Birnbaum, R. (1995). The determination of sensory deficits in children with hemiplegic cerebral palsy. *Journal of Child Neurology, 10*(4), 300–309.

Deutsch, J. E., Guarrera-Bowlby, P., Myslinski, M. J., & Kafri, M. (2015). Is there evidence that active videogames increase energy expenditure and exercise intensity for people poststroke and with cerebral palsy? *Games for Health Journal, 4*(1), 31–37. https://doi.org/10.1089/g4h.2014.0082

Dunne, A., Do-Lenh, S., Laighin, G. O., Chia, S., & Bonato, P. (2010). *Upper extremity rehabilitation of children with cerebral palsy using accelerometer feedback on a multitouch display*. Paper presented at the Engineering in Medicine and Biology Society (EMBC) Annual International Conference of the IEEE, Buenos Aires, Argentina, 31 August – 4 September 2010.

Geerdink, B., Levesley, M. C., Bhakta, B., Clarke, M., Spinty, S., Cnossen, F., & Richardson, R. (2004). Force feedback joystick therapy for children with cerebral palsy. In *Proceedings of the 2nd Cambridge Workshop on Universal Access and Assistive Technology* (Technical Report CUED/C-EDC/TR129, pp. 81–90).

Henschke, M., Hobbs, D., & Wilkinson, B. (2012). Developing serious games for children with cerebral palsy: Case study and pilot trial. In *Proceedings of the 24th Australian Computer-Human*

Interaction Conference, Melbourne, Victoria, 26–30 November 2012, pp. 212–221. https://doi.org/10.1145/2414536.2414574

Herbert, D. L., Barnett, A. G., White, R., Novak, I., & Badawi, N. (2016). Funding for cerebral palsy research in Australia, 2000–2015: An observational study. *BMJ Open, 6*(10), e012924. https://doi.org/10.1136/bmjopen-2016-012924

Hobbs, D., Henschke, M., Wilkinson, B., & Reynolds, K. (2012). *Game on! Accessible gaming for children with disabilities*. Paper presented at the 9th Australian Rehabilitation and Assistive Technology Association (ARATA) National Conference, Sydney, 22–24 August 2012.

Hobbs, D., Russo, R., Hillier, S., & Reynolds, K. (2014). Tactile sensory impairments are common in the hands of children with cerebral palsy – Preliminary results from a cohort study. *Developmental Medicine and Child Neurology, 56*(S2), 20. Paper presented at the 7th Biennial Scientific Conference of the Australasian Academy of Cerebral Palsy and Developmental Medicine (AusACPDM), Hunter Valley, New South Wales, 11–14 March 2014.

Hobbs, D. A., Walker, A. W., Wilkinson, B. H., Hughes, M. B., Wesson, B. R., Hillier, S. L., Russo, R. N., & Reynolds, K. J. (2015) Using a trans-disciplinary and trans-institutional team approach and co-design principles to develop an accessible serious gaming system for children with limited hand function. In K. Christer (Ed.), *Proceedings of the 3rd European Conference on Design4Health*, Sheffield Hallam University, United Kingdom, 13–16 July 2015. https://research.shu.ac.uk/design4health/wp-content/uploads/2015/07/D4H_Hobbs_et_al.pdf

Impact for CP. (2021). *About CP*. https://impact.cerebralpalsy.org.au/about-impact/about-cp/. Accessed 28 Jan 2021.

Li, W., Lam-Damji, S., Chau, T., & Fehlings, D. (2009). The development of a home-based virtual reality therapy system to promote upper extremity movement for children with hemiplegic cerebral palsy. *Technology and Disability, 21*(3), 107–113.

Monfraix, C., Tardieu, G., & Tardieu, C. (1961). Disturbances of manual perception in children with cerebral palsy. *Developmental Medicine and Child Neurology, 3*(6), 544–552. https://doi.org/10.1111/j.1469-8749.1961.tb10419.x

Odding, E., Roebroeck, M. E., & Stam, H. J. (2006). The epidemiology of cerebral palsy: Incidence, impairments and risk factors. *Disability and Rehabilitation, 28*(4), 183–191.

Pearson, E., & Bailey, C. (2007). *Evaluating the potential of the Nintendo Wii to support disabled students in education*. Paper presented at the ASCILITE: Australasian Society for Computers in Learning in Tertiary Education, Nanyang Technological University, Singapore, 2–5 December 2007. https://www.ascilite.org/conferences/singapore07/procs/pearson-poster.pdf

Preston, N., Weightman, A., Gallagher, J., Levesley, M., Mon-Williams, M., Clarke, M., & O'Connor, R. J. (2016). A pilot single-blind multicentre randomized controlled trial to evaluate the potential benefits of computer-assisted arm rehabilitation gaming technology on the arm function of children with spastic cerebral palsy. *Clinical Rehabilitation, 30*(10), 1004–1015. https://doi.org/10.1177/0269215515604699

Reddihough, D. (2011). Cerebral palsy in childhood. *Australian Family Physician, 40*(4), 192–196.

Rosenbaum, P., Paneth, N., Leviton, A., Goldstein, M., & Bax, M. (2007). A report: The definition and classification of cerebral palsy April 2006. *Developmental Medicine and Child Neurology, 49*(s2), 8–14.

Sandlund, M., McDonough, S., & Hager-Ross, C. (2009). Interactive computer play in rehabilitation of children with sensorimotor disorders: A systematic review. *Developmental Medicine and Child Neurology, 51*(3), 173–179. https://doi.org/10.1111/j.1469-8749.2008.03184.x

Sandlund, M., Dock, K., Häger, C. K., & Waterworth, E. L. (2012). Motion interactive video games in home training for children with cerebral palsy: Parents' perceptions. *Disability and Rehabilitation, 34*(11), 925–933. https://doi.org/10.3109/09638288.2011.626489

Sharan, D., Ajeesh, P. S., Rameshkumar, R., Mathankumar, M., Paulina, R. J., & Manjula, M. (2012). Virtual reality based therapy for post operative rehabilitation of children with cerebral palsy. *Work, 41*(Suppl 1), 3612–3615. https://doi.org/10.3233/wor-2012-0667-3612

Staiano, A. E., & Flynn, R. (2014). Therapeutic uses of active videogames: A systematic review. *Games for Health Journal, 3*(6), 351–365. https://doi.org/10.1089/g4h.2013.0100

Story, M. F. (1998). Maximizing usability: The principles of universal design. *Assistive Technology, 10*(1), 4–12.

Sweetser, P., & Wyeth, P. (2005). GameFlow: A model for evaluating player enjoyment in games. *Computers in Entertainment, 3*(3), 1–24.

Tachdjian, M. O., & Minear, W. L. (1958). Sensory disturbances in the hands of children with cerebral palsy. *Journal of Bone and Joint Surgery, 40-A*(1), 85–90.

Tizard, J. P. M., & Crothers, B. (1952). Sensory disturbances in hemiplegia in childhood. *Transactions of the American Neurological Association, 56*, 227–229.

Tizard, J. P. M., Paine, R. S., & Crothers, B. (1954). Disturbances of sensation in children with hemiplegia. *Journal of the American Medical Association, 155*(7), 628–632.

Van Heest, A. E., House, J., & Putnam, M. (1993). Sensibility deficiencies in the hands of children with spastic hemiplegia. *Journal of Hand Surgery. American Volume, 18*(2), 278–281.

Walker, A. W., & Hobbs, D. A. (2014). An industrial design educational project: Dedicated gaming controller providing haptic feedback for children with cerebral palsy. *The International Journal of Designed Objects, 7*(3), 11–21.

Wigfield, M. E. (1966). Cerebral palsy: Altered sensation, astereognosis and sensory perception in relation to vocational training and job performance. *Clinical Orthopaedics and Related Research, 46*, 93–110.

Wilkinson, B. G., & Hobbs, D. A. (2015). *Usability evaluation by typically developing children of a custom game system designed for children with cerebral palsy*. Paper presented at the 12th international conference on applied computing, Maynooth, Greater Dublin, Ireland, 24–26 October 2015.

Wingert, J. R., Burton, H., Sinclair, R. J., Brunstrom, J. E., & Damiano, D. L. (2008). Tactile sensory abilities in cerebral palsy: Deficits in roughness and object discrimination. *Developmental Medicine and Child Neurology, 50*(11), 832–838.

Chapter 9
Designing a General Open Authorable Digital Ecosystem for Educational Games to Support Special Learning Needs

Nikolas Vidakis, Eirini Christinaki, Efthymios Syntychakis, and Georgios Triantafyllidis

Introduction

Increasingly, experts, teachers, parents, and students look to technology as a complimentary support for their educations. Currently, ample researches have been done in serious games that cover matters related to education, therapy for communication, psychomotor treatment, and social behavior enhancement. Michael Zyda (2005) defines a serious game as: "*a mental contest, played with a computer in accordance with specific rules that uses entertainment to further government or corporate training, education, health, public policy, and strategic communication objectives.*" Serious games for education and health can be combined in a series of impairments such as autism or attention and concentration deficits.

Educational gaming is a great platform that helps in motivating students to learn and is designed to teach students about a specific subject and/or skill. Prensky in (2001) argues that children are naturally motivated to play games. Educational games are interactions that teach students goals, rules, adaptation, problem-solving, and interaction, all represented as a narrative. Such games give them the fundamental needs of learning by providing enjoyment, passionate involvement, structure, motivation, ego gratification, adrenaline, creativity, interaction, and emotion. "*Play has a deep biological, evolutionarily, important function, which has to do specifically with learning*" (Prensky, 2001).

N. Vidakis (✉) · E. Christinaki · E. Syntychakis
Department of Informatics Engineering, Technological Educational Institute of Crete, Heraklion, Crete, Greece
e-mail: nv@ie.teicrete.gr; echrist@ics.forth.gr; info@hmu.gr

G. Triantafyllidis
Medialogy Section, AD:MT, Aalborg University, Copenhagen, Denmark
e-mail: gt@create.aau.dk

E. Brooks, D. J. Brown (eds.), *Virtual Reality Games for Rehabilitation*, Virtual Reality Technologies for Health and Clinical Applications,
https://doi.org/10.1007/978-1-0716-3371-7_9

In general, computer games and other digital technologies such as mobile phones and the Internet seem to stimulate playful goals and to facilitate the construction of playful identities. This transformation advances the ludification of today's culture in the spirit of Johan Huizinga's *Homo Ludens* (Huizinga, 1955). In this context, this ludification of today's culture can be also used in educational activities to strengthen the motivation and the engagement of the students as well as in rehabilitation to maintain patient motivation and interest.

Moreover, the narrative of an educational game plays an important role in its success. The story is the root of the whole gaming experience. Up to now, educational games are usually created with a closed architecture and a single narrative, resulting to fail in providing a more personalized or customized learning procedure.

In this chapter, we introduce the IOLAOS framework for serious games (Vidakis et al., 2014) that can be applied in a wide range of cases (from no conditions to severe) and ages (from toddlers to elderly people). IOLAOS aims to combine ludology and narratology improvements to provide efficient educational and therapy gaming for all.

Regarding the game narrative, IOLAOS suggests a fully authorable editor (implemented using the *Unity* game engine (2014)), with which experts can create templates and carers can shape and customize the template-based games according to specific needs for a more personalized education or rehabilitation. It is important that such customizations can be performed easily and without the reliance on software developers. The editor is also open. This means that new templates can be added easily for creating new games serving new educational or rehabilitation goals.

Regarding the ludic approach, IOLAOS features the use of a natural user interface (NUI). NUI is a human-computer interface that allows humans to communicate with the computer using standard modes of human communication, such as speech or gestures, and to manipulate virtual objects in a fashion similar to the way humans manipulate physical objects. During the last few years, technology has been improved rapidly and allowed the creation of efficient and low-cost applications featuring these interfaces.

One of the characteristics of a successful NUI is thus the reduction of cognitive load on people interacting with it. This is an important feature that makes it a suitable interface in developing, for example, successful learning applications for children. In our design, a NUI (instead of a restricted human-computer interface) is used to enhance playfulness and thus establish a ludic interface. NUI features and focuses also on the kinesthetic factor (gestures, movements, etc.), which is an important element in achieving this playfulness of a ludic interface. For example, it is much more "fun" in a game to drive a car with your hands naturally, compared to pressing some keyboard keys. And this is even more important and critical when the target group is children.

Besides the NUI-based interface, ludic design for the game has been also employed in order to improve playfulness, maintain patient motivation and interest, make the educational games more attractive for the children, and aim to improve the learning and rehabilitation procedure.

Briefly, the IOLAOS project:

- Introduces an open authorable narrative editor for creating templates and customizing educational and rehabilitation (healthcare) games, without the reliance on software developers
- Employs a twofold ludic approach for both the interface (NUI) and the game design
- Aims to a creation of more personalized games that support the educational and rehabilitation activities better

As a proof of concept for the IOLAOS project, a work scenario is presented in this chapter, for creating an educational game for teaching preschoolers with autism spectrum conditions (ASC) to improve their skills in recognizing facial expressions (Christinaki et al., 2014). Facial expressions give important clues about emotions and provide a key mechanism for understanding, identifying, and conveying them. Children with ASC often fail to recognize the qualitative differences and associations between various expressions of emotions (Hobson, 1986). Due to limited social and emotional understanding, they do not know how to adequately interact with other people – a problem which sometimes leads to inappropriate behaviors. Studies have reported that individuals with ASC experience difficulties in recognizing expressions while in youth and experience problems recognizing emotions as adults (Rump et al., 2009).

Treatment approaches and rehabilitation aim to improve social interaction, conquest communication, and control inappropriate behavior. Children with ASC are more likely to initiate positive interaction after treatment (Bauminger, 2002). Education is also considered as a solution for the socio-emotional deficits, and training is claimed to improve face processing abilities and strategies in autism (Faja et al., 2007). A variety of educational interventions have been proposed for children with autism, and many proponents have claimed developmental improvement and other benefits (Eikeseth, 2009).

In this context, this chapter also presents how IOLAOS platform can be used in order to create an educational game featuring playfulness both in playing (NUI) and in designing the game, along with a customized narrative of the game, which can be edited according to the needs. Our aim is twofold: (a) to teach facial emotion recognition to preschoolers with ASC and (b) to enhance their social interaction.

The rest of the chapter is organized as follows: In section "Background", a brief presentation of similar existing work in creating educational games is presented. Section "The IOLAOS platform" focuses on the proposed open architecture of the IOLAOS project. To illustrate the concepts of the proposed architecture, section "Representative scenario" presents the scenario for teaching preschoolers with ASC about expression recognition and how is this possible by using the IOLAOS framework. Finally, section "Conclusion and future work" describes conclusions and discusses future work.

Background

Educational games for children have been widely used in supporting learning inside and out of school, and as a result a growing interest has appeared for the potential of digital games to deliver effective and engaging learning experiences (Hwang & Wu, 2012). There is a variety of computer games and software that intend to assist users to achieve various educational goals. A well-known educational software is the project Scratch from MIT Media Lab (Resnick et al., 2009), a programming language for learning to code. With Scratch users can program their own interactive stories, games, and animations by putting together images, music, and sounds with programming command blocks. Monterrat et al. (2012) in their study claimed that game modding as an educational activity could be interesting not only to learn programming but for any kind of learning. Their pedagogical tool allows people without game design skills to modify and share digital games. It allows a learner to become a teacher by designing an educational game that others can use to learn. Their main idea is that if learning a game helps students to acquire knowledge, then being able to change the game can provide students with the ability to deeply learn the content.

Narrative architecture and ludic design are two major approaches in contemporary video game theory. They both play important roles in teaching and learning as parts of educational gaming. Lester et al. (2013) described the design issues and the empirical findings about motivation in narrative-centered learning environments. They found a strong connection between narrative and educational games, and they claimed that a narrative-centered learning environment is a promising approach for fostering positive learning gains, as well as for promoting student motivation. On the other hand, Padilla-Zea et al. (2014) included digital storytelling in an educational video game and introduced narrative elements to foster the students' motivation in learning processes by integrating specific educational models and ludic aspects. They claimed that ludic tasks in educational games are important elements to maintain students' interest, motivation, and immersion.

During the last decade, researchers have begun to explore the use of computer technologies dedicated to ASC as intervention tools for improving and eliminating different deficits. In a recent review, Wainer and Ingersoll (2011) examined innovation computer programs as educational interventions for people with ASC. They focused on studies describing programs to teach language, emotions, or social skills. Their analysis showed that those tools are promising strategies for delivering direct intervention to individuals with ASC. Bernardini et al. (2014) proposed a serious game for children with ASC to practice social communication skills; they used an intelligent virtual character that acts both as a peer and as a tutor on a number of different learning activities. These activities can be selected manually by a human operator (practitioner, parent, or other carer) through a graphical interface. Their experimental results showed encouraging tendencies by relating the effectiveness of the children's interaction with the virtual character acting as a social partner to them. Porayska-Pomsta et al. (2013) suggest an intelligent and authorable environment to assist children with ASC in gaining social interaction skills. Their tool contains an intelligent agent and a play environment that allows teachers and parents to become cocreators and tailor the game according to the needs of the individual children in their care. Although the design and creation of personalized games is crucial for children with ASC, as reported by the authors, limitations in the agent's intelligence (agent inability to deal with inappropriate or unexpected behavior from the user) contradict the structured, stable, and predictable learning environment that is also crucial. The importance of active family participation in interventions and their collaboration in the research process has also been examined. Wright et al. (2011) conducted a qualitative study to consider a tool to facilitate intergenerational family relationships. Their study examined social engagement among families with a child with ASC and the vital importance of the families in technology-based programs that promote social engagement and self-esteem for children with high-functioning autism. Their findings support technology as a tool to facilitate family and social engagement in children with ASC. Current studies have also gone considerably beyond the simple use of computers. Diverse technology-based interventions have been employed for empowerment and skill acquisition. Recent reviews (Ramdoss et al., 2011; Grynszpan et al., 2014) have shown that there is a growing number of interventions and report a variety of technologies such as interactive DVDs and virtual reality programs (Parsons & Cobb, 2011).

Ludology and narratology can also be considered as two important elements when creating educational games for children with ASC. Game narrative can provide context that assists children to apply the skills learned within the game. Ludology in both the interface and the game design also can engage children with autism in playful interactions and strengthen their motivation. Foster et al. (2010) have suggested embedding interactive narrative in multimodal learning environments for social skill improvement of children with ASC. Castelhano et al. (2013) studied therapeutic activities for children with developmental disabilities with the use of multisensory stimulation environments and documented its perception concerning ludic content and play and the computer-mediated ludic activity. The main theme that emerged from their study regarding playfulness was that the computer-mediated ludic experience is perceived as useful for intervention.

In general, educational computer games for children that combine ludology and narratology can provide an effective and engaging learning experience. Hence, developing learning environments that are both storytelling and play-based by combining narrative and ludicity may empower children to achieve great impact, improve deficits, and gain new skills.

The IOLAOS Platform

The initial design of IOLAOS platform focuses on setting up the operational model for carrying out the codification of educational theories and learning styles as well as the generation of ludic, narrative, and educational games according to the needs, abilities, and educational goals. This design exhibits several novel characteristics, which differentiate an IOLAOS-based game from other forms of educational computer games and platforms. First of all, IOLAOS is not only concerned with educational computer games, but instead, it seeks to provide a guided learning environment for both educators and children, that is, storytelling and play-based, by combining narrative and ludic for harnessing knowledge. Consequently, its primary focus is to enable educators and children with the use of ludology and narratology to perform learning tasks and provide an effective and engaging learning experience. To achieve this, IOLAOS builds on a range of technologies, including semantic web, game engines, and advanced human-computer interaction. Secondly, IOLAOS adopts a knowledge-based, reuse-oriented, and natural user interaction model to attain high quality during the performance of learning tasks.

The Architecture

The proposed architecture has been designed in order to support a game platform that fulfills the requirements of customized narratives, ludic interfaces, and ludic game designing. The narrative is created by the expert and edited by the teacher according to the learning needs and goals by using the template codification and template customization modules of the suggested architecture. The ludology is supported in two ways: first, by creating and customizing ludic-based designed games through the template codification and game compilation components and, second, by employing natural user interfaces to the playing process that enhance the playfulness of the game.

The system architecture (Fig. 9.1) consists of four distinct components that collaborate together to (a) codify all different elements of educational theories and learning styles available and to create templates which are then offered to game developers; (b) compile games through a three-step process, namely, *template customization*, *game creation*, and *utilization definition*; (c) manage learning session and play room attributes; and (d) administer all necessary elements, users and their roles, game engine parameters, etc. Peripheral to the system architecture is knowledge derived from educational theories, learning styles, and classroom practices. The components of our architecture are the *Template Codifier*, the *Game Compiler*, the *Play Room*, and the *System Administration*. The following paragraphs describe in more detail the abovementioned architectural components.

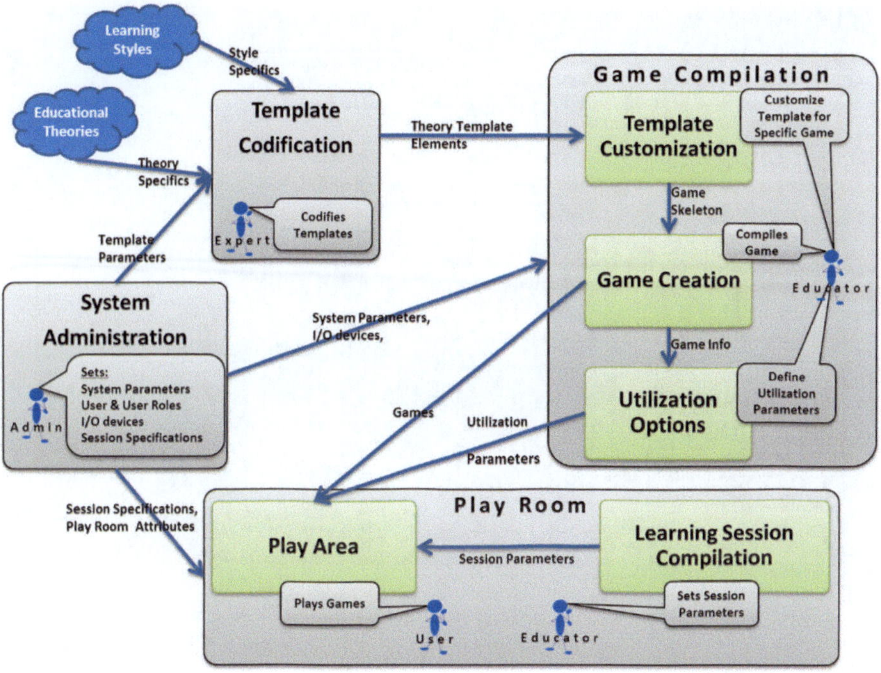

Fig. 9.1 System architecture

System Administration Component

The *System Administration* component (Figs. 9.1 and 9.2) of the system is responsible for managing system attributes, template parameters, game elements, artifacts and behaviors, session attributes, input/output modalities, and user accounts and roles.

The Template Codification Component

The *Template Codifier* component (Figs. 9.1 and 9.3) of the system is accountable for systemizing/codifying the various elements of the educational theories and learning styles. This is achieved by imprinting the theory's elements using a tabbed stepwise process by the expert. Apart from the first steps that imprint basic information about the theories, the process has no strict order of step execution. The template codification process that has been developed in IOLAOS in different tabs (Fig. 9.3) gives the user the capability to define the theory's elements in an organized and clear manner. The imprinting of the educational theories and learning styles is performed by the role "Expert." The different groups of data that have been developed in IOLAOS for imprinting the theory's elements are as follows: "Template Basic Info," "Style Basic Info," "Target Group," "Scenery Basics," "Audio/Motion," "Play Environment," "Rewarding," "Feedback," and "Evaluation" (Fig. 9.3).

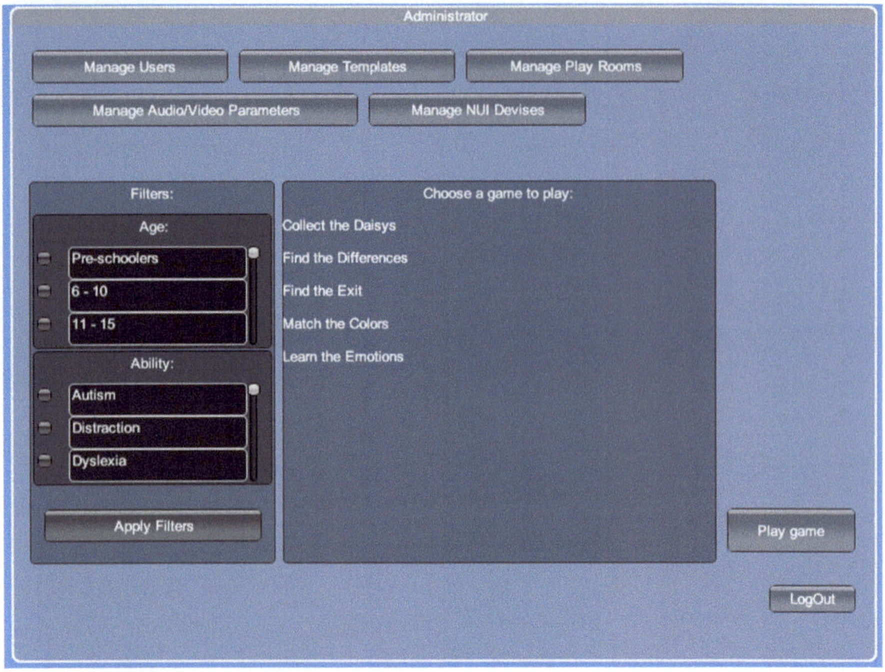

Fig. 9.2 IOLAOS administrator main screens

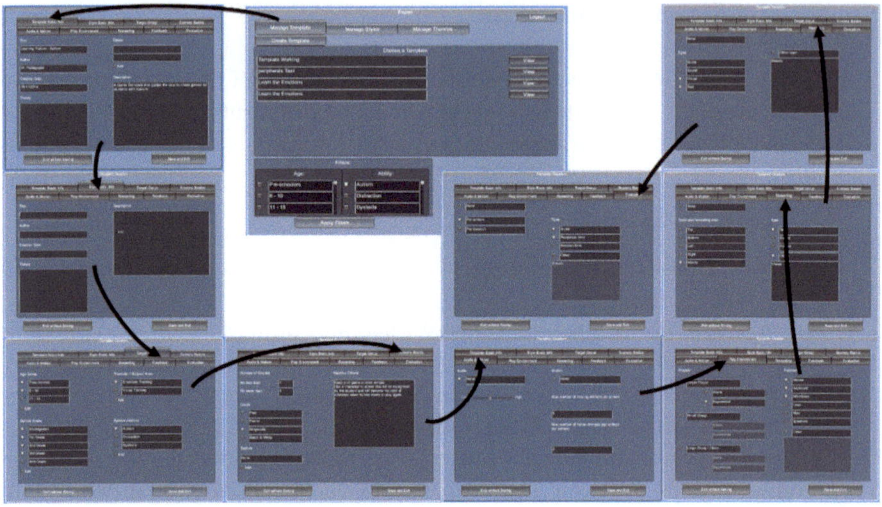

Fig. 9.3 The IOLAOS template codification and customization

In more detail, the theory's imprinting elements elucidate in:

- *Template Basic Info* records general data such as Title, Description, Theory based upon, Template Author, Creation Date, etc.
- *Style Basic Info* records data concerning the learning style such as Title, Description, Theory based upon, Template Author, Creation Date, etc.
- *Target Group* records data concerning player details, abilities, and thematic areas such as Age Group, School Grades, Thematic/Subject Area, Special Abilities, etc.
- *Scenery Basics* deals with data concerning the storytelling that is involved in the game. Such data includes Number of Scenes, Color Information, Texture, Motion, Narrative Criteria, etc.
- *Audio/Motion* records data concerning the use of sound and image input/output modalities such as Audio (yes, no, scalable), Motion (yes, no, number and frequency of moving artifacts), etc.
- *Play Environment* documents data with reference to the type of game (i.e., single player, small group, etc.), the environment played (i.e., supervised or not supervised), and the peripherals used (i.e., classic I/O devises, NUI devices, etc.).
- *Rewarding* deals with data concerning the rewarding of the player such as type of rewarding (i.e., textual, sound, movie, puzzle, etc.).
- *Feedback* records all necessary information about feedback before, during, and after the game flow (i.e., text, sound, movie, score, etc.).
- *Evaluation* deals with data concerning the evaluation of the player (i.e., evaluate per level or per game or per game section, etc.) as well as the evaluation type.

The Game Compilation Component

The *Game Compiler* component (Fig. 9.1) of the system consists of the *Template Customization*, the *Game Creation*, and the *Utilization Options*. It is responsible for providing the "Educator" with the necessary tools to set up a ludic educational game. In other words, it gives the "Educator" the possibility to (a) customize the generic template set up by the "Expert" at the *Template Codification* component in such a way that suits the specific game requirements (Fig. 9.3) needed according to the target user group abilities and goals to be achieved, (b) create a ludic game with the use of the tools provided by the IOLAOS platform, and (c) to define game utilization parameters such as Free Use, Registered User Only, etc.

In more detail, at the "Template Customization" step of the "Game Compilation" component of the architecture, the user chooses a predefined abstract educational template that suits its game criteria and proceeds to tailor this abstract template to the specific necessities of its current game. Figure 9.4 shows the IOLAOS platform elements that enable the user to tailor the abstract educational template discussed above. Elaborating at the first screen of Fig. 9.4, the user chooses game creation which triggers a series of actions before the actual game construction (Fig. 9.5). Initially, the user chooses the predefined abstract educational template (top right screen, Fig. 9.4) and then tailors the template (bottom screen, Fig. 9.4) to suit the

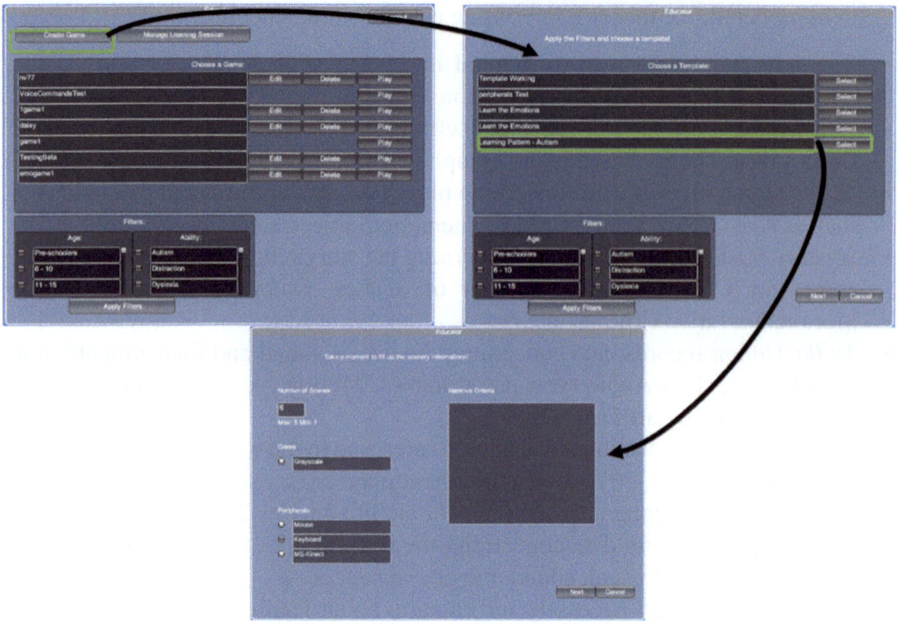

Fig. 9.4 The IOLAOS Template Customization

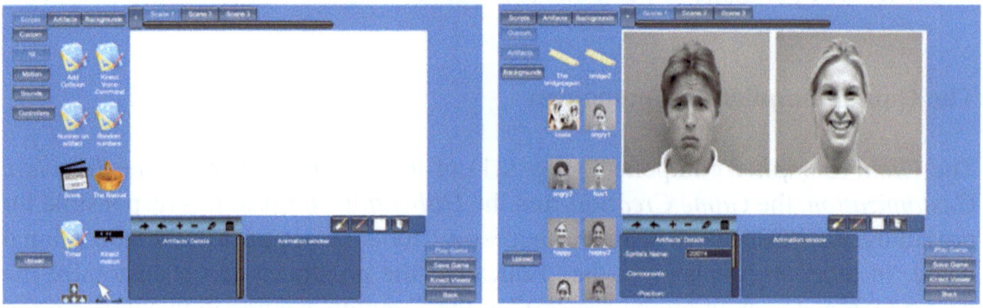

Fig. 9.5 The IOLAOS Game Creation. The face stimuli used and presented are from the CAlifornia Facial Expressions (CAFE) dataset. (Dailey et al., 2001)

specifics of its game within the educational boundaries that the chosen abstract template stipulates.

Once the abstract template has been customized, the user proceeds to construct the actual game with the use of the game creation editor provided by the IOLAOS platform. The game editor provides the user with a number of tool sets that allow a ludic, stepwise, effortless, straightforward, and uncomplicated game creation. This assemblage of tool sets includes the following: (a) a game object tank with predefined game objects, scripts, and backgrounds as well as facilities for custom object creation; (b) game scene management facility with scene navigation, addition, and deletion; (c) game canvas management with gridding, sizing, locating

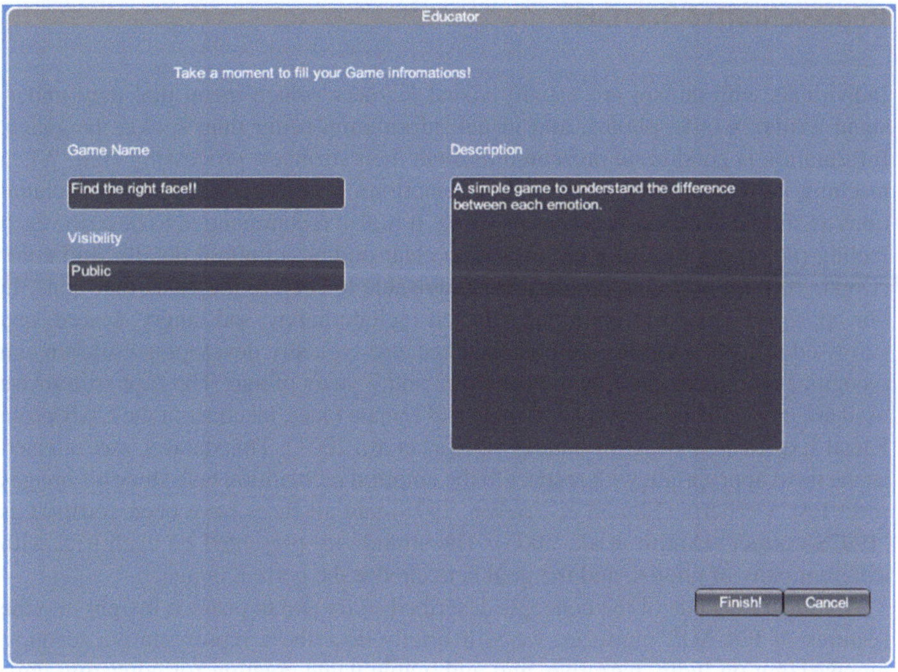

Fig. 9.6 The IOLAOS Utilization Options

options, etc.; and (d) game construction previewing facilities (see left screen of Fig. 9.5).

Upon completion of the game construction, the user proceeds at the final step of the "Game Compilation" component, namely, the "Utilization Options" (Fig. 9.6). At this step utilization options such as game visibility (public or private), target game players, etc. are defined.

The Play Room Component

The *Play Room* component (Fig. 9.1) is responsible for setting up the appropriate space for playing games and consists of "Learning Session Compilation" and "Play Area."

The *Learning Session Compilation* provides the "Educator" the ability to fully manage learning sessions according to individual, group, or class requirements every time she/he needs to run an educational game. In particular the "Educator" can determine (a) Players and/or Group, (b) Marking/Evaluation Specifics/ Procedure, (c) Session Statistics, and (d) Session parameters. She/he can also save incomplete learning sessions in order to be completed in the future.

The *Play Area* deals with the game runtime specifics such as save, load, single player or multiplayer parameters, etc.

Representative Scenario

Individuals with autism are usually visual learners, which mean that they understand written words, photos, and visual information better than spoken language. Information is good to be presented through their strongest processing area. When teaching individuals with autism about emotions, it is important to keep explanations as simple and as concrete as possible. It is also recommended to describe each feeling pictorially by using pictures with clear outline, minimal details, and color (Dodd, 2005). For young children it is advisable to keep to the basic emotions. In our approach, the basic emotions selected include happy, sad, angry, scared, and surprised. Those emotions were chosen because typically developing children can recognize and understand them between 2 and 7 years of age. The face stimuli we used are grayscale photographs of male and female faces, taken from the CAlifornia Facial Expressions (CAFE) dataset (Dailey et al., 2001). This dataset was selected as the most appropriate with respect to the emotion recognition task since all images meet FACS criteria (Ekman & Friesen, 1978) and all faces have been certified as "FACS-correct" (Smith et al., 2005). The stimuli are presented on each trial with different pairs of photos, and the goal is to choose the correct image.

To illustrate some of the concepts described so far and to provide insight into the features of IOLAOS platform, we will briefly describe a representative scenario emphasizing on ludic, narrative, and authorable game creation for educating children with autism diagnosis. Our reference scenario is summarized in Exhibit 9.1. For more details see (Christinaki et al., 2013).

Exhibit 9.1

The game begins with an instruction page where the child is informed what is going to happen, what she/he has to do, and how she/he can do it. A two-hand gesture which is performed by moving both hands above the head is required to start the game. In the first level, children should learn labeling emotions by correlating emotion terms with images. The stimuli are presented on each trial with different pair of photos, and the goal is to choose the correct image among the two. Selecting the left image (the orientation of the image is decided by looking toward the screen) requires a one-hand gesture which is performed by moving the left hand above the head. Selecting the right image (the orientation again of the image is decided by looking toward the screen) requires a one-hand gesture which is performed by moving the right hand above the head. Upon correct answer the "$\surd$" symbol appears on top of the image, while upon incorrect answer, the "x" symbol appears on top of the image. Moving to the next play area requires a two-hand gesture, which is performed by moving both hands above the head. In the second level they should learn to recognize emotions from their description and their association with facial features. In the third level they should learn to identify the causes of various feelings in different situations, obtained through the use of social stories. At the end of the game, there is a congratulations message.

Play Game

At the previous section we have described the "Game Compilation" process based on our representative scenario. This section elaborates on playing the game by children with autism diagnosis in their school settings and in supervision by a kindergarten teacher. Detailed results and findings about our survey on preschoolers with ASD which are analyzed into emotional state versus game performance, emotional state versus surroundings, concentration and game performance, and NUI device and game acknowledgement can be found at (Christinaki et al., 2014).

The game environment is kept simple in order to avoid children's distraction. Individuals with autism are reported to have enhanced perception of details (Ashwin et al., 2009) which may cause distraction. For these reasons the selected educational template denotes the use of black context presented on a white background and grayscale stimuli. Black and white contrast may also help to increase and retain child's attention and keep them focused on the screen.

The game begins with an instruction page (Fig. 9.9, top left scene) where the child is informed what is going to happen, what she/he has to do, and how she/he can do it. Apart from the text on the screen, audio instructions are also provided. Audio cues are important as the information presented is clear and age-appropriate. When the child feels ready, she/he can choose to start the game. The game provides a structure learning environment which consists of three different levels with increasing difficulty (Fig. 9.9, scenes labeled "SADNESS," "ANGER," "HAPPINESS"). Breaking the teaching intervention into small learning steps makes the task easier to perform. In the first level (Fig. 9.10, scene labeled "SADNESS"), children should learn labeling emotions by correlating emotion terms with images. In the second level (Fig. 9.10, scene labeled "ANGER"), they should learn to recognize emotions from their description and their association with facial features. In the third level (Fig. 9.10, scene labeled "HAPPINESS"), they should learn to identify the causes of various feelings in different situations, obtained through the use of social stories. Those three levels provide recognition, matching, observation, understanding, and generalization of facial emotions.

Computer-based interventions that use a keyboard or a mouse for interaction might cause problem with the younger children which may not be able to use a computer. Our gesture-based interaction approach moves the control of computer from a mouse and keyboard to the motions of the body via new input devices.

Our game is designed to use non-touch-based NUI and to be controlled by hand gestures. The gestures are translated into control commands. The player has three possible actions in all game states, to choose left or right image and move to the next play area. These basic actions are implemented with efficient and easy-to-use gestures. Moving to the next play area requires a two-hand gesture which is performed by moving both hands above the head. Selecting the left image requires a one-hand gesture which is performed by moving the left hand above the head. Respectively, selecting the right image requires a one-hand gesture which is performed by moving the right hand above the head.

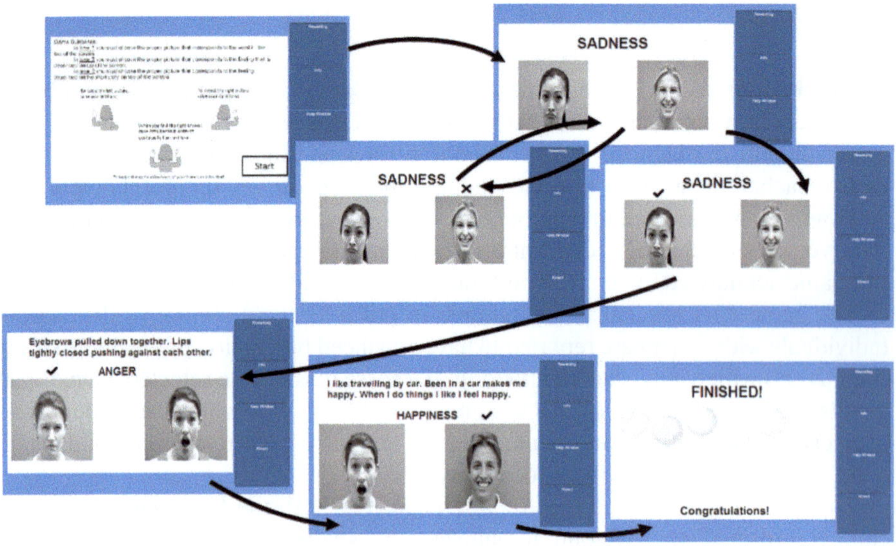

Fig. 9.10 Representative scenario (Christinaki et al., 2013). The face stimuli used and presented are from the CAlifornia Facial Expressions (CAFE) dataset. (Dailey et al., 2001)

During the game, if the player selects the correct or incorrect stimuli, the system will inform the player that she/he gave the correct or incorrect answer. Each answer provides an audio and a visual feedback such as operation-related sounds and appropriate marks above the selected image ("√" for correct answer and "x" for wrong answer). A voice telling "Bravo" rewards the player for the correct answer, and a voice telling "Try again" encourages the player to try again when the user provides an incorrect answer. There are no other sound effects because individuals with ASD may suffer from auditory sensitivity (Gomes et al., 2008), may demonstrate oversensitivity to certain sounds even at low volume, and may feel discomfort when exposed to certain sounds (Tan et al., 2012).

Conclusion and Future Work

In this chapter we have attempted to sketch the organizational underpinnings of the IOLAOS – a pilot effort aiming to build an open authorable framework for educational games for children by combining ludology and narratology. Our primary design target is to set up an operational model for carrying out the codification of educational theories and learning styles as well as the generation of ludic, narrative, and educational games according to the needs, abilities, and educational goals and to support this model with appropriate software platform and tools.

Ongoing work covers a variety of issues of both technological and educational engineering character. Some of the issues to be addressed in the immediate future include the following: (a) elaborate on the learning session compiler, (b) further explore learning styles and educational theories in collaboration with expert and educator professional associations, (c) run various use cases in vivo with the guidance and involvement of expert and educator professional associations, (d) enhance ludology aiming not only to children experience but also to experts and teachers, and (e) introduce further involvement of multimodal NUI devices so that the roles between game player and machine are reversed and the player performs gestures, sounds, grimaces, etc. and the machine responds. Moreover, IOLAOS could also offer valuable contribution to develop effective games for rehabilitation. Based on the work scenario presented in this chapter, we have demonstrated the feasibility of using this platform to create serious games that combine education and health. Therefore, this operational model must be further studied.

References

Ashwin, E., Ashwin, C., Rhydderch, D., Howells, J., & Baron-Cohen, S. (2009). Eagle-eyed visual acuity: An experimental investigation of enhanced perception in autism. *Biological Psychiatry, 65*(1), 17–21.

Bauminger, N. (2002). The facilitation of social-emotional understanding and social interaction in high-functioning children with autism: Intervention outcomes. *Journal of Autism and Developmental Disorders, 32*(4), 283–298.

Bernardini, S., Porayska-Pomsta, K., & Smith, T. J. (2014). ECHOES: An intelligent serious game for fostering social communication in children with autism. *Information Sciences, 264*, 41–60.

Castelhano, N., Silva, F., Rezende, M., Roque, L., & Magalhães, L. (2013). Ludic content in multisensory stimulation environments: An exploratory study about practice in Portugal. *Occupational Therapy International, 20*(3), 134–143.

Christinaki, E., Vidakis, N., & Triantafyllidis, G. (2013, September). Facial expression recognition teaching to preschoolers with autism: A natural user interface approach. In *Proceedings of the 6th Balkan conference in informatics* (pp. 141–148). ACM.

Christinaki, E., Vidakis, N., & Triantafyllidis, G. (2014). A novel educational game for teaching emotion identification skills to preschoolers with autism diagnosis. *Computer Science and Information Systems, 11*(2), 723–743.

Dailey, M. N., Cottrell, G. W., & Reilly, J. (2001). *CAlifornia Facial Expressions (CAFE)*. [Online]. Available http://www.cs.ucsd.edu/users/gary/CAFE/

Dodd, S. (2005). *Understanding autism*. Elsevier Australia.

Eikeseth, S. (2009). Outcome of comprehensive psycho-educational interventions for young children with autism. *Research in Developmental Disabilities, 30*(1), 158–178.

Ekman, P., & Friesen, W. V. (1978). *Facial action coding system*. Consulting Psychologists' Press.

Faja, S., Aylward, E., Bernier, R., & Dawson, G. (2007). Becoming a face expert: A computerized face-training program for high-functioning individuals with autism spectrum disorders. *Developmental Neuropsychology, 33*(1), 1–24.

Foster, M. E., Avramides, K., Bernardini, S., Chen, J., Frauenberger, C., Lemon, O., & Porayska-Pomsta, K. (2010, October). Supporting children's social communication skills through interactive narratives with virtual characters. In *Proceedings of the international conference on multimedia* (pp. 1111–1114). ACM.

Gomes, E., Pedroso, F. S., & Wagner, M. B. (2008). Auditory hypersensitivity in the autistic spectrum disorder. *Pró-Fono Revista de Atualização Científica, 20*(4), 279–284.

Grynszpan, O., Weiss, P. L. T., Perez-Diaz, F., & Gal, E. (2014). Innovative technology-based interventions for autism spectrum disorders: A meta-analysis. *Autism, 18*(4), 346–361.
Hobson, R. P. (1986). The autistic child's appraisal of expressions of emotion. *Journal of Child Psychology and Psychiatry, 27*(3), 321–342.
Huizinga, J. (1955). *Homo ludens. A study of the play element in culture*. Beacon.
Hwang, G. J., & Wu, P. H. (2012). Advancements and trends in digital game-based learning research: A review of publications in selected journals from 2001 to 2010. *British Journal of Educational Technology, 43*(1), E6–E10.
Lester, J. C., Rowe, J. P., & Mott, B. W. (2013). Narrative-centered learning environments: A story-centric approach to educational games. In *Emerging technologies for the classroom* (pp. 223–237). Springer.
Monterrat, B., Lavoué, E., & George, S. (2012, October). Learning game 2.0: Support for game Modding as a learning activity. In *Proceedings of the 6th European conference on games based learning* (pp. 340–347).
Padilla-Zea, N., Gutiérrez, F. L., López-Arcos, J. R., Abad-Arranz, A., & Paderewski, P. (2014). Modeling storytelling to be used in educational video games. *Computers in Human Behavior, 31*, 461–474.
Parsons, S., & Cobb, S. (2011). State-of-the-art of virtual reality technologies for children on the autism spectrum. *European Journal of Special Needs Education, 26*(3), 355–366.
Porayska-Pomsta, K., et al. (2013). Building an intelligent, authorable serious game for autistic children and their carers. In *Advances in computer entertainment* (pp. 456–475). Springer.
Prensky, M. (2001). Fun, play and games: What makes games engaging. *Digital Game-Based Learning, 5*, 1–05.
Ramdoss, S., et al. (2011). Use of computer-based interventions to teach communication skills to children with autism spectrum disorders: A systematic review. *Journal of Behavioral Education, 20*(1), 55–76.
Resnick, M., et al. (2009). Scratch: Programming for all. *Communications of the ACM, 52*(11), 60–67.
Rump, K. M., Giovannelli, J. L., Minshew, N. J., & Strauss, M. S. (2009). The development of emotion recognition in individuals with autism. *Child Development, 80*(5), 1434–1447.
Smith, M. L., Cottrell, G. W., Gosselin, F., & Schyns, P. G. (2005). Transmitting and decoding facial expressions. *Psychological Science, 16*(3), 184–189.
Tan, Y. H., Xi, C. Y., Jiang, S. P., Shi, B. X., Wang, L. B., & Wang, L. (2012). Auditory abnormalities in children with autism. *Open Journal of Psychiatry, 2*(1), 33–37.
Unity Game Engine. *Unity Game Engine – Official Site*. [Online] http://unity3d.com. (Cited: February 5, 2014).
Vidakis, N., Christinaki, E., Serafimidis, I., & Triantafyllidis, G. (2014). Combining ludology and narratology in an open authorable framework for educational games for children: The scenario of teaching preschoolers with autism diagnosis. In *Universal access in human-computer interaction. Universal access to information and knowledge* (pp. 626–636). Springer.
Wainer, A. L., & Ingersoll, B. R. (2011). The use of innovative computer technology for teaching social communication to individuals with autism spectrum disorders. *Research in Autism Spectrum Disorders, 5*(1), 96–107.
Wright, C., et al. (2011). SketchUp™: A technology tool to facilitate intergenerational family relationships for children with autism spectrum disorders (ASD). *Family and Consumer Sciences Research Journal, 40*(2), 135–149.
Zyda, M. (2005). From visual simulation to virtual reality to games. *Computer, 38*(9), 25–32.

Chapter 10
How Does the Alteration of an Avatar's Proportions Affect Experience and Performance When Controlling It?

Mark Palmer, Sophie Pink, and James Smith

Introduction

Videogames have traditionally been played through the use of game controllers manipulated using movements of the hands and fingers, such as joysticks, keyboards and mice or game pads. Up until 2010 a series of alternative control mechanisms for various games consoles were developed (Microsoft's Kinect™, Sony's EyeToy™ and Move™ and Nintendo's Wii™) which have moved the field towards motion sensing input devices, transforming the body into a 'natural user interface'. Other sensors have been introduced with consumer VR headsets, but these have largely reproduced the tracking capacity found in devices such as the Wii™ remote and Move™. The pursuit of an embodied approach to virtual worlds can be traced back to Ivan Sutherland's notion of 'The Ultimate Display' (Sutherland, 1965):

> The ultimate display would, of course, be a room within which the computer can control the existence of matter. A chair displayed in such a room would be good enough to sit in. Handcuffs displayed in such a room would be confining, and a bullet displayed in such a room would be fatal.

This is because our experience of the physical world has formed our expectations of how we might interact with it. In this way the invisibility of a 'natural user interface' is in a large part because the virtual accommodates these expectations. Whilst our design of objects and interactions in the physical world has slowly adapted to varying needs, the introduction of natural user interfaces requires virtual worlds to adapt

M. Palmer (✉) · J. Smith
Department of Computer Science and Creative Technologies, University of the West of England, Bristol, UK
e-mail: Mark.Palmer@uwe.ac.uk; James.smith@uwe.ac.uk

S. Pink
IBM Client Innovation Centre, Hampshire, UK
e-mail: Sophie.pink-cic-uk@ibm.com

E. Brooks, D. J. Brown (eds.), *Virtual Reality Games for Rehabilitation*, Virtual Reality Technologies for Health and Clinical Applications,
https://doi.org/10.1007/978-1-0716-3371-7_10

too. In the move towards natural interfaces, we need to consider the ways in which the body informs our sense of self and our interactions with the world.

In examining the importance of the body in forming our cognition of the world, Gallagher states that:

> If the self is anything [...] it is nonetheless and first of all this, an embodied self. (Gallagher, 2005, p. 3)

He argues that we generally have a body image which is strongly tied to the physical self. However, the body image is itself made up from the 'body percept' and the 'body schema'. As we experience growth from infant to adult, the continuous alteration of the size and shape of our body requires us to adapt to this constant growth, and as a result, he asserts that the *body percept* and *body schema* are fluid mechanisms.

What defines the 'body image' has long been a point for discussion. Sir Henry Head (1920) first coined the term for the aspect of 'body image' most related to movement the body schema and described it as a model within the brain which organises and alters 'the impressions produced by incoming sensory impulses in such a way that the final sensation of position, or of locality, rises into consciousness charged with a relation to something that has happened before'. This description is taken further in Gallagher's work (and subsequent investigations into the psychology of movement) to be a pre-noetic filter through which body actions are performed. The body percept, meanwhile, can be considered as the mental image that is actively formed within the mind when one considers one's own 'owned' body.

The fluidity of the body percept has been demonstrated through experiments which show that the body percept is malleable even when the body is at rest, for example, with the rubber hand illusion (Botvinick & Cohen, 1998). Further studies have also shown that it is possible to achieve the illusion of 'ownership' of a different body, even from the third-person perspective, provided that the participant is given a plausible viewpoint from which to see the fake body as 'themselves' (Petkova et al., 2011).

Building upon this work, it has been shown that participants can also experience changes to their body, as has been shown through the perceived elongation of their arm. This was achieved using head-mounted displays (HMDs) and the manipulation of third-person viewpoints of participants (Preston & Newport, 2012). Likewise, other medically recognised conditions offer insights into the roles of different senses in the construction of the body schema and body percept. Sight seems to play a key role in constructing the body percept (Petkova et al., 2012) as those individuals born with congenital blindness do not experience a modified rubber hand illusion (in which sight is not used), whilst non-blind individuals do. Likewise, a patient that lost her somatosensory signals (Farrer et al., 2003) needed to close her eyes to perform a simple manipulation task when her hand was not visible. This may be symptomatic of overreliance on vision for performing manipulation tasks after the loss of somatosensory signals. That is, the visual sense was overwhelming all other senses and she needed to cut off this input to concentrate on less intense senses.

Whilst the rubber hand illusion (RHI) has demonstrated plasticity of the body image, it has also been shown that this may be a far more everyday and necessary feature of experience at the level of the body schema than we might at first imagine. This is because it has been demonstrated that tools can become incorporated into peripersonal space and the body schema (Berti & Frassinetti, 2000). In sport, this can been seen in the ways in which a racquet or sword can become an 'extension' of the forearm and the ways that players deal with the surrounding space, but this can also be seen in other limbs such as the way sprung stilts become an extension of the legs.

Given the implications of the RHI and tool use, in this chapter we will examine the consequences of each prior to considering the design of the tests conducted. We will then consider the results of these tests and reflect on these prior to considering their consequences in terms of the design of avatars for natural interfaces.

The Rubber Hand Illusion

The RHI was an experiment performed by Botvinick and Cohen (1998) which demonstrated that it was possible for the human mind to believe that an inanimate, foreign object was actually that person's real hand. Since then virtual 'mediated' environments have also provided adequate feedback for this experience to occur within virtual reality (IJsselsteijn et al., 2006; IJsselsteijn & Haans, 2008), and such environments have been described as 'a powerful and versatile tool we can use to teach us something fundamental about the structure of perception and the workings of the brain' (Ibid, p. 5).

Botvinick and Cohen's original report was entitled 'Rubber hands 'feel' touch that eyes see' and it is interesting how further studies have emphasised the importance of sight in the creation of the illusion; indeed Tsakiris and Haggard at one point asserted that visual and tactile data is a *necessary* condition for the RHI (2005). In contrast Ehrsson et al. (2005) felt it was *...clearly important to find out whether an illusory feeling of ownership can be induced in the absence of visual input...* This was investigated by blindfolding participants, and instead of brushing the hand, they moved the subject's own hand to touch the rubber hand whilst simultaneously touching the participants' remaining hand in the 'same' place. Using this method it was discovered that the illusion could be generated using synchronous touching *without* the need for a visual representation. However, it has since been shown (Petkova et al., 2012) that sight may still 'play' a significant role even when participants are blindfolded. This involved a comparison between participants who had been blind since birth and a group of aged matched sighted participants. It was discovered that participants who were congenitally blind did not experience the illusion whilst sighted participants did. Additionally blind participants stated the illusion was 'totally absurd' or that 'they could not even imagine the illusion'. As a possible explanation for the lack of the illusion in the blind group, it was noted that behavioural studies have shown those who have been blind since birth do not appear to map somatosensory sensation in external coordinates the way the sighted do (Röder et al., 2004, 2007; Azanon et al., 2010; Yamamoto & Kitazawa, 2001). The lack of visual experience appears to affect the way other sensations work together, influencing the way the body is perceived.

Further experiments have shown that 'ownership' requires that the object that is to be 'owned' should be at an orientation (Tsakiris & Haggard, 2005) and distance (Preston, 2013) from the body to be plausible as a part of the body. With reference to Gallagher's concepts of the body image, this would appear to be the 'plausable' alteration of the body percept, incorporating the object into it. At the same time, the real body part becomes 'disowned' (Moseley et al., 2008). It might be the case that the RHI requires that for an object to become 'owned', it must be human-like in shape and size (Yuan & Steed, 2010). However, this was challenged due to evidence that ownership of a tabletop (Armel & Ramchandran, 2003) and 'empty space' is possible (Guterstam et al., 2013), although it is certainly easier for ownership to occur in human-like objects (Kilteni et al., 2012).

Although the RHI seems to require a 'plausible' point of view for the ownership effect to occur (Petkova et al., 2011), it appears that the mind understands when an everyday point of view means that the object being viewed cannot possibly belong to oneself, but accepts that HMDs and cameras allow for an apparently foreign body (as seen through a third-person perspective) to be your own. Elongation and distortion of limbs has also been shown to occur from this perspective by Preston and Newport (2012). Using a camera to provide a view of the participant from 2 m behind, they then fed this into a HMD which was worn by the participant. Their arm was then pulled 'vigorously upwards' whist the image from the camera was distorted to show their limb being elongated to twice its normal length. Participants reported that they had been watching themselves and had seen their arm being stretched with the result that they felt it was longer. This resulted in them overestimating the reach of the 'stretched' arm compared with their other arm. Participants were also asked to touch where they believed their opposing wrist to be whilst their eyes were closed; in this instance no significant changes between 'stretched' and 'unstretched' conditions were detected. Preston and Newport believed that this demonstrated that although ownership had been demonstrated, there was no effect upon the body schema. However, two things should be noted in relation to this conclusion. Given that the schema is postulated to be a mechanism involved with turning intentions of body movement into action, the absence of arm movement in the creation of the illusion might have significantly contributed to the schema remaining unaffected. The lack of an effect on the schema might also be an illustration of the importance of vision in dynamically affecting the schema.

The concept of 'ownership' is often referred to when discussing the RHI. It is suggested that 'levels' of ownership can develop, although work in this regard had tended to focus upon 'proprioceptive drift' as a measure of determining this (Kilteni et al., 2012). 'Proprioceptive drift' is a measure of how far away from the actual position or orientation a person believes their limb to be. However experimentation has shown that proprioceptive drift can occur without ownership, bringing this measure into doubt (Rohde et al., 2011). This was demonstrated by using asynchronous tactile feedback to 'remove' the feeling of ownership, whilst proprioceptive drift remained unaffected. It was speculated (ibid.) that separate mechanisms may be at work for the two phenomena, although both may be caused by similar multi-sensory inputs.

Although not conclusive this survey illustrates a number of things. The illusion can occur, whether or not ownership is a concurrent phenomenon. The illusion can occur in such a way that it may be manifest through the ownership of objects that are not a part of the body, and given this, it affects the participants' perception of where 'their' limb is in space. Vision plays an important role in the formation of the illusion, although this need not be 'active' in that it appears to have affected the way other senses are utilised. In addition if vision is involved, it is not necessary to possess a first-person perspective but the view provided should be plausible; and such plausibility can incorporate technology such as cameras and HMDs. In addition the perception of the shape of the limb can be altered. If the body image is in part constituted from the body schema, the way in which objects that are not 'owned' are incorporated into the schema, it may be an important factor in affecting the perception of our body and this is what we will examine next.

Peripersonal and Extrapersonal Space

If grasped objects do not become an 'owned' incorporation of the body (as seen in the RHI), then it is likely to be considered as a tool. Fake hands 'owned' through the illusion extended peripersonal space around them when the illusion occurs (Makin et al., 2008) and tools also extend this region of peripersonal space to the location around the tool itself (Berti & Frassinetti, 2000).

It has been observed that there may be a distinction between the processes or regions of the brain involved with the handling of near (peripersonal) and far (extra-personal) spaces; in itself the distinction between these spaces is based upon human action and the spaces within which particular actions occur. Peripersonal space is defined as the space within which things are in hand reaching distance and extrapersonal space being that which is beyond our reach and requires some form of locomotion to be able to grasp an object. What interested Berti and Frassinetti were cases where those who had suffered strokes showed dissociation between near and far spaces, manifesting spatial neglect in only one or the other of those spaces (Halligan & Marshall, 1991; Cowey et al., 1994; Vuilleumier et al., 1998).

A task used to establish the degree of neglect suffered by patients involves subjects bisecting a line in near and far spaces. Berti and Frassinetti reported the case of patient P.P., who, having suffered a stroke, showed dissociation between near and far spaces where neglect occurred in a line-bisection test in near space, but where P.P. could perform this task without impediment in extrapersonal space by using a light pen. They predicted that if the bisection of the line in 'far' space were to be executed with a tool such as stick, the extended representation of the body should now include that 'far' space as 'near'. The outcome of this would then be that the same neglect that had occurred in near space would now be seen in 'far' space. The result was as predicted and when a stick was used instead of a light pen, the line was misperceived in the same way as it was when within near space; far had indeed become near. As a result of this, it seems the simple use of a tool is enough to incorporate it into the space defined by the body. In fact, Berti and Frassinetti define the coding of near and far spaces as a dynamic process; as such it is something which is necessarily plastic.

We can of course see examples of tool extensions that can be found in every day such as the use of a badminton racquet or hockey stick, which would be considered extensions of the forearm, or of skis, which would be extensions of the feet. This kind of elongation is very rare in parts of limbs which are attached at both ends – for example, the upper arm – because tools tend to be extensions of limb extremities. Tools affect the body schema as they require adaptation to be able to use them effectively as they cause the body to behave differently when moving (Cardinali et al., 2009).

It is believed that objects within peripersonal space are mapped onto an egocentric referencing space and used in action simulation (Ter Horst et al., 2011). Action simulation is a simulated movement action that is created without actually performing the action (Gallese, 2005). This means that actions have been mentally constructed prior to performing the touching or grasping action for those objects that are within peripersonal space. This would insinuate that the action must, however, have been formed using the body schema, a body schema which has learned how to function through the use of the physical body. Even the imagination of using a tool is enough to incorporate the tool into the body schema (Baccarini et al., 2014).

Tool use can also extend peripersonal space into a virtual setting provided that the user of the tool is familiar with how the tool behaves (Gozli & Brown, 2011). This would indicate that, if the user should perceive the avatar as a tool, peripersonal space would be extended around it – provided that they are familiar with how the avatar moves. To this extent the use of 'player' movements through devices such as the Kinect will mean that it is highly likely that an extension of peripersonal space will occur. What then becomes an issue is whether, and if so to what degree, do any changes between the user's and the avatar's proportions might affect or break such a connection, much in the way that we saw that the incongruous positioning of the rubber hand could disrupt the RHI.

Experimental Design

As a result of these issues, it was predicted that distorting the limb proportions of an avatar whilst viewing it from the third-person perspective would affect the percept and schema of the individual controlling it. This would be due to the interactions and 'natural' motions which are used to control the avatar being filtered through the user's body schema and extended peripersonal space; in turn it is likely such an effect would be influenced by feedback provided via the use of an avatar with differing proportions. It is predicted that such feedback would suggest that the user's 'habitual' schema would be in error, demanding arm movement correction, without providing any real-world sensation of elongated or shortened arms. It was decided to perform a simple initial evaluation of this hypothesis through participants performing simple reaching and touching tasks. These tasks would be measured to ascertain the effectiveness of participants' motions whilst also seeking qualitative evidence of any changes in perception that participants experienced. However, the design of these tests needed to take into account a number of the factors highlighted through the examination of the RHI and tool use.

The Perspective of the Experiment

Typically, for an object to be seen as 'belonging' to oneself, the first-person perspective is used (Botvinick & Cohen, 1998; Yuan & Steed, 2010; Petkova et al., 2011; Kilteni et al., 2012). However, in the virtual world, the first-person perspective is limited to specific genres of games (such as first-person shooters), none of which presently use full-body interaction (some use motion tracking 'shortcuts' for actions such as grenade throwing, although given these are used with a controller possessing a simple button press to achieve the same end, the notion of a shortcut is somewhat stretched). This is most likely to be due to effective full-body interaction requiring the sight of the avatar's entire body for effective feedback. The first-person perspective is limited in this regard as its field of view of the avatar's body provides few opportunities for any feedback to be visible when compared to a third-person perspective.

In the ownership experiments which were investigating ownership from the third-person perspective, the use of HMDs (head-mounted displays) was typical. However, this would usually involve passive or reclining positions (Petkova et al., 2011; Preston & Newport, 2012) which would affect the ability to receive any substantial feedback through movement due to its lack. Virtual reality headsets such as the Oculus Rift™ would offer the ability to provide the user with a 3D view of the environment. This would have an advantage over a flat 2D screen which loses this aspect of depth perception, but given the nature of the active movement that would be taking place, there was a danger that disorientation or tripping might occur due to the HMD's occlusion of the physical environment, thereby becoming a health and safety issue. In fact, placing the user into a situation where they would have to consider two environments simultaneously due to such a hazard would most likely detract from the very issues that were to be investigated. Although various forms of 3D systems exist for use with 2D displays (utilising shutter glasses or polarised projection), the active nature of the tasks would require the tracking of the participant's point of view. Given that the investigation was based around the use of systems available to gamers in domestic environments, it was decided that the projection of the virtual environment onto a large projection screen in front of the participant was the most appropriate method, given that if control of the avatar were to affect users in 2D, it would be highly likely its use in 3D would be similar if not more pronounced. The chosen method would also allow the user to clearly see the avatar and the screen would fill the forward view of participants, assisting in immersion with the task.

To interact within the virtual world from a third-person perspective, an avatar of some form would be required for these interactions. Humans can take the perspective of other individuals or viewpoints, finding it less cognitively taxing the closer to their own viewpoint (Kessler & Thomson, 2010). Given the decision not to use a HMD, these interactions would not be viewed from a first-person perspective, a viewpoint that allowed for as natural an opportunity for interaction needed to be sought. Viewpoints of this sort are normal within games using a third-person viewpoint, and on this occasion, a particular concern was the possible occlusion of the objects that were to be placed within the environment for participants to interact with.

To achieve an appropriate viewpoint it was decided that to reduce cognitive load and to test the traditional third-person perspective used in videogames, the experiment's viewpoint must be from behind. In addition, it would need to be slightly above the avatar's 'head' to reduce occlusion of the objects to be interacted with.

Due to issues of the Kinect'sTM accuracy in tracking the legs and feet, which can potentially result in movements where none were performed, the decision was made that the view would not include the avatar's legs or lower torso given that the depiction of such movements might disrupt the relationship between user and avatar that was being examined. As a result of this the interactions asked of participants would be simple reaching and touching activities. However, there were additional reasons influencing this decision.

Peripersonal Space and Action Simulation – Or How the Avatar Might Extend the Action Simulation Area

As has been noted peripersonal space can be experienced within both the real (Berti & Frassinetti, 2000) and virtual worlds (Gozli & Brown, 2011). The limitations on the virtual world mean that eventually, as learning occurs, peripersonal space will develop using any tool (Gamberini et al., 2008). This is significant as action simulation occurs upon objects within peripersonal space (Ter Horst et al., 2011).

Action simulation occurs when the mind goes through the preliminary steps of imagining an action taking place (Gallese, 2005). These simulations make use of the same neural pathways as those employed to perform the action being imagined, or simulated, but some mechanism prevents them from actively being performed overtly (Jeannerod, 2001).

Given this, regardless of whether the avatar is owned or used as a tool, *both* outcomes would extend the region of peripersonal space around it (Berti & Frassinetti, 2000) and into the virtual environment. Objects in extrapersonal space do not experience action simulation and, as a result, require more time to grasp or touch given that an intermediary action is required to place them within peripersonal space. As a result of this, the tests were designed so that the virtual objects users would interact with would be placed just within their reaching distance. It was expected that once participants realised that these were within the reaching distance of the avatar (being provided this opportunity through warm-up exercises), they would then begin to simulate the actions of touching them.

However, given that the avatar might be treated as a tool, extending peripersonal space into the virtual environment, it was also the case that altering the length of limb extremities might lead to participants performing the tasks as they might do if provided with a tool. As a result of this it was decided to vary the length of the upper arms of the avatar, allowing for a lengthening of limbs that would not normally be encountered through tool use.

Experimental Setup

As a result of these considerations the primary experiment consisted of tasks being performed through a virtual avatar, projected onto a screen in front of participants. This avatar would be created using the Kinect's skeleton data gathered from the participant, including limb lengths and relative joint angles (see Fig. 10.1).

The Kinect™ was centrally positioned in front of the projector screen. It was then elevated to a position where it could be as high as possible without interference from the light being projected onto the screen: approximately 1.5 ms above the floor.

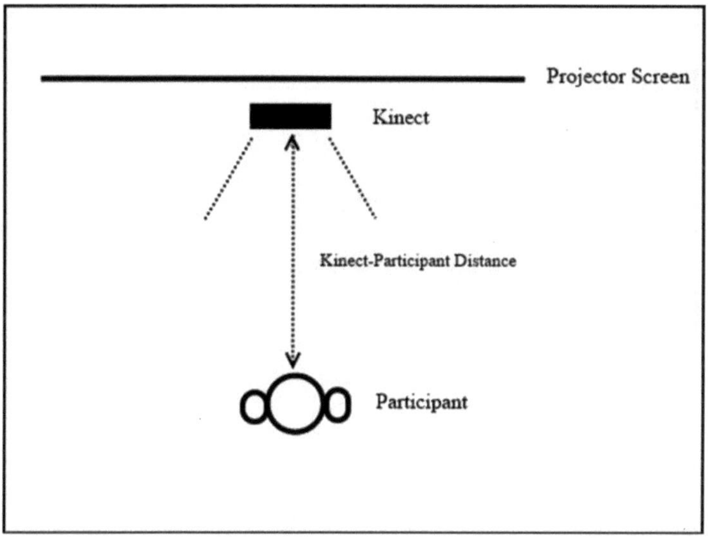

Fig. 10.1 Diagram showing where the participants stood relative to the equipment

A 30 cm square box was marked on the floor that was 2 m (the Kinect-Participant Distance) directly in front of, and central to, the position of the Kinect device. This distance was chosen in accordance with Microsoft's Kinect's documentation (Microsoft, 2013). Participants were asked to stand within this box for the duration of the tasks, facing towards the Kinect and the projector screen.

The Kinect™ device was used to calibrate the proportions of the avatar for individuals. Whilst standing in a squared Y position in front of the device (shown below), with their arms at approximately 90 degrees to their torso, elbows are bent so that their hands are raised roughly level with their ears (Fig. 10.2). This allowed the relative lengths of the limbs to be captured and the avatar altered so that it shared the relative dimensions of the participant.

Participants were kept unaware as to the precise purpose of the experiment prior to performing the tasks. Five unmodified warm-up tasks were allowed for each participant before data was recorded. The aim of these warm-ups was to remove the early period of training from the data. It was assumed that when the experiments first began, participants would be new to the tasks and would not be performing as well as they would be at the end of the tasks. The warm-ups were intended to alleviate some of this learning curve. The same unmodified proportions were used as the 'normal' condition for the experiments, whilst the 'control' condition changed the colour of the avatar's joints but kept the same proportions as the 'normal' condition, the purpose being to test whether any significant differences between results were being caused by changes to the avatar's appearance, rather than subsequent alterations in arm length.

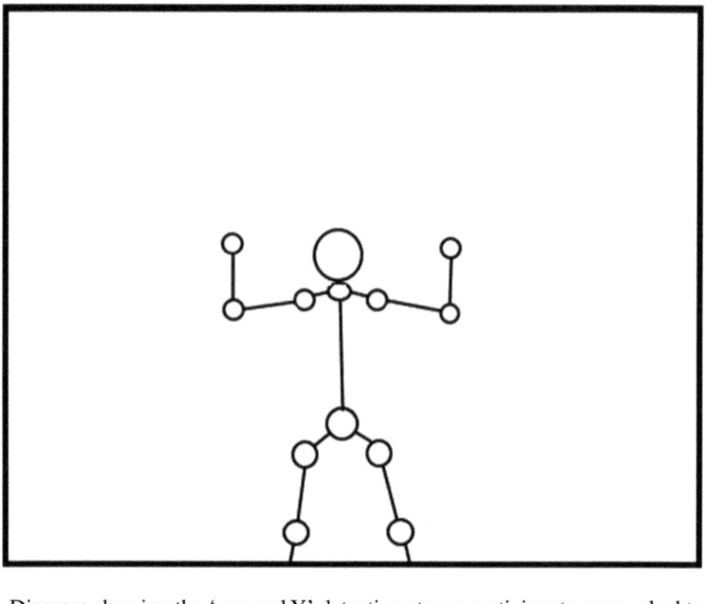

Fig. 10.2 Diagram showing the 'squared Y' detection stance participants were asked to perform

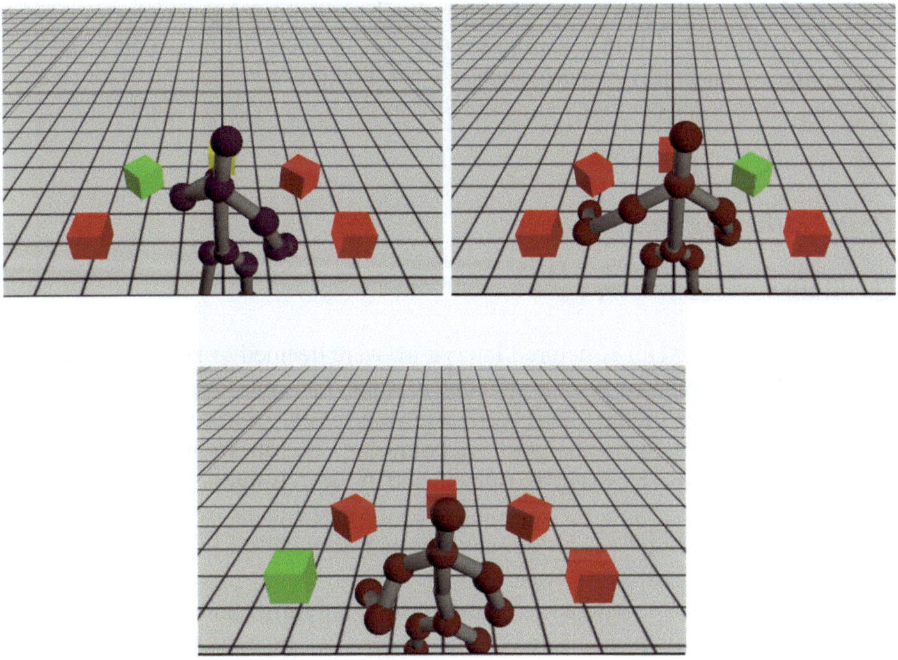

Fig. 10.3 (Left) The control avatar being used to touch the cubes. (Right) The 40% longer upper arm length condition. (Bottom) An avatar with a 20% increase in upper arm length being used

There were three modified conditions, each affecting the length of both of the avatar's upper arms' length: a 20% increase, a 40% increase and a 60% increase (Fig. 10.3).

Each task required participants to move in such a way that the avatar touched a sequence of the five virtual cubes that appeared around it. One of the cubes would appear green, indicating that it was the cube the participant should attempt to touch, whilst the remaining cubes were red. Once the green cube was touched, a randomly selected red cube would turn green and the touched green cube would turn red. This would continue for 25 s – a point being awarded for touching a green cube and a point deducted for touching a red cube.

Participants were given 20 such tasks to perform. Each task was identical except for the lengths of the avatar's upper arms and the coloured order of the boxes.

Ten tasks were performed in a row at the beginning of the experiment, after which the participants were asked to complete a questionnaire on their experiences of performing the tasks. After the questionnaire was complete, the remaining 10 tasks were then performed. Once these were finished, there was a short semi-structured interview, asking more extensive and subjective questions on the experiential aspects of the tasks.

Ethical approval was received before experiments began. Participants were requested via university e-mail. An open appointment system was made available, allowing those taking part to declare their details and allocate themselves a time to take part. Participants were also asked to declare any pre-existing conditions which might affect their safety or performance when making vigorous arm movements. However, there were no pre-existing conditions declared by participants.

Data Gathering and Analysis

Qualitative

Questionnaires and semi-structured interviews were deemed to be the most appropriate methods for gathering the qualitative data. The questionnaire allowed for feedback to be given on the Likert scale, allowing for only a fixed range of answers that could be quantitatively analysed and compared. The questionnaires followed a similar structure to those used in the rubber hand illusion (Botvinick & Cohen, 1998).

The semi-structured interviews would keep the participants' feedback to areas of interest without forcing 'yes' or 'no' answers and would allow them to elaborate on the experiences in their own words.

The decision was made to issue questionnaires for participants to fill in after ten tasks so that the participants had had a chance to experience the potential effects of the experiment before they completed them, but this was also done to limit the contamination of responses given in the semi-structured interviews at the end. Ten further tasks would then be performed after the questionnaires had been filled in, before the semi-structured interviews.

There were several ways in which the outputs from the interviews might have been analysed. Interpretative phenomenological analysis (IPA) and thematic analysis and grounded theory are common techniques that are used.

It was decided that thematic analysis would provide the greatest flexibility in analysing the data, taking into consideration the number of participants that took part in the experiment.

Quantitative

Participants received a score and an accuracy value for each task that they performed. A point was received each time that the avatar touched the correct cube, and a point lost for touching an incorrect cube. Accuracy results were based upon the total percentage of touches which were made correctly.

The data gathered of both the score and accuracy were analysed separately for a normal distribution using the Kolmogorov-Smirnov (KS) test for normality. Failure to reject the KS test's null hypothesis indicated the requirement for non-parametric analysis of the data. Friedman's two-way analysis of variance was performed as a result, and, due to a significant result, this was then followed by Wilcoxon signed-rank comparisons between groups.

Results

There were 31 participants in total, 11 of which were female. Two of the participants reported themselves to be left-handed.

Participants were selected through a university staff email, requesting volunteers for the experiment, and all were automatically accepted. They were left as naïve to the purpose of the experiment as ethically possible.

Qualitative Results

Questionnaires were given to participants halfway through the tasks. The questions that were asked were as follows:

1. I felt as if I were present within the virtual environment.
2. I felt that the avatar always accurately reflected my bodily proportions.
3. I felt as if the avatar was mimicking or copying my actions.
4. It felt as though the avatar was my real body.
5. At times my arms felt as if they were shorter.
6. I felt as if I were controlling the avatar.
7. At times my arms felt as if they were longer.
8. My movements felt less coordinated than normal.

The results indicated that participants felt as if they were both controlling the avatar, and that at times the avatar was copying them. They also indicate that many participants felt less coordinated in controlling the avatar than they would if they were performing the tasks physically (Fig. 10.4).

There were several control questions within the questionnaire that were not followed up on, including whether participants felt that the avatar was their real body or if they felt as if they were present within the virtual environment.

Interestingly, participants tended to positively report that they experienced their arms to be shorter rather than longer, despite the increase in arm length; however, the difference was not statistically significant. If the experiments were to show this effect, however, it would most likely be caused by the front block being harder to touch for some than others. This would lead to the perception from time to time that they could not reach as far as they thought they could.

Semi-structured Interviews

Participants were requested to take part in semi-structured interviews at the end of their experiments. In this situation they were given a few questions to answer:

- Were any of the tasks harder or easier than the others?
  - Did movements feel awkward?

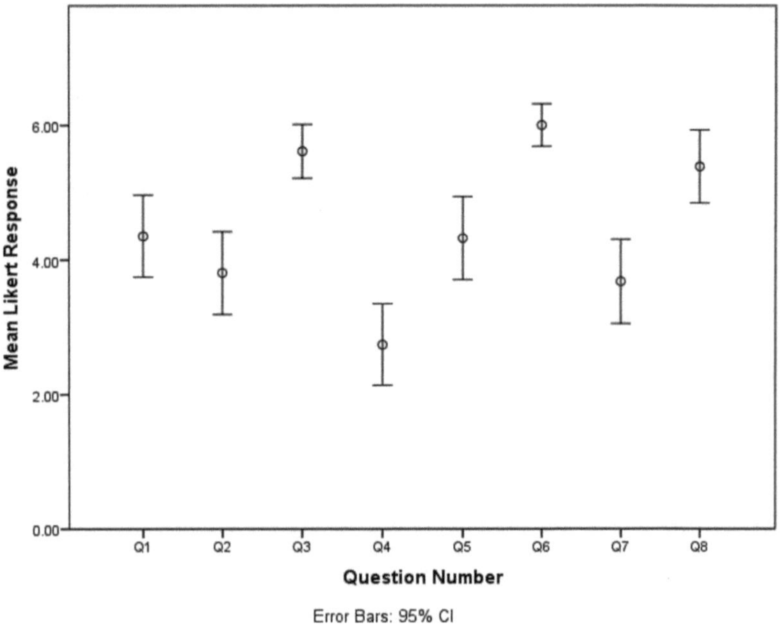

Fig. 10.4 The mean responses from participants on the Likert scale

- Did you notice any effects on your perceptions of your own body as a result of the tasks you were asked to perform?
  - Did limbs feel as if they were longer/shorter or less/more manoeuvrable than before?
- Did it feel as if you were controlling the avatar, or that the avatar was copying your movements?
  - Was this different in different situations?

As the experiments went on, and in conjunction with the feedback that some participants provided during the tasks, if it became clear that there were some avenues of investigation which were not being explored, another question was also asked of the participants.

- Did the cubes appear to become larger or smaller, or closer or further away?

The responses to the questions gave rise to several interesting themes.

Because of the design of the experiment, some of the shorter participants found that it was difficult to reach the front cube with the unmodified avatar arm lengths. When questioned at the end of the experiment, six participants reported that they felt as if their own arms were shorter than expected on those occasions when they found it hard to reach that cube.

There were six participants who reported that they felt 'uncoordinated' or 'clumsy' with one participant likening it to 'clunky bits of iron, or something'.

Although the cubes were stationary for the entire experiment (and could be seen against the grid of the virtual floor), nine participants reported that they felt as if the cubes around them were coming closer on some tasks. One participant reported that after the questionnaire in the middle of the experiment they had realised what was happening and no longer experienced this as happening. One more participant reported that they felt as if only the front cube were moving, when they found it difficult to reach.

One participant reported during the experiments that they felt as if they were being 'trapped' by the cubes, and as if they could not move their arms much for fear of touching one of the virtual cubes.

Six participants reported that they noticed no or very little difference between tasks. Most reported that *something* was changing which resulted in them performing worse in some tasks and better in others, but mentioned that it was either a rare thing, or that they did not know what was causing it.

From those results, many participants were experiencing some form of alteration to how they perceived either themselves or the virtual environment changing because of the modification to the upper arm lengths.

Quantitative Results

The results of this first experiment give evidence that under the experimental design that was chosen, the 20% increase in arm length seemed to be more optimal than the other increased arm lengths. This was seen as a statistically significant difference in both score and accuracy over the 40% and 60% conditions, but not over the unmodified arm lengths.

To analyse the data, the mean of each participant's scores and accuracy for each condition was calculated. These means were then tested for normality using the Kolmogorov-Smirnov test (see Tables 10.1 and 10.2).

As the null hypothesis for the Kolmogorov-Smirnov test for normality is that the data is not normally distributed, non-parametric tests were required to analyse the data.

Table 10.1 Kolmogorov-Smirnov test for normality on score data

–	*N*	Mean	Std. dev.	Minimum	Maximum	K-S Z	Asymp. sig. (two-tailed)
Normal	31	18.9194	5.15444	8.50	26.50	.799	.546
Control	31	18.6210	5.23246	8.00	26.25	.789	.562
20%	31	19.5645	6.39041	5.75	28.50	.896	.399
40%	31	17.8387	7.29342	−2.00	27.25	1.112	.169
60%	31	17.1048	6.75579	2.25	26.50	.966	.308

Table 10.2 Kolmogorov-Smirnov test for normality on accuracy data

–	*N*	Mean	Std. dev.	Minimum	Maximum	K-S Z	Asymp. sig. (two-tailed)
Normal	31	67.6374	18.09942	25.65	90.94	1.067	.205
Control	31	66.1413	19.15797	23.52	91.69	.896	.399
20%	31	65.9313	22.07425	13.14	92.38	1.026	.243
40%	31	59.3242	25.22878	−3.74	94.26	1.053	.217
60%	31	57.4374	25.49640	5.16	88.87	.968	.306

Friedman's two-way ANOVA was performed on the score (chi-square = 13.093, $df = 4$, $p = .011$) and accuracy (chi-square = 14.452, $df = 4$, $p = .006$). These tests suggest that there is a statistically significant difference between at least two groups for both the score and the accuracy.

Score Data

The score data were analysed (Table 10.3) using two-tailed Wilcoxon signed-rank related sample ($\alpha = 0.05$, $N = 31$) tests performed between groupings to ascertain where the significant differences are located.

As shown in Table 10.3, no significant differences are seen between the normal (*N*) and control (*C*) group ($Z = -.471$, $p = 638$), giving evidence that any differences were not solely due to alterations to the representation of the avatar upon the screen.

Significant differences were found to exist between the *N* and 60% ($Z = -2.251$, $p = .024$) conditions' scores, highlighting the difference in ability to perform the tasks between the participants' normal arm lengths and an extraordinarily increased one.

The graph (Fig. 10.5) displays that the 20% increase in arm length resulted in a higher score compared to the other groups, but not in a higher success rate compared to the control and normal arm lengths. The highly significant difference that was identified between the 20% and the 40% ($Z = -3.589$, $p < .001$) and 60% ($Z = -3.656$, $p < .001$) groups not only provides evidence that a 20% increase in upper arm length appears to be more productive, but also suggests that with a larger sample size there may have been a significant difference seen between the 20% and normal conditions as well.

No significant difference was shown between the 40% and 60% groups ($Z = -1.245$, $p = .213$), suggesting either that the cubes were at a similarly awkward distance for any increase in upper arm length above 20% or that the avatar was similarly foreign to control beyond 20%.

It can be concluded that the 20% group of tests resulted in a higher average score compared to the other groups of experiments, but this higher average was not necessary because of improved accuracy. It may be possible that the 20% increase allowed participants to manoeuvre their arms more easily and quickly than any of the other conditions due to the increased arm length being small enough that it could still be incorporated into the normal schema, as if tool use had occurred, whilst still receiving the benefit of increased reach.

Accuracy Data

As shown in Table 10.4, the accuracy data were also analysed using two-tailed Wilcoxon signed-rank related sample tests ($\alpha = 0.05$, $N = 31$). Statistically significant differences were identified between the *N* ($Z = -2.783, p = .005$ and $Z = -2.841, p = .004$), *C* ($Z = -2.312, p = .021$ and $Z = -2.499, p = .012$) and 20% ($Z = -3.723, p < .001$ and $Z = -3.508, p < .001$) groups, when compared with the 40% and 60% groups, respectively. This would strongly indicate that there was little difference in difficulty between the participants' normal arm lengths and the 20% increased condition (Fig. 10.6). However, beyond this value participants were finding that controlling the limbs in a precise fashion became increasingly difficult.

No statistically significant differences were identified between the 40% and 60% conditions, although it is inconclusive as to whether this is because participants were finding them equally as difficult to control, or that there was insufficient time within experiments for any differences to become evident.

The lack of a difference between the normal and control conditions' accuracy refutes the idea that any differences in results might come solely from the fact that changes were taking place.

Tables and Figures

Table 10.3 The Wilcoxon signed-rank pairwise comparisons of mean scores per condition

Pair	Z	Sig. (two-tailed)
Normal-control	−.471	.638
Normal-20%	−1.333	.182
Normal-40%	−1.441	.150
Normal-60%	−2.251	.024
Control-20%	−1.766	.077
Control-40%	−.667	.505
Control-60%	−1.688	.091
20–40%	−3.589	.000
20–60%	−3.656	.000
40–60%	−1.245	.213

Table 10.4 The Wilcoxon signed-rank pairwise comparisons of mean accuracy per condition

Pair	*Z*	Sig. (two-tailed)
Normal-control	−.676	.499
Normal-20%	−.627	.531
Normal-40%	−2.783	.005
Normal-60%	−2.841	.004
Control-20%	−.176	.860
Control-40%	−2.312	.021
Control-60%	−2.499	.012
20–40%	−3.723	.000
20–60%	−3.508	.000
40–60%	−.627	.531

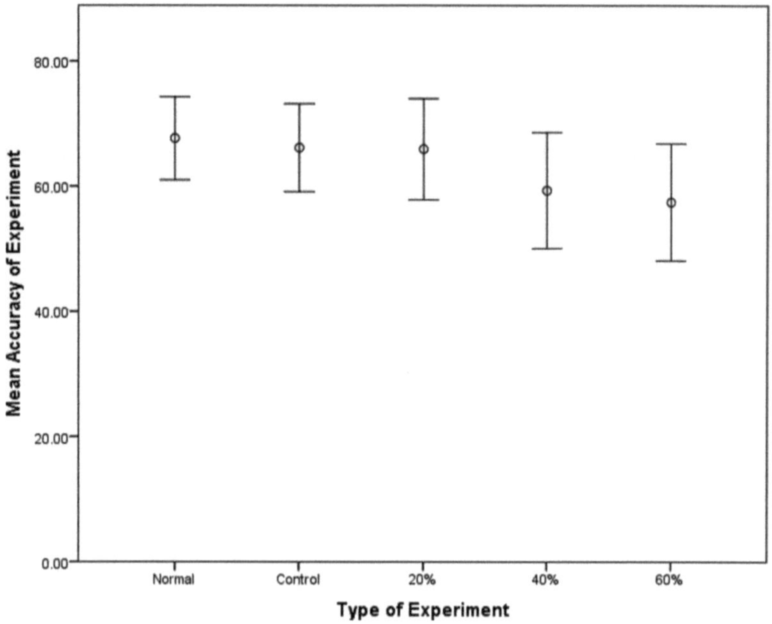

Fig. 10.5 An error bar graph showing the 95% confidence intervals of mean experiment scores per condition

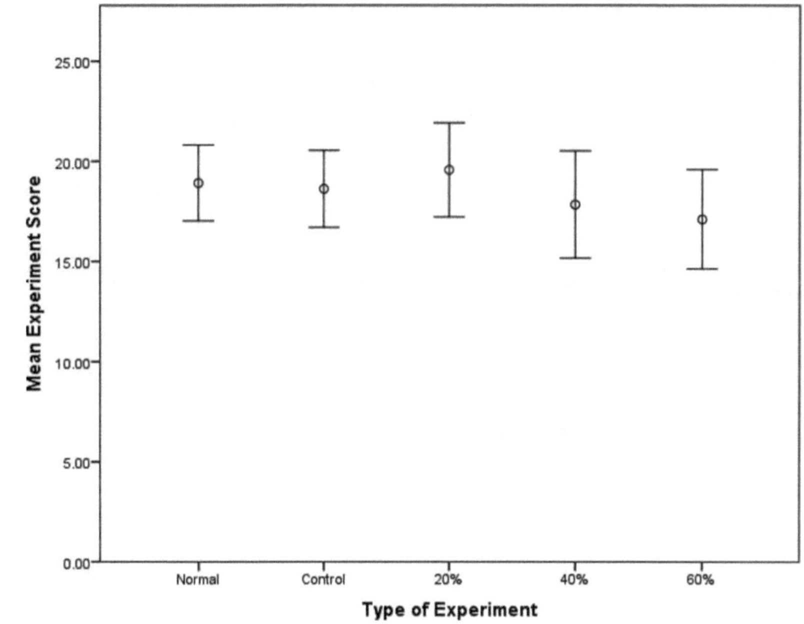

Fig. 10.6 An error bar graph showing the 95% confidence intervals of mean experiment accuracy per condition

Discussion

Participants scored significantly higher and more accurately when they used the avatar with a 20% increase in arm length, over arm lengths which were longer. Whilst the differences between the normally proportioned arm lengths and the 20% increase in arm length were not statistically significant, there is the suggestion that participants performed better with the additional length to their upper arms.

The likely reason for this increase is due to the increased ease with which it allowed participants to reach the cubes, without adding too much change in how they must perform the actions, akin to what might be considered to be day-to-day tool use. In contrast more noticeable changes to movement would have been required with longer arm lengths. The larger limb extensions may have caused the limbs to be 'too long' for the comfortable touching of the cubes. This awkwardness seems to have outweighed the advantage of being able to move the arms a shorter distance to achieve the same goal.

It can be concluded that, given blocks which are at a distance which may be just out of reach, an improved performance can be achieved by lengthening the arms by a small amount. Further increases in arm length do not improve performance and in fact inhibit it. This is interesting because most of our habitual touching tasks involve objects which are well within arm's reach, so our habitual actions should have lent themselves towards the handling of tasks that are within easy reach rather than at arm's length. Lengthening the arms of an avatar beyond the proportions of the user's body also created an experience of their arms feeling uncomfortably flexible or rigid.

Limitations

There were limitations to the experiment. Mostly this is due to the cubes always being a fixed distance away from the participants, regardless of height or normal arm reach. This may have resulted in the 20% increase in arm length being optimal for that distance, and if the cubes were further away, then a further increase may have been optimal.

In turn this might also have been an outcome of the avatar having been adapted to the proportions of the user, which might have been overcome by the inclusion of a typical game avatar for comparison to the tests that were conducted.

Conclusion and Future Work

Altering the length of an avatar's limbs relative to users' own limb lengths affected the performance of users. Users also perceived these changes in a variety of ways, either through changes in the perception of their own body, the avatar through which they perform these interactions or through changes in the environment with which they are interacting.

Further work needs to be performed to determine the extent to which the limitations of the tests were a factor in the results of this experiment. However, it currently appears that unintended consequences of avatar design choices that do not consider users' bodies could introduce discomfort into the user experience as well as influencing effectiveness in controlling it. To this extent the use of such systems in a therapeutic setting, without the use of appropriately proportioned avatar and appropriately calibrated environment, may be problematic. However, given an adequate understanding of these factors, it may be possible to utilise the plasticity afforded by such systems to affect altered movements. Given this, new therapeutic treatments for injuries may then become a possibility by encouraging some motions over others.

As a result, further investigation into the potential influences resulting from alterations to the avatar upon the perception of users' bodies would be needed. This would allow the examination of the potential extent of such interventions, and this should begin by examining the way that movements through space are affected rather than just looking at 'headline' efficiency of those movements. Areas for additional investigation might include the manipulation of the width of limbs, thereby altering the sense of mass in the users' own limbs. The potential for this is clear given that work by the Hearing Body Project (Tajadura-Jiménez et al., 2014) has shown that this is possible simply through the use of sound.

The scope of such plasticity also needs investigating. It may be that beyond a certain level, it becomes impossible to accommodate and learn how to control the new limb, or it may be that it will eventually be possible to learn how to control any alteration provided.

With the release of more affordable HMDs and virtual reality headsets aimed at the mass market and gaming community, the first-person perspective is an area that will require further investigation. Although only small parts of the avatar are visible in this perspective, the effects of the avatar may still be of consequence. The nausea that is often reported through the use of such systems might have some of its origins in the inappropriate representation of the body affecting the perception of the body and virtual environment; interestingly earlier explorations of VR provided examples with significantly lower frame rates and resolutions, but that also provided experiences that avoid nausea. Work that succeeded in doing this made use of an embodied means to navigate space (Davies' *Osmose* (1995) and *Ephémère* (1998)), albeit without the representation of the body and the interactions that are now expected within modern VR environments.

References

Armel, K. C., & Ramachandran, V. S. (2003). Projecting sensations to external objects: Evidence from skin conductance response. *Proceedings of the Royal Society of London, Series B: Biological Sciences, 270*(1523), 1499–1506.

Azanon, E., Longo, M. R., Soto-Faraco, S., & Haggard, P. (2010). The posterior parietal cortex remaps touch into external space. *Current Biology, 20*, 1304–1309.

Baccarini, M., Martel, M., Cardinali, L., Sillan, O., Farnè, A., & Roy, A. C. (2014). Tool use imagery triggers tool incorporation in the body schema. *Frontiers in Psychology, 5*, 492.

Berti, A., & Frassinetti, F. (2000). When far becomes near: Remapping of space by tool use. *Journal of Cognitive Neuroscience, 12*(3), 415–420.

Botvinick, M., & Cohen, J. (1998). Rubber hands 'feel' touch that eyes see. *Nature, 391*, 756.

Cardinali, L., Frassinetti, F., Brozzoli, C., Urquizar, C., Roy, A. C., & Farnè, A. (2009). Tool-use induces morphological updating of the body schema. *Current Biology: CB, 19*(12), R478–R479.

Cowey, A., Small, M., & Ellis, S. (1994). Left visuo-spatial neglect can be worse in far than in near space. *Neuropsychologia, 32*(9), 1059–1066.

Davies, C. *Osmose* (1995) and *Ephémère* (1998). http://www.immersence.com/

Ehrsson, H., Holmes, N., & Passingham, R. (2005). Touching a rubber hand: Feeling of body ownership is associated with activity in multisensory brain areas. *The Journal of Neuroscience, 25*(45), 10564–10573.

Farrer, C., Franck, N., Paillard, J., & Jeannerod, M. (2003). The role of proprioception in action recognition. *Consciousness and Cognition, 12*(4), 609–619.

Gallagher, S. (2005). *How the body shapes the mind.* Oxford University Press.

Gallese, V. (2005). Embodied simulation: From neurons to phenomenal experience. *Phenomenology and the Cognitive Sciences, 4*(1), 23–48.

Gamberini, L., Seraglia, B., & Priftis, K. (2008). Processing of peripersonal and extrapersonal space using tools: Evidence from visual line bisection in real and virtual environments. *Neuropsychologia, 46*(5), 1298–1304.

Gozli, D. G., & Brown, L. E. (2011). Agency and control for the integration of a virtual tool into the peripersonal space. *Perception (London), 40*(11), 1309–1319.

Guterstam, A., Gentile, G., & Ehrsson, H. H. (2013). The invisible hand illusion: Multisensory integration leads to the embodiment of a discrete volume of empty space. *Journal of Cognitive Neuroscience, 25*(7), 1078–1099.

Halligan, P. W., & Marshall, J. C. (1991). Left neglect for near but not far space in man. *Nature, 350*(6318), 498–500.

Head, H. (1920). *Studies in neurology* (p. 2). Oxford University Press.

IJsselsteijn, W. A., & Haans, A. (2008). Touch, tools, and telepresence: Embodiment in mediated environments. *Proceedings of SPIE, 6806*(1). https://doi.org/10.1117/12.785308

IJsselsteijn, W. A., de Kort, Y. A. W., & Haans, A. (2006). Is this my hand I see before me? The rubber hand illusion in reality, virtual reality, and mixed reality. *Presence Teleoperators and Virtual Environments, 15*, 455–464.

Jeannerod, M. (2001). Neural simulation of action: A unifying mechanism for motor cognition. *NeuroImage, 14*(1), S103–S109.

Kessler, K., & Thomson, L. A. (2010). The embodied nature of spatial perspective taking: Embodied transformation versus sensorimotor interference. *Cognition, 114*(1), 72–88.

Kilteni, K., Normand, J. M., Sanchez-Vives, M. V., & Slater, M. (2012). Extending body space in immersive virtual reality: A very long arm illusion. *PLoS One, 7*(7), e40867.

Makin, T. R., Holmes, N. P., & Ehrsson, H. H. (2008). On the other hand: Dummy hands and peripersonal space. *Behavioural Brain Research, 191*(1), 1–10.

Microsoft Corporation. (2013). *Kinect for windows human interface guidelines v.1.7.* [online] Available http://download.microsoft.com/download/B/0/7/B070724E-52B4-4B1A-BD1B-05CC28D07899/Human_Interface_Guidelines_v1.7.0.pdf

Moseley, G. L., Olthof, N., Venema, A., Don, S., Wijers, M., Gallace, A., & Spence, C. (2008). Psychologically induced cooling of a specific body part caused by the illusory ownership of an artificial counterpart. *Proceedings of the National Academy of Sciences, 105*(35), 13169–13173.

Petkova, V. I., Khoshnevis, M., & Ehrsson, H. H. (2011). The perspective matters! Multisensory integration in ego-centric reference frames determines full-body ownership. *Frontiers in Psychology, 2*, 35.

Petkova, V. I., Zetterberg, H., & Ehrsson, H. H. (2012). Rubber hands feel touch, but not in blind individuals. *PLoS One, 7*(4), e35912.

Preston, C. (2013). The role of distance from the body and distance from the real hand in ownership and disownership during the rubber hand illusion. *Acta Psychologica, 142*(2), 177–183.

Preston, C., & Newport, R. (2012). How long is your arm? Using multisensory illusions to modify body image from the third person perspective. *Perception, 41*(2), 247–249.

Röder, B., Rösler, F., & Spence, C. (2004). Early vision impairs tactile perception in the blind. *Current Biology, 14*, 121–124.

Röder, B., Kusmierek, A., Spence, C., & Schicke, T. (2007). Developmental vision determines the reference frame for the multisensory control of action. *Proceedings of the National Academy of Sciences, 104*, 4753–4758.

Rohde, M., Di Luca, M., & Ernst, M. O. (2011). The rubber hand illusion: Feeling of ownership and proprioceptive drift do not go hand in hand. *PLoS One, 6*(6), e21659.

Sutherland, I. E. (1965). The ultimate display. *Proceedings of IFIP, 65*(2), 506–508.

Tajadura-Jiménez, A., Tsakiris, M., Marquardt, T., & Bianchi-Berthouze, N. (2014). *Action sounds change the mental representation of arm length: Effects of kinaesthesia and sense of agency.* Poster presentation at the 15th International Multisensory Research Forum, Amsterdam, The Netherlands, 10th–14th June 2014.

Ter Horst, A. C., Van Lier, R., & Steenbergen, B. (2011). Spatial dependency of action simulation. *Experimental Brain Research, 212*(4), 635–644.

Tsakiris, M., & Haggard, P. (2005). The rubber hand illusion revisited: Visuotactile integration and self-attribution. *Journal of Experimental Psychology. Human Perception and Performance, 31*(1), 80–91.

Vuilleumier, P., Valenza, N., Mayer, E., Reverdin, A., & Landis, T. (1998). Near and far visual space in unilateral neglect. *Annals of Neurology, 43*(3), 406–410.

Yamamoto, S., & Kitazawa, S. (2001). Reversal of subjective temporal order due to arm crossing. *Nature Neuroscience, 4*, 759–765.

Yuan, Y., & Steed, A. (2010). Is the rubber hand illusion induced by immersive virtual reality? In *Virtual reality conference (VR), 2010 IEEE* (pp. 95–102).

Chapter 11
Videogames for Players with Visual Disabilities

Jaime Sánchez

Introduction

For people who are blind, navigation through unfamiliar spaces can be a complex task compared to a sighted person. To achieve orientation and mobility (O&M) (Konstantinosa et al., 2015; Sánchez & Tadres, 2010), people who are blind need to use other resources to receive feedback from the environment, such as sounds and textures.

If children who are blind do not receive orientation and mobility instruction, blindness will be synonymous with difficulty in navigation. According to Goldman (1969), it is necessary to establish navigation training programs to allow people who are blind, as soon as possible, to become aware of their body, experience new situations causing actions related to spatial knowledge and awareness of its location in space that may become complex, and thus move independently.

As the collection of environmental information in people who are blind is based on different sensory channels than sight, the integration of this information is different when creating mental representations of the environment (Aubert et al., 2022). For example, learning the environment through touch means having to rely on sequential observations and building a mental image from its components and not from the whole (Anirudha et al., 2015; Pawluk et al., 2015; Agrawal & Singh, 2020).

This sequential capture coming from touch contrasts with identification by sight, which allows sighted people an identification of the objects and space more quickly. However, da Silveira Nunes and Lomonaco (2008) point out that the perception of space and objects by the person who is blind occurs by joining tactile sensations, kinesthetic, and auditory allied to mental experiences already made by that person.

J. Sánchez (✉)
Center for Advanced Research in Education CARE & Department of Education, University of Chile, Santiago, Chile
e-mail: jsanchezi@uchile.cl

E. Brooks, D. J. Brown (eds.), *Virtual Reality Games for Rehabilitation*, Virtual Reality Technologies for Health and Clinical Applications,
https://doi.org/10.1007/978-1-0716-3371-7_11

The lack of vision, by itself, is not an impediment to development, but requires different forms of interaction and learning for the construction of knowledge and the development of skills such as orientation and mobility (Zhao et al., 2018; Siu et al., 2020; Crandall & Karado, 2021).

In general, people with visual disabilities, properly trained, can navigate and have a representation of the environment (Façanha et al., 2020; Williams et al., 2014). In the case of children who are blind, whose learning process of O&M skills is in development, it may be difficult to process spatial information if they have not had enough experience to determine their own position and relationship to objects using the rest of their senses through virtual environments. Also, children who are blind can become familiar with real-life, unfamiliar, closed spaces before physically navigating them (Giudice et al., 2020; Guerreiro et al., 2019, 2020). The user's interaction with these virtual environments can occur through spatialized sound- and audio-based interfaces (Sánchez & Elías, 2007; Sánchez et al., 2009, 2010b) and/or through haptic-based interfaces (Sánchez & Espinoza, 2011; Sánchez & Mascaró, 2011; Sánchez et al., 2010a). During this interaction, the user receives information from the virtual environment that facilitates his navigation through these spaces in the real world, as the experiences enhance the user's orientation and mobility skills (Lahav & Mioduser, 2008a, b; Sánchez & Espinoza, 2011).

In addition to this, serious videogames contribute significantly to the development of various cognitive abilities in both sighted and visually impaired learners (Sánchez & Elias, 2007; Sánchez & Espinoza, 2011; Sánchez et al., 2010a, b; Yuan, 2009; Yuan & Folmer, 2008).

Based on this, it is relevant to research how the development of O&M skills is fomented in learners who are blind, through tools that integrate the characteristics of serious videogames and virtual environments. This chapter presents the design, implementation, and cognitive impact evaluation of three audio- and haptic-based videogames for learners who are blind. The objective of these videogames was to develop O&M skills in learners who are blind, supporting the construction of a mental map of the virtual space navigated through the integration of its audio and haptic components.

Related Work

If real-life surroundings are represented through virtual environments, it is possible to create several training applications that allow a user who is blind to interact with the elements in the simulated environment during navigation (Sánchez et al., 2009, 2010b). Videogames, when integrated with virtual training environments, represent an important tool for the development of various abilities and O&M skills (Squire, 2003; Steinkuehler, 2004). For example, AbES (Sánchez et al., 2009, 2010b) allows the creation of videogames that integrate virtual environments, focused on the mental construction of real and fictitious environments by users who are blind navigating through virtual environments, using the keyboard of a computer to execute actions and receive audio feedback to support O&M.

Various virtual environments have been designed to train people who are blind and to assist them with the development of O&M skills (Lahav & Mioduser, 2008a; Lumbreras & Sánchez, 1999; Sánchez et al., 2009). To navigate through an environment, it is necessary to have access to the information that can be recovered from the environment, to then filter out useful information in a way that is coherent and comprehensible for whoever needs it. It is for this reason that in the case of people who are blind, the use of virtual environments and appropriate interfaces allows them to improve their O&M skills (Sánchez et al., 2010a). These kinds of interfaces can be, for example, haptics or audio based. Such resources can also be used for recreational purposes.

Overall blind children learn their environment using their own perception and experience. A factor in this learning is the motivation to interact with the environment and explore their physical properties (Warren, 1994). It is suggested that from early age they receive O&M training to develop skills that enable them to travel safely and efficiently.

It is also possible to allow for a user, either blind or sighted, to interact with a software program or videogame by using the movement of his own body as input, increasing the degree of interactivity, and encouraging mobility (Lange et al., 2010). MOVA3D is a videogame in which a real-life, closed space is represented virtually, through which the user navigates by turning around his own axis, over a specially adapted carpet that detects movement (Sánchez et al., 2010a).

Haptic interfaces have come to represent a significant contribution to the cognitive development of learners who are blind. There is previous evidence from work with interfaces that provide force feedback by using different technologies and provide the user with differing haptic sensations, generating a higher degree of realism in the user's interaction with virtual environments (Sánchez, 2008). Using Novint Falcon and Sensable Phantom haptic devices, a learner who is blind can recognize surfaces, objects, and graphics by just using his hands (Lutz, 2006; Sánchez & Espinoza, 2011; Sánchez & Mascaró, 2011; Yu & Brewster, 2002). In this way, the user receives haptic feedback, which allows him to recognize objects, walls, and hallways in the virtual environment (Lahav & Mioduser, 2004, 2008a, b; Sánchez & Espinoza, 2011; Sánchez & Mascaró, 2011).

A simple and low-cost way to detect the user's movement is to utilize the Wiimote controller of the Nintendo Wii console, and specifically there is evidence of a "finger-tracking" system by using the Wiimote (Williams, 2010). Research has also been done regarding the use of virtual environments that people who are blind can explore by using Nintendo Wii devices, with audio and haptic feedback, facilitating and supporting the construction of cognitive maps and spatial strategies (Evett et al., 2009). As such, it is relevant to research the development and use of serious videogames based on audio and haptic interfaces that integrate virtual training environments in which users who are blind interact through their own body movement, allowing for the development of O&M skills.

Due to the impossibility of obtaining information through sight, people who are blind must employ other senses, such as touch, to be able to perceive their surroundings (Lutz, 2006). In this way, it has been possible to establish two categories of perceptions used by people who are blind (Ballesteros, 1993): (i) tactile perception, which is information perceived exclusively by the skin, and (ii) kinesthetic perception, which is information provided by muscles and tendons. The combination of both concepts, to benefit a person who is blind regarding the acquisition of information, is called haptic perception (Ballesteros, 1993; Oakley et al., 2000).

Jütte (2008) discusses the use of haptic perception in health-related applications, citing, for example, the development of prostheses for patients with spinal cord injuries, which can result in an extended reach of the human hand. In the case of people who are blind, it is possible to simulate, through a virtual environment, a return to what was originally based on visual channels, providing a perception of space as the user interacts with the application.

Unlike the sense of sight, the functionality of haptic perception lays in the codification of the various properties of elements, objects, and substances such as hardness, texture, temperature, and weight. Such properties are difficult to quantify through the sense of sight (Travieso, 2007).

Haptic interfaces have been provided using devices that can create feedback through interaction with muscles and tendons (Lahav & Mioduser, 2008b). This provides for the feeling of applying force over a certain object (Lahav & Mioduser, 2008b). More recently, research on haptic interfaces has become increasingly relevant, and the use of the Novint Falcon device with videogames for training and rehabilitation has enjoyed growing attention (Reuters, 2009). This device is reasonably useful for representing virtual environments and provides force feedback in such a way that when it is used the user can feel the volume and force of a virtual object in his hand (Sánchez et al., 2009).

In most of these systems, information is sought intentionally by the user that touches a game object (active touch) rather than receiving it unintentionally (passive touch).

Several studies (GauBert et al., 2011, 2012; Heller et al., 2001; Norman et al., 2004) have sought to compare vision with haptic perception, showing that for the perception of properties that are visible, such as a bumpy texture or porosity, haptic perception is able to match or even overcome visual perception in terms of specificity (Travieso, 2007; Hu et al., 2006) and match it in the spatial perception of objects (Rosa & Ochaita, 1993). From this it can be gathered that the use of haptic perception is feasible as an alternative form of providing contextual information on volumes and objects (Sarmiento, 2003).

Diverse studies have been presented that include the use of haptic perception by people who are blind in various contexts (De Felice et al., 2005; Homa et al., 2009; Huang, 2009; Murphy et al., 2007; Yu et al., 2000; Yu et al., 2003). In the context of O&M, one study is that of Lahav and Mioduser (2002), who present and evaluate an application that allows for the construction of a virtual environment based on the design of a layout formed by using geometric shapes. Once the design phase has been concluded, the user who is blind can interact with the virtual environment thanks to the use of a haptic device. The user takes on an aerial perspective of the environment, for which reason the feedback that the user receives is equivalent to having a hard model of the environment and tracing possible paths by using a pencil, in which collisions are transmitted through the sense of touch (Lahav & Mioduser, 2002). The use of haptic perception as a strategy for understanding visual information was also discussed by Kim (2010), who points to the importance of the idea that the heterogeneous needs of users must be considered in the design of assisted technology. This author researches the individual differences between various users' capacities for the use of haptic perception, mainly related to age differences and visual disability. She also discusses more accessible and applicable design approaches for users with visual disability based on haptic user interfaces.

Another alternative for providing information to people who are blind is through audio-based interfaces. Using audio-based cues, a person who is blind is encouraged to perceive sounds, interpret them, and convert them into guidelines for its orientation in space and to be able to locate objects of interest in the same way as a sighted person (Crossan & Brewster, 2006). This kind of interface requires careful design, as it is necessary to assure that the end user does not feel saturated by an excessive amount of information (Loomis et al., 2005). One example of audio-based virtual environments can be seen in the videogame AbES (Sánchez et al., 2009). This videogame expands on the concept of the fictitious corridors used in its predecessor AudioDoom (Lumbreras & Sánchez, 1999), to generate an audio-based virtual representation of real environments, thus serving as a videogame that allows for O&M training (Sánchez et al., 2009). Together with a three-dimensional interface, the use of audio allows to increase the potential for various forms of interaction between the user and the computer. Frauenberger and Noisternig (2003) present an audio-based virtual reality system that allows the user to explore a virtual environment using only his sense of hearing. Jain (2012) performed empirical evaluations of various approaches through which spatial information on the environment is transmitted using audio cues. Audio-based applications are also being developed for mobile devices with users who are blind as the target audience. One example of this is a puzzle game in which the pieces with images originally used for puzzles are replaced with randomized musical patterns (Carvalho et al., 2012).

Audio- and Haptic-Based Videogames

MovaWii

MovaWii was proposed based on these interface elements, consisting of the virtual representation of a real-life plaza through audio and haptic interfaces, in which a learner who is blind has the objective of finding a lost jewel by using the Wiimote controllers.

In navigating through a virtual plaza searching for the jewel, the learner must be able to avoid various obstacles in addition to sectors that are off limits. To find the jewel, the player can consult a compass, which indicates in which direction the jewel is located. To change direction, the learner must stand and turn about his own axis to the degree considered necessary, and the game automatically detects the player's change in direction.

MovaWii was developed using C# language and .NET Framework 4.0, through Microsoft Visual Studio 2010 Ultimate development environment. To integrate the characteristics of the Wiimote controller into the videogame, the WiimoteLib v1.7 library was utilized.

Interfaces

Audio Interface The audio interface consists of a set of iconic sounds associated with the objects and actions performed by the user. Every time the user moves forward, a sound representing a step is heard; similarly, when the player bumps into objects or obstacles, a sound representative of a collision is heard. In order to provide the player with an audio clue regarding the location of the jewel, an alarm sound is used that increases in volume as the players gets closer to the jewel and decreases in volume as the players moves farther away from it. In addition, there is a component of recorded speech using AT&T's free web Text-to-Speech engine. These recorded speech phrases are used to indicate to the player the direction in which the jewel is located when he consults the compass. Also, speech was recorded that is used to provide feedback regarding the relative direction in which the player has advanced compared to the previous direction in which the player had moved.

Haptic Interface This consists of vibration feedback provided by the Wiimote controller that the player holds in his hand and which acts as a cane for the user who is blind. Every time the player bumps into an object, he feels an intermittent vibration in his hand. In addition, when the player moves his hand and no longer holds the controller in the position of the "cane" (at least 45° between the axis of the body and that of the arm), he feels a continuous vibration in his hand to alert him that the cane is not in an appropriate position for use.

Graphic Interface This interface was designed so that a facilitator (an aide who provides on-site support during the interaction with the videogame) can observe the player's location when navigating through the virtual environment. The interface consists of a bird's-eye view of the virtual space (see Fig. 11.1), in which it is possible to distinguish the navigable areas (beige-colored areas in Fig. 11.1) and non-navigable areas (all that is not beige) in the plaza represented by the game, in addition to the user's position and direction at any given moment (red dot), as well as the location of the jewel (yellow dot).

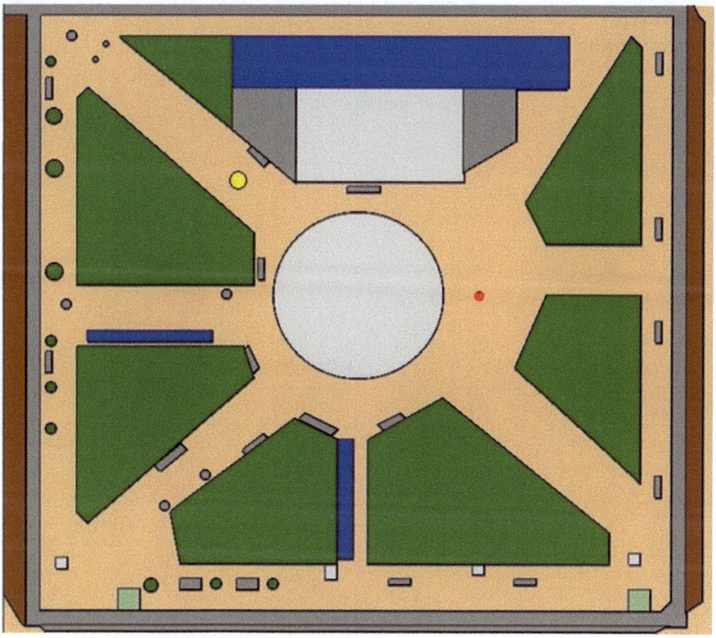

Fig. 11.1 Graphic interface of the videogame

Interaction

The videogame virtually represents a real, physical place, through which learners who are blind must navigate to find a lost jewel. This real-life, physical place consists of a plaza that is made up of navigable sectors, sectors that are off limits, and obstacles such as trees, playground equipment, light posts, and benches. To model the virtual environment, two public plazas were used: the Ovalle Plaza in Santiago, Chile, and the Plaza Izidor Handler in Viña del Mar, Chile. These plazas were diagrammed and scaled with their respective components, to incorporate them into the videogame. It is important to point out that as part of the videogame's design, the grass was considered as an obstacle (or restricted area), to limit the learners' movements. This allows learners who are blind to navigate only over the graveled and paved paths, as in each of the respective plazas such paths are clearly demarcated.

To navigate through the physical surroundings, a user has to use the clock orientation system (Sánchez & Elías, 2007), turning around his own axis according to the indications provided by the software. To detect the user's turns, a wireless bar with infrared LEDs was utilized together with a Wiimote controller (see Fig. 11.2). The Wiimote controller hangs from the ceiling in the room where the software is utilized, so that the infrared detection area is facing downwards. The user must stand directly below the controller, wearing a jacket that has the wireless infrared bar attached to the back. In this way when the user turns, the infrared LEDs turn with him, and the Wiimote controller detects the variation in the position of the infrared

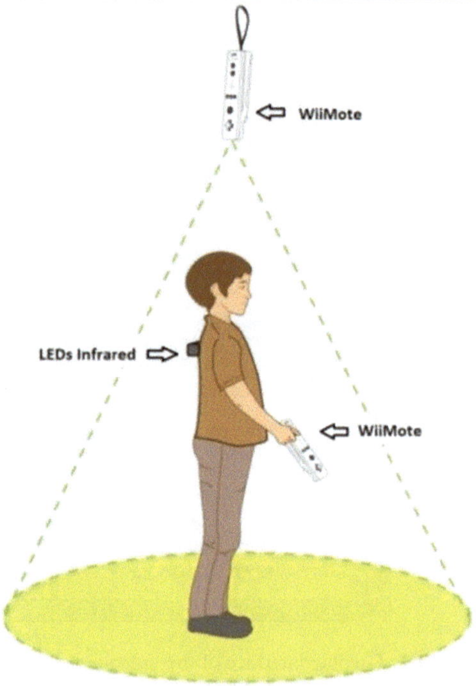

Fig. 11.2 Hardware montage to interact with the videogame

LEDs. To aid the user in determining the correct position in which it is necessary to stand, a plastic circle was placed on the floor that serves as a guide to demarcate the space where the players must stand in order to be appropriately detected by the Wiimote controller.

In addition the use of a second Wiimote controller was incorporated, which the player holds in his hand and uses like a cane for users who are blind (see Fig. 11.2). Using two specific buttons (the A and B buttons), the user can consult the compass (obtaining a clue regarding the clock direction to which he must turn in order to find the jewel) and move forward a step in the user's current direction (direction that is detected by the other Wiimote based on the position of the LEDs). It is important to point out that these actions can only be performed if the learner is holding the Wiimote controller at an angle that is like the common use of a cane (at least 45°, between the axis of the body and that of the arm).

Audio Haptic Maze

Audio Haptic Maze (AHM) is a videogame based on AbES (Sánchez et al., 2009) and was designed for use by users who are blind either autonomously or with the supervision of a facilitator in contexts of research and practice. The game includes the use of both audio- and haptic-based interfaces that can be used together or separately. AHM is a first-person videogame in which the user must escape from a maze. To fulfill the mission, the player must find treasure chests dispersed throughout several corridors and rooms in the maze, which contain keys and treasures. The keys have geometric shapes that correspond to certain doors in the maze. The user must pick them up and try them out one at a time, until he identifies which key can be used to open the doors needed to get out of the maze. To add another entertaining component to the game, the score of the game increases with each treasure that the player finds. The time that the player takes to get out of the maze is also a factor, in which the shorter amount of time taken implies a higher score.

The videogame was developed utilizing C++ language in the Microsoft Visual Studio .NET 2010 development environment, in which GLUT libraries were used for the graphic display, OpenAL was utilized for the use of spatial audio, and the SDK of the Novint Falcon was used to generate haptic feedback.

Interfaces

AHM includes different interfaces to provide feedback to the user and information to the facilitator.

Audio Interface The audio interface is utilized by the user who is blind. AHM uses spatialized sound to represent the ambience of the corridors. For example, if the user has a corridor to the left, he can hear an ambience sound through the left-hand channel. The same kind of interaction is possible with other objects such as doors and keys, which are also represented by certain audio cues. All the actions in the virtual environment have a particular sound cue associated to them. For example, if the user walks, a step sound cue can be heard. Examples of other possible actions are to bump into an object, turn in a specific direction, and pick up an object. In addition to this audible feedback, verbal audio is used to indicate certain situations. For example, when the user picks up a key, the context of the game changes, and the user is informed through verbal audio so that he can now listen to a sequence of beeps indicating the number of vertices on the key.

Through the audio description, the system transmits information on the environment that would normally be understood visually in real time. This procedure aids the users in creating points of reference that help him to determine places and objects, as well as the distribution of these objects throughout the virtual environment. Based on this information, the user can construct a mental map of the AHM environment.

Haptic Interface The haptic interface is utilized by the user who is blind. By using the haptic device, the user can control a 3D cursor inside the virtual environment. All of the audio-based feedback is emulated by using haptics. Thus, haptic textures are used to represent distinct objects on the map, so if the user touches a wall with the 3D cursor, the haptic feedback of that object's texture will be different compared to that associated with touching a door. Also, the user will be able to identify shapes

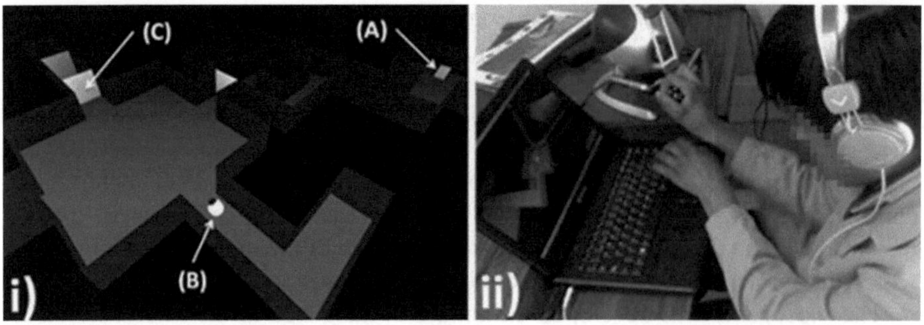

Fig. 11.3 (i) AHM graphic interface, used by the facilitator. (ii) A user who is blind interacting with the videogame

within the map. Regarding the feedback for actions, like walking or turning left or right, force feedback is applied, such as a vibration in the direction of the user's movement. In this way, if the user decides to walk forward, there is a vibration to the front and corresponding vibrations to either side if the user turns left or right. In this way, the audio-based information is complemented by haptic perception, facilitating the user's interaction with the system/environment.

Graphic Interface The graphic interface, used by the facilitator, represents the current state of the game, using a third person perspective to show where the user who is blind is in real time. Figure 11.3.i represents a screenshot of the graphic interface of AHM with the elements that can be found on the map, in which (A) represents a treasure chest, which can have a key or a treasure inside; (B) represents the character controlled by the user; and (C) represents a door in the maze.

Interaction

The interaction with the videogame is carried out using a standard computer keyboard, a Novint Falcon haptic device, and earphones (see Fig. 11.3, ii).

In the case of the audio-based interface, the entirety of the user's immersion is achieved using stereo sound, in order to provide information regarding the location of objects, such as walls and doors, in the virtual environment. In this way, the user can create a mental model of the spatial dimensions of the environment. In navigating, the user can interact with each of the previously mentioned elements, and each of these elements provides feedback that helps the user to become oriented in the environment.

The Novint Falcon device was used for haptic feedback, which works as a three-dimensional pointer that allows for an interaction with 3D volumes, generating force feedback.

Audiopolis

The Audiopolis videogame was designed to represent in principle any urban environment for navigation by blind learners. This environment can be real or fictitious, being relevant in that a person who is blind can experience the space to better understand it. Various elements and co-experiencing components of a city can be included in the environment such as streets, opens spaces, and buildings. In Audiopolis, a bank, museum, jewelry store, hospital, restaurant, shops, city hall, parks, plazas, library, bookstore, school, university, hotel, supermarket, houses, apartment, and office buildings can all be included in the virtual environment.

The videogame was developed with C++ programming language using the Visual Studio 2010 development software. To program the audio routines the OpenAl Utility Toolkit (ALUT) was utilized which requires the use of the OpenAl library. For graphic representation, the OpenGl library was used. Finally, for haptic modeling, the Novint Falcon Hdal library was used.

Interfaces

The videogame possesses three interface options for interaction (haptic, audio, and haptic plus audio) which operate in combination with the graphic interface. The latter graphic interface is designed for use by the facilitators that support the experiment.

Audio Interface This interface has two main modes: environmental and instructive. The environmental component consists of a set of sounds that simulate both the indoor and outdoor environments in which the player is located. It also serves to provide information that allows learners to recognize the shapes of different geometric objects. The instructive component is made up of questions that provide clues and the instructions from the main menu, such as quit, save game, etc. In addition, during the game the player can query his or her current position or ask for the direction in which he or she is facing. All of this is answered through the audio interface.

Haptic Interface The Novint Falcon device was used as a haptic-based interface. With this device, we sought to simulate haptic information that could be obtained through direct touch (i.e., with the hands) and indirect touch (i.e., with a cane). The force feedback generated by the Falcon provides information regarding the physical characteristics of the place where the user is located. As the player moves about through the city (by pressing the arrow keys on the device and by dragging the cane on the floor to feel different textures that signal different paths), the user can find his or her way on a route with different levels. The player can also identify objects (e.g., a cube) by exploring their shape using the device. In this case, an object is modeled in 3D and the haptic control simulates a hand.

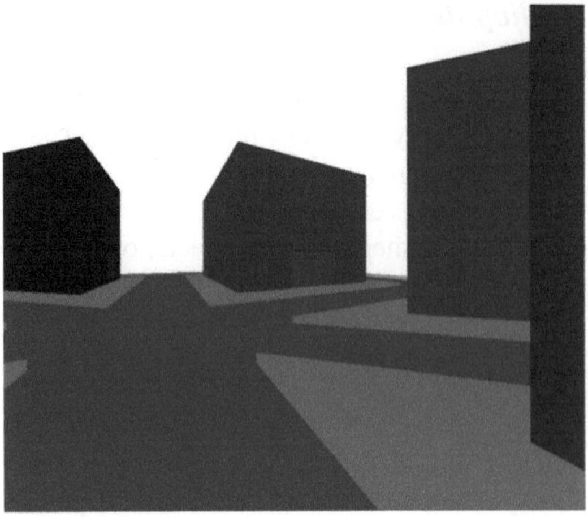

Fig. 11.4 Graphic interface of audiopolis

Haptic and Audio Interface This interface combines the two previously mentioned sensory inputs to provide the user with more robust information regarding position and to provide more ample support for navigation tasks.

Graphic Interface This interface represents a high contrast rendering of the virtual environment so that the facilitator can observe where and at what point in the game the blind learner is and help the user if necessary (see Fig. 11.4).

Interaction

The videogame is played from a first-person perspective. The user can move freely throughout the environment, including forward, backward, and turning left and right. The user recognizes the various surfaces through which he is traveling either through audio or haptic feedback, as well as the various obstacles while moving through the virtual city. Through virtual exploration, the users can familiarize themselves with the entire map and established routes.

Turn angles of 30° were defined as well as a standard length of each step taken as the user moves through the environment.

The game consists of three different levels of difficulty: easy, medium, and advanced. These different levels are determined by the degree of difficulty of the geography of the corresponding virtual city. To do this, the city was divided into three sectors. Level 1 considers tasks in sector 1. Level 2 considers tasks in sectors 1 and 2. Finally, level 3 considers tasks in sectors 1, 2, and 3 (see Fig. 11.5). Each level implies a gradually more difficult access, presenting streets with different addresses and having available a wider number of buildings to explore.

For each level, the map of the city expands out on four sides, leaving more free space for the player to move about. In addition, the map integrates new elements that increase the level of complexity as the user moves through the environment.

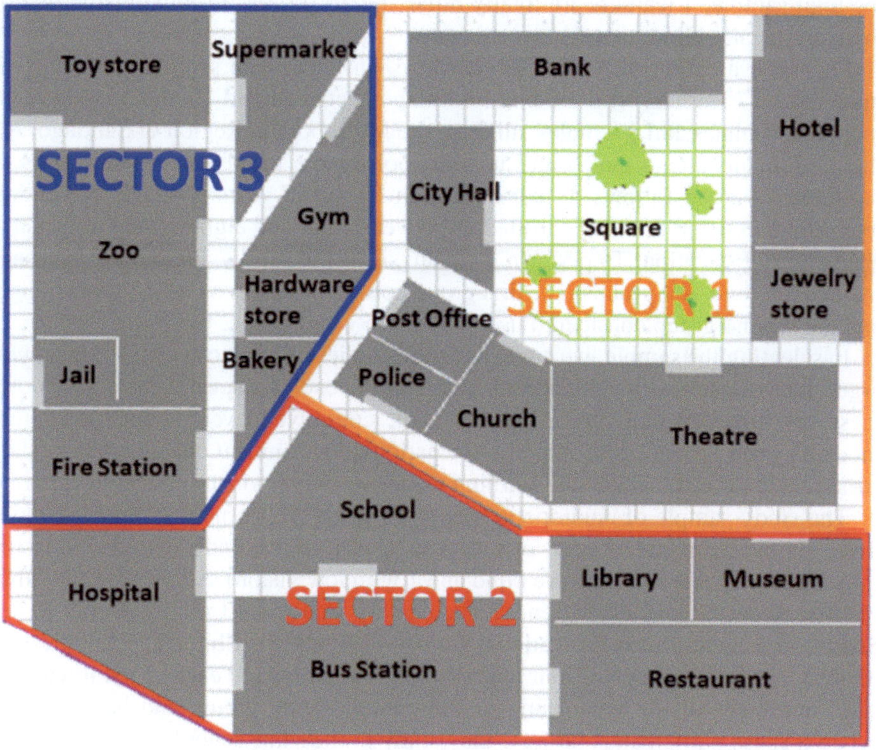

Fig. 11.5 Audiopolis level map

There are three stages within each level. In each stage a thief steals an object, and the goal of the game is to find the thief. In each stage, the player begins at the scene of the crime and must find three different places within the city while "chasing" the thief. The player must also solve a series of questions that are presented to receive the next clue and continue moving throughout the city. Once the stolen object has been found, the player passes on to the next stage.

Cognitive Evaluation

Sample

The sample selected for the use of MovaWii was made up of 20 learners (7 female; 13 male), in which 11 of them are between 6 and 8 years old, from the first years of primary school at the Santa Lucia Educational Center in the city of Santiago de Chile. The 9 remaining users are between 9 and 15 years old, from primary school at the Antonio Vicente Mosquete Institute in the city of Viña del Mar, Chile. Among the total sample, 4 learners are totally blind and 16 possess residual vision. All of them are legally blind.

For the evaluation of Audio Haptic Maze, an intentional sample was selected, made up of 7 learners who are blind with ages between and 10 and 15 years old, including 4 males and 3 females, all from the Metropolitan Region of Santiago. All the participants attend the Santa Lucia School for the Blind. The requirements to participate were as follows: 1. being between 10 and 15 years of age, 2. presenting total blindness, and 3. being enrolled in between third and eighth grade of General Elementary Education. To perform the analysis of the results, the sample was segmented into two user groups. The first group considered users of 10–12 years of age, and the second group considered users of 13–15 years of age.

In selecting the sample, we considered the studies of Espinosa et al. (1998), who argue that the spatial knowledge of a person depends on several factors. Among these are the personal characteristics (age, cognitive development, perceptual modality used for encoding spatial information), environment characteristics (size, structure), and factors related to learning processes in relation to spatial information.

The study sample of Audiopolis was made up of 12 learners (8 females and 4 males) between 10 and 15 years of age, with special educational needs due to visual impairment (11 learners who are blind and 1 with low vision). All were from within the first or second cycles of General Elementary Education from the Helen Keller School and Santa Lucia Educational Center in Santiago, Chile. The sample was divided into three groups of four learners and randomized to each of the three possible interfaces of the videogame (audio group, haptic group, and haptic+audio group). These participants, because they study in the same schools, take part in the same methods to teach people who are blind to construct spatial concepts.

Instruments

The instruments of evaluation utilized were created by a group of special education teachers who specialize in children who are blind and are integrated members of the research team.

Evaluation Guidelines for O&M Skills (MovaWii)

This is an evaluation instrument that serves for the gathering of data and the collection of information regarding O&M skills. The Evaluation Guidelines was utilized as both a pre-test and post-test during the study and is made up of five dimensions: sensory-perceptual development, psychomotor development, development of techniques without mobility aides, development of initial cane techniques, and development of concepts. In order to evaluate these dimensions, 40 items were evaluated on a scale from 0 to 2, in which 0 implies that the item was not achieved (NA), or that the learner was unable to perform the requested behavior; a value of 1 corresponds to an item in process (IP), or that the behavior requested of the learner was inconsistent; and a value of 2 corresponds to an achieved item (A), which implies that the learner performed the requested behavior successfully.

The dimensions measured by the Evaluation Guidelines for O&M Skills are:

Sensory-Perceptual Development Made up of the subdimensions audio sensory-perceptual development and tactile kinesthetic sensory-perceptual development. These dimensions allowed the researchers to measure the development of audio senses (audio recognition and discrimination, origin of sounds, direction and following of sounds) and tactile senses (recognition of textures, perception of obstacles).

Psychomotor Development This dimension allowed researchers to measure motor activities regarding O&M, in addition to navigation through real and virtual spaces.

Development of Techniques Without Mobility Aides This dimension allowed researchers to measure the use of information that can be extracted autonomously from the environment and which depends on the user's own behavior and the way in which the information is used for mobility.

Development of Initial Cane Techniques This dimension allowed researchers to measure the learners' skills in using the mobility cane as an aide for navigating through open or closed, real or virtual environments.

Development of Concepts Made up of the subdimensions development of geometric concepts, development of spatial concepts, development of environmental concepts, and development of temporal concepts. These dimensions allowed the researchers to measure the conceptualization of parameters and concepts needed to attend to and understand instructions, actions, and situations within the virtual environment and later in the real-life environment.

Questionnaire (MovaWii)

This is an evaluation instrument made up of five questions: (1) What did you like about today's activities? (2) What did you not like about today's activities? (3) What was difficult for you to do? Why? (4) What was easy for you to do? Why? (5) What did you learn today? The criteria considered for the construction of these questions were satisfaction with the intervention, which is related to questions 1 and 2; complexity of the intervention, which is related to questions 3 and 4; and learning from the intervention, which is related to question 5.

This questionnaire was administered after each cognitive task solved by the user, by reading the questions to them and recording their responses. The purpose of this instrument was to collect the learners' opinions regarding the experience of their interactions with the videogame interfaces.

Evaluation Guideline for Transfer from Virtual to the Real-World Environment (MovaWii)

This is an instrument to support the observation of the activity designed to transfer what was achieved in the virtual experience to the real-world environment. In this guideline, the same dimensions from the Evaluation Guidelines for O&M skills were used. However, this guideline is made up of some additional items (44 in total), which were used to evaluate these dimensions on a scale of 0 to 2 points, in which the values for 0, 1, and 2 correspond to the same criteria described in the Evaluation Guidelines for O&M Skills.

This guideline was administered during the observation of the video recordings that were made of all the movements made by each participating user in the corresponding plaza, according to the version of the videogame that they worked with. The Evaluation Guideline for Transfer to the Real-World Environment served to demonstrate the transfer of the lessons and tasks learned by the users during the virtual interaction with the videogame to their navigation through the real plaza.

O&M Skills Checklist (Audio Haptic Maze)

In order to study the degree of the videogame's impact, together with the cognitive tasks performed, on the development of the participants' O&M-related skills, an O&M skills checklist was created for children with visual disability between 10 and 15 years of age. The validation of the instruments was performed by these teachers applying the O&M skills checklist to users who are blind other than those involved in the sample, to detect errors in comprehension and the measurement of results.

This evaluative instrument was applied individually to each user at the beginning and at the end of the cognitive intervention, in order to determine in what way the use of the videogame had affected the development of O&M skills. The dimensions contained within this instrument are:

Sensory Perception The perception of information through the auditory and haptic channels is evaluated, considering the fact that sensory capacities are the primary functions that are developed to pick up on, integrate, and react to information and stimulus from the environment.

Tempo-Spatial Development The users' knowledge regarding their position in space is evaluated, in being able to understand the distribution and location in space of various elements based on their own bodies, while at the same time being able to establish a relation between these aspects to navigate through the space.

O&M Skills The skills regarding navigation based on O&M training is evaluated, either through use of the cane as a technical aide to detect obstacles in the environment or not. The purpose of this was to show whether the users can navigate both real and virtual environments based on these techniques, thus validating them for facilitating and strengthening their navigation.

Interviews (Audiopolis)

Two interviews were carried out: one in-depth and the other structured. The in-depth interview was applied to analyze the O&M difficulties that the subjects faced in their daily lives. In addition, it sought to understand how they perceived the contribution of the audio- and haptic-based videogame to the development of their O&M skills. This was determined through statements that were evaluated on an appreciating numeric scale with four frequency categories: never, almost never, sometimes, and always. This information was also complemented by a section with open-ended questions. The objective of the structured interview was to understand the perception that the subjects have of themselves regarding their O&M skills and other variables such as their motivation and self-esteem.

O&M Test (Audiopolis)

The O&M test was designed to estimate the level of knowledge related to this specific area of learning. The dimensions included were (i) sensory development (SD) containing 35 indicators which included the subdimensions audio sensory development (ASD) with 12 indicators and haptic sensory development (HSD) with 23 indicators, (ii) tempo-spatial development dimension (TSD) containing 24 indicators, and (iii) O&M technique (O&MT) dimension containing 12 indicators, grouping together 71 indicators in total. The evaluation criteria for each indicator were Achieved (A), In Process (IP), and Not Achieved (NA), with scores of 2, 1, and 0, respectively.

Tasks

MovaWii Training Tasks

In the first training task, the objective was to incorporate the clock orientation system, which is a metaphor utilized within the O&M training skills and which consists of situating the user within an analogue clock so that directions are associated with the position of the hour hands in which the user turns (see Fig. 11.6). In this way, if it is desired that the learner moves to the right, he is instructed to "turn to 3 o'clock"; if the user is to turn left, he is instructed to "turn to 9 o'clock"; and if it is desired that the user moves backwards, he is instructed to "turn to 6 o'clock."

In the second training task the users interacted with the hardware devices, specifically on exploring and utilizing the Wiimote controller buttons associated with

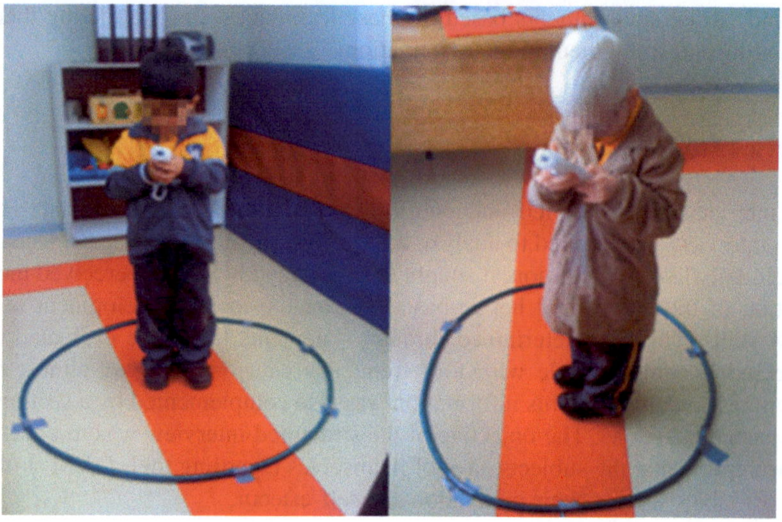

Fig. 11.6 Training activities

certain actions in the virtual environment. Based on these tasks, an experimental laboratory was implemented in a room, consisting of a laptop computer, two Wiimote controller devices, and speakers.

MovaWii Cognitive Tasks

Cognitive tasks 1 and 2 corresponded to the perception of and relation to iconic elements. These tasks consisted of the learners relating the audio and haptic stimuli to actions and/or elements that make up part of the interaction within the videogame, in addition to the use of these clues for moving about through the virtual space.

Cognitive tasks 3 and 4 corresponded to the dynamics of the interaction with the videogame. The objective of these tasks was for the learners to establish a tempo-spatial structuring of the virtual environment and to determine the distances within the virtual plaza regarding the elements that they encounter while navigating.

Cognitive tasks 5, 6, and 7 correspond to navigation activities and the representation of the navigated environments. These tasks were based on the work performed during tasks 1, 2, 3, and 4, with the objective of integrating this knowledge into the planning of navigational routes.

Tasks Regarding the Comprehension of Dynamic Components (Audio Haptic Maze)

These tasks sought to develop and/or strengthen O&M skills in learners who are blind, based on the use of Audio Haptic Maze and its audio- and/or haptic-based interfaces. These tasks were subdivided into:

Integration of Elements In this task, it was sought to integrate each of the audio and/or haptic elements used in the videogame into the user's mental map, to establish the dynamics of the videogame that are related to movement.

Establishment of Distances and Sizes on the Map This task sought to solidify the establishment of the relationship of equivalence between one step and one cell. The maze is made up of a certain number of cells, corresponding both to rooms and hallways. By integrating knowledge of this dynamic, the user can establish distances to doors and keys and can determine the size of the various environments by counting the cells while moving from one place to another.

Directionality and Movement on the Map This task sought to strengthen the establishment of relations between the segments on the map and the direction in which the learners are facing and moving, so that the user can locate the various elements on the map. In addition, players were asked to delimit their movements regarding the direction that they took, mainly in order to verify whether or not they noticed when they moved forwards or backwards or turned in one direction or another.

Composition and Distribution of the Map This task was related to all the map-based sessions and sought to work on the identification of hallways, rooms, elements represented using audio and/or haptics, and the search for these elements based on the character's location on the map.

Map Appropriation and Navigational Tasks (Audio Haptic Maze)

These tasks were centered on establishing a mental representation of the navigated environment based on the videogame's dynamics that strengthen the establishment of relationships useful for orientation and mobility in the virtual space. The maze in the videogame was divided into different sectors (see Fig. 11.7), which determined the following tasks:

Sector A This task sought to establish the number of hallways, rooms, and/or elements available in this area. In addition, it sought to establish the direction of movement, relationships of distance and size pertaining to the elements, hallways, and rooms, to facilitate the formation of movement strategies. Afterwards, each player was asked to represent the space he had navigated with representative material of the elements of the videogame.

Sector B This task had as an objective that through the audio- and/or haptic-based interfaces, the players would move through sector B in the maze, locating the different hallways and elements. After navigating this sector of the maze, each player was asked to represent the space that had been navigated, describing the route taken and the elements that the player had located on that route, in addition to describing whether the user was walking down a hallway or through a room.

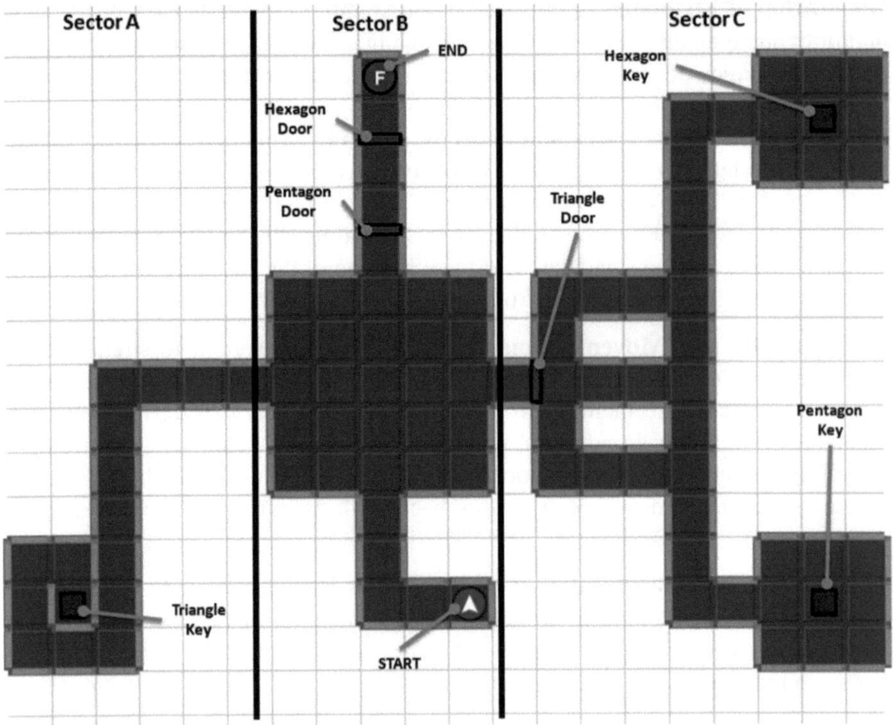

Fig. 11.7 Sectors within the maze of Audio Haptic Maze

Elements and Size Dynamics This task consisted of comprehending the videogame's dynamic regarding the execution of actions and the interaction with various elements in the videogame such as doors and differently shaped keys that could be used to open specific doors. Based on this, the learner had to resolve problems such as inferring the need to find a specific key to open a particular door, understanding if he was walking down a hallway or through a room, determining the number of steps taken when moving about, and based on the latter, establishing the size of the space in which the user is located. In addition, the users had to comprehend the functionality of the Novint Falcon and the buttons on the keypad and learn to orient themselves based on audio and/or haptic cues, to determine and identify the elements within the videogame.

Sectors A, B, and C, Directionality, and Movement The objective of this task was to establish the relationships of movement performed by the player when moving through the three sectors of the maze, using the respective interface assigned to each work group. Each user had to identify each sector (based on characteristics that had already been established during prior navigational exercises) and the directions and elements located both in a hallway and in a room. Once the route had been navigated, each player was asked to represent the space that had been navigated with representative material, requiring knowledge of the number of cells for each hallway and room, and the elements such as intersections, doors, treasure chests, and keys.

Total Navigation of the Map This last task was based on navigating freely throughout the entire maze, applying all the strategies and dynamics involved in the videogame that are needed in order to successfully complete the mission of opening all of the doors and navigating between the three sectors of the virtual environment. In addition, the need to establish the directions in which the learner was moving was emphasized, as well as the need to establish the relationships of size regarding hallways and rooms, the relationship between the audio and haptic elements of the videogame as associated with concrete objects, and the verbal description of everything the player had identified and the routes taken. In this task, the learners were also asked to graphically represent the environment that had been navigated, adding arrows to indicate the directions that had to be followed to move from one sector to another.

Audiopolis Training Tasks

The training tasks were designed to introduce the participants to the concepts and components used in the videogame. The training tasks were (i) clock technique, to learn heading cues used in the videogame; (ii) geometric shapes, to develop the interpretation of the shapes used during the interaction with the videogame; and (iii) the elements of the videogame, to introduce the participant to the integrated use of all the elements involved in the videogame.

Audiopolis Cognitive Tasks

The cognitive tasks were focused on developing specific O&M skills based on the software interface. The cognitive tasks were as follows: (i) level 1, perception and dynamics; (ii) level 1, movement, directionality, and distribution; (iii) level 1, establishment of distances; (iv) level 2, perception and dynamics; (v) level 2, movement, directionality, and distribution; (vi) level 2, establishment of distance; (vii) level 3, perception and dynamics; (viii) level 3, movement, directionality, and distribution; and (ix) level 3, establishment of distances. Furthermore, the total integration of the game level was scored for (x) game 1, (xi) game 2, and (xii) game 3.

The objective of the cognitive tasks is related to the perception of the virtual space through sound, haptics, or both, depending on the interface used. Furthermore, movement, directionality, and distribution were promoted using turns connected to the clock system. In this way, users would learn to perceive places and how these places were in spatial relation to one another. In the case of the cognitive tasks regarding the establishment of distances, the purpose was to work on the structuring of Audiopolis and the relation between steps and distance. This means that a higher number of steps implied a longer distance between one place and another.

Procedure

MovaWii Procedure

Before the intervention with the videogame, the Evaluation Guidelines for O&M Skills instrument was administered to learn of the initial state of each user's O&M skills. Afterwards, two training tasks were performed during independent work sessions in which each task lasted 45 min per learner.

Once the training tasks were performed, the learners performed seven cognitive tasks through the use of the videogame, during 7 different 45-min sessions. Once each of these tasks had been completed, the questionnaire was administered to each learner. After each task, the learners had to represent a mental map of the virtually navigated plaza by using concrete materials (Lego blocks and play dough). In this way, the facilitator was able to demonstrate the users' progress regarding their mental constructions of the social environment represented by the videogame.

Afterwards, a work session was performed with the learners in which the O&M skills instrument was administered to compare the results obtained before having participated in the intervention with the videogame. In this way, it was possible to evaluate the impact that the videogame had on the users' navigation through the virtual environment.

After finalizing these tasks with the use of the videogame and the evaluation of its impact on the learners' navigation through the virtual world, a cognitive task designed for the transfer of the skills learned virtually to the real-world environment was applied (see Fig. 11.8).

To perform this task, the learners were taken to the real-world environment corresponding to the plaza that they had navigated virtually in the videogame. Each learner was asked to replicate the movements and routes navigated in the videogame to complete the requested missions, according to the mental map of the environment that they had constructed based on their experience interacting with the videogame. Each learner's experience was filmed, recording all his movements. Once this activity was completed, the questionnaire was applied to each learner.

Afterwards, each of the video recordings was analyzed to identify and describe various practices and behaviors, successful performances, and difficulties displayed during the movements through the real plaza. To achieve this, the Evaluation Guideline for Transfer to the Real-World Environment was used to support the observation of the recordings. With this information, three main successfully completed tasks were established for each student, as well as the three main tasks that were the most difficult for each learner.

Audio Haptic Maze Procedure

Initially, the O&M skills checklist was applied as a pre-test, in 45-min sessions with each user. During these sessions, the users were provided with a set of materials in order to perform some of the actions required by the instrument (see Fig. 11.9).

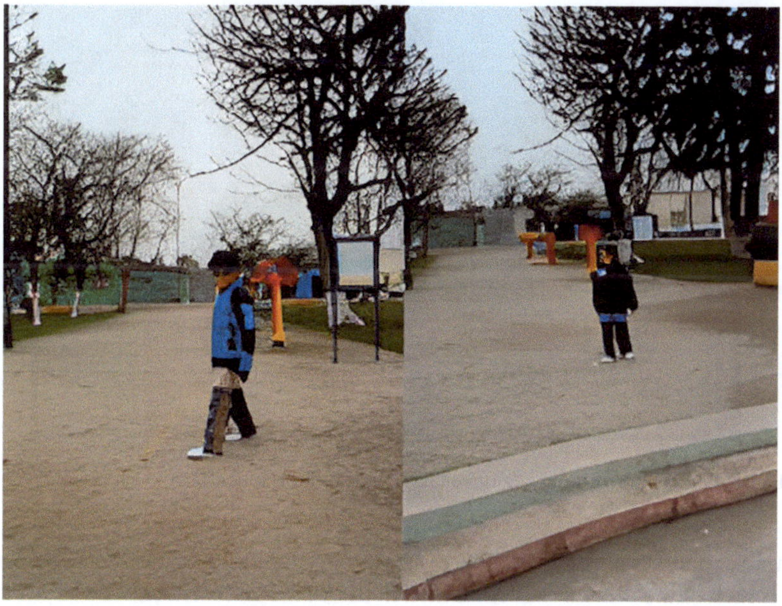

Fig. 11.8 Cognitive task for transfer from virtual to the real-world environment

Fig. 11.9 Activities performed by the user during the pre-test

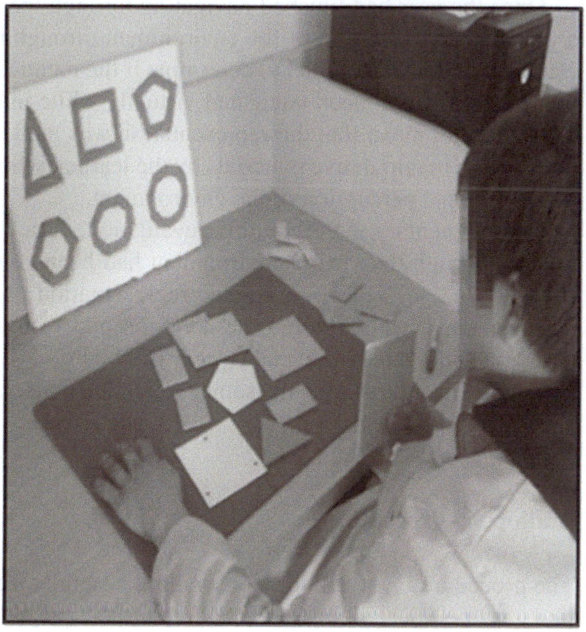

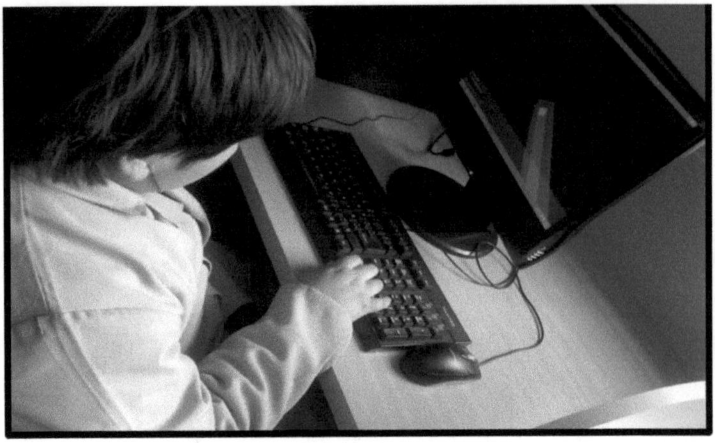

Fig. 11.10 Learner performing cognitive tasks with Audio Haptic Maze

In a second stage, the users performed cognitive tasks using the videogame in which each of the dimensions contained in the O&M skills checklist was worked on (perceptual development, temporal-spatial development, O&M skills) to strengthen the development of these skills by using AHM (see Fig. 11.10). This stage involved a total of twelve, 40-min sessions with each user.

Once the user had finished navigating through the maze, he was asked to create a graphic representation of the environment through representative material of the elements of the videogame, to determine if the mental image created coincided with the spaces that had been navigated virtually while interacting with the videogame. This does not mean that the representation was made through a freehand drawing, but through manipulative materials by the learner, who should place them according to his personal perception of the environment.

Complementary to the cognitive evaluation, during each work session, once navigation through the virtual environment had been completed, each user was asked (in order of age) to form a graphic representation of the virtual environment they had navigated, to determine the adoption and restructuring of the mental model based on audio and haptic cues (see Fig. 11.11).

Finally, in a third stage the same O&M skills checklist used in the first stage was applied as a post-test.

Audiopolis Procedure

The procedure involved all the users in the sample. In addition, two special education teachers specializing in visual impairment played the role of facilitators. These teachers aided the users and recorded their use of the instruments.

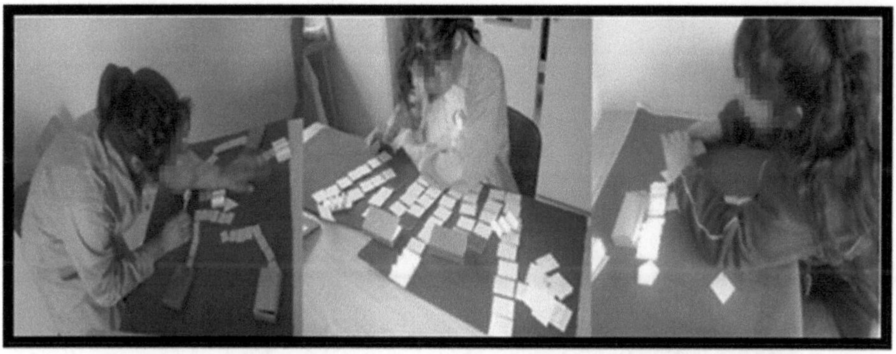

Fig. 11.11 Learners forming graphic representations of the environments navigated

The work was carried out in three stages: (i) initiation, before working with the software; (ii) process, during the development of the activities using the computer games; and (iii) finish, at the end of the process.

In the phase prior to the use of the software, the O&M test was applied as a pre-test to record the subjects' initial baseline skills. Interviews were also conducted with the participants. Afterwards, the users performed the three training tasks related to the skills that they needed to master before using the videogame.

During the process of the intervention with the videogame, the users performed the 12 cognitive tasks taking 1 session per task (see Fig. 11.12). Each session involved carrying out a series of activities according to the previously described dimensions and in accordance with the three levels of complexity included in the videogame.

Finally, in the final stage, the O&M test was applied to the users as a post-test, to determine whether there was any change on the previously evaluated skills.

Results

MovaWii Results

The criteria considered for the construction of the questionnaire were translated into three categories (satisfaction, complexity, and learning), used to classify the users' opinions after having performed the cognitive tasks. As such, 17 common themes were identified among the opinions, which can be associated with the 3 categories for the classification (see Table 11.1).

The students demonstrated great satisfaction with the activities in the videogame, especially looking for the jewel, which is the object used to represent achieving the goal of the videogame (48.1%). Other significant themes for which satisfaction was expressed were the use of the hour hands of the clock as a means for developing the cognitive tasks (37.2%) and the use of the various technologies included in the

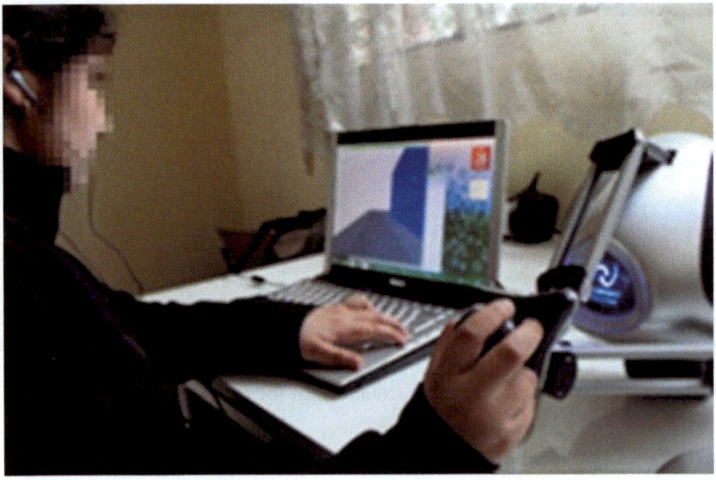

Fig. 11.12 A user performing a cognitive task: playing Audiopolis.

Table 11.1 Percentage frequencies for satisfaction, complexity, and learning during the intervention

Themes	Satisfaction [%]	Complexity [%]	Learning [%]
Looking for the jewel	48.1	9.6	6.4
Finding the jewel	18.6	0.0	3.8
Losing	1.0	0.0	0.0
Using the cane	0.0	1.1	0.0
Turning	17.1	19.3	11.4
Hours on the clock	37.2	25.7	29.2
Walking	6.2	12.8	10.2
Cardinal directions	12.4	9.6	54.6
Technology (WiiMote, jacket)	31.0	10.7	11.4
Playing MovaWii	27.9	0.0	6.4
Everything	7.8	0.0	0.0
Nothing	1.6	17.1	3.8
Representing the map	7.8	0.0	12.7
Bumping into objects	14.0	5.4	3.8
Numbers	3.1	2.1	7.6
Sounds	6.2	0.0	0.0
Use of the compass	0.0	1.1	0.0

initiative, such as the Wiimote used as a cane, the jacket with the infrared LED bar, and the use of the buttons on the Wiimote to make decisions (31.0%).

Regarding the elements that were complicated to use (complexity), the learners displayed a lack of knowledge regarding the hours on the analogue clock (25.7%). As such, the action of "turning" was the second most difficult aspect (19.3%). These two aspects are directly related to the way of using the clock system as a mechanism for spatial location and orientation. The opinion that "nothing" caused any difficulties was expressed in 17.1% of the opinions.

Finally, in the category related to learning, the users valued a set of elements learned throughout the cognitive tasks performed in the intervention. One of these elements corresponds to the cardinal directions (54.6%), which are related to the possibility of identifying north, south, east, and west as references for playing the game and navigating when walking. This theme is followed by learning the hours of the clock (29.2%), which is related to the use of the clock system for O&M. Finally, there is "representation of the map" (12.7%), which corresponds to the capacity to transfer the actions performed in the virtual environment to a physical representation of the desired navigation.

On the other hand, the results obtained from the pre-test and post-test were analyzed using a Student's t-test for related samples, for each of the dimensions contained in the instrument utilized (see Table 11.2).

In comparing the averages obtained for the pre-test and the post-test in the differing dimensions analyzed, it was found that the audio sensory-perceptual development ($t = -3.322, p < 0.05$), technique without mobility aides ($t = -4.841, p < 0.05$), initial cane techniques ($t = -2.629$, $p < 0.05$), geometric concepts ($t = -3.337$, $p < 0.05$), spatial concepts ($t = -3.488$, $p < 0.05$), environmental concepts ($t = -3.107$, $p < 0.05$), and temporal concepts ($t = -2.517$, $p < 0.05$) dimensions presented statistically significant differences, displaying in all cases an increase in the average obtained on the post-test compared to the pre-test.

For the tactile kinesthetic sensory-perceptual development and psychomotor development dimensions, no statistically significant differences were found between the pre-test and post-test.

In performing a global analysis regarding O&M skills, an increase in the average of the post-test was found compared to the pre-test for the Global O&M Skills indicator ($t = -5.697$, $p < 0.05$), and this difference was found to be statistically significant.

Table 11.2 Summary of the statistical Student's t-test results

Indicator	Mean pre-test	Mean post-test	T	p
Audio sensory-perceptual development	1.667	1.883	−3.322	.004
Tactile kinesthetic sensory-perceptual development	1.825	1.800	.252	.804
Psychomotor development	1.900	1.936	−.925	.367
Development of techniques without mobility aides	1.280	1.590	−4.841	.000
Development of initial cane techniques	1.175	1.575	−2.629	.017
Development of geometric concepts	1.163	1.738	−3.337	.003
Development of spatial concepts	1.530	1.750	−3.488	.002
Development of environmental concepts	1.733	2.000	−3.107	.006
Development of temporal concepts	1.850	1.933	−2.517	.021
Global O&M skills	1.602	1.801	−5.697	.000

The increases in the indicators for which the differences are statistically significant show that the videogame and its associated activities influence O&M skills.

Based on the statistical results, a more in-depth analysis of the dimensions for which the increases were statistically significant was performed, incorporating the analysis of the video recordings and the data obtained from the evaluation guidelines for transfer from the virtual to the real-world environment. The analysis of the video recordings was performed in accordance with two criteria: the performances achieved, or those that the learners executed successfully, and the less-achieved performances, or those that the learners did not perform adequately.

In the audio sensory-perceptual development dimension, the results of the statistical analysis indicated that throughout the experience with the use of the interfaces defined for the intervention, aspects such as following direction and discrimination of sounds were improved among the participating students. The analysis of the video recordings showed a transfer of audio sensory-perceptual aspects in the learners' performances during the experience navigating through the real-world plaza, which obtained a 23.5% frequency among the most-achieved performances.

The development of techniques without mobility aides dimension, which corresponds to the skills that learners use to turn and walk in different directions using the clock system (which is to say locating and orienting oneself using the hour hands on a clock as a reference), increased significantly after the interaction with the interfaces included in the intervention experience. During the cognitive task for transfer to the real-world environment, it was observed that the learners showed some difficulties in performing turns (19.3% of the performances less achieved). However, the students pointed to a high degree of learning regarding the cardinal directions and their use as a means of orientation. This learning emerged as a process of reconceptualization of the use of the 12:00-, 3:00-, 6:00-, and 9:00-h hand positions as points of reference for north, east, south, and west, respectively.

For the development of initial cane techniques dimension, the statistical analysis showed that the interaction with the interfaces included in the intervention allowed learners to develop and/or improve skills for the use of the cane as a means of mobility. In this way, aspects such as the handle, the position of the arm, movement, navigating, and tracking displayed significant progress after having participated in the experience with the videogame. During the cognitive task for transfer from virtual to the real-world environment performed by the learners, it was observed that the use of the cane as a means of tracking and navigating reached a frequency of 11.8% among the most-achieved performances.

Regarding the concepts development dimension, the statistical analysis related to the subdimension for the development of spatial concepts showed an improvement in the learners' abilities to use the cardinal directions and those related to forward, back, sideways, and oblique as references for orientation and navigation. In addition, the results regarding the development of geometric concepts subdimension showed an improvement in the learners, related to the comprehension of that which is vertical, horizontal, a curved line, an oblique line, a straight line, a circle, a square, and a triangle. Finally, the results related to the development of environmental concepts subdimension showed an improvement in the learners regarding the connection of being positioned either along the edge of the environment or in the center, in addition to being able to calculate distances. During the performance of the cognitive tasks for the transfer from the virtual to the real-world environment, a higher degree of difficulty was observed related to the transfer of concepts and especially environmental and some geometric concepts, reaching a frequency of 17.9% of the least achieved performances.

Audio Haptic Maze Results

The results obtained from the evaluation of the 10–12-year-old age group from the sample showed an increment in the pre-test/post-test performance means in all dimensions. Based on a t-test that was performed with this data, it was found that the differences in the pre-test/post-test means for the "sensory perception" (pre-test mean = 65.75 points; post-test mean 70.75 points; range of scores from 0 to 72 points) and "tempo-spatial development" (pre-test mean = 24.45 points; post-test mean = 28.75 points; range of scores from 0 to 34 points) dimensions were not statistically significant. However, for the "O&M skills" (pre-test mean = 32.31 points; post-test mean = 48.75 points; range of scores from 0 to 52 points) dimension, the difference between the two means was statistically significant ($t = -4323$; $p < 0.05$).

The results obtained for the evaluation of the 13–15-year-old age group from the sample showed increments in their pre-test/post-test performance means in all dimensions as well. Based on a t-test that was performed with this data, it was found that the differences in the pre-test/post-test means for the "tempo-spatial development" (pre-test mean = 33.33 points; post-test mean = 34.00 points; range of scores from 0 to 34 points) and "O&M skills" (pre-test mean = 34.00 points; post-test mean = 43.76 points; range of scores from 0 to 44 points) dimensions were not statistically significant. However, for the "sensory perception" (pre-test mean = 59.00 points; post-test mean = 68.00 points; range of scores from 0 to 68 points) dimension, the difference between the two means was statistically significant ($t = -5197$; $p < 0.05$).

Also, the users were able to navigate through all the areas that make up the maze design, making intelligent decisions regarding what direction to follow to go from point A to point B based on the information provided.

Results of a behavioral analysis of the 13–15-year-old user's navigations through the environment using behavioral analysis and Path Analyzer confirmed that users integrate both interfaces to completely navigate all the areas on the map of the maze in the virtual environment.

As for the graphic representations of the users' mental maps after having finished the navigation sessions, these representations included all the elements involved in the videogame's virtual environment but lacked precision regarding specific dimensions and the orientation of the corridors and rooms (see Fig. 11.13). The problem associated with spatial dimensions is due to the users' tendency to perform a

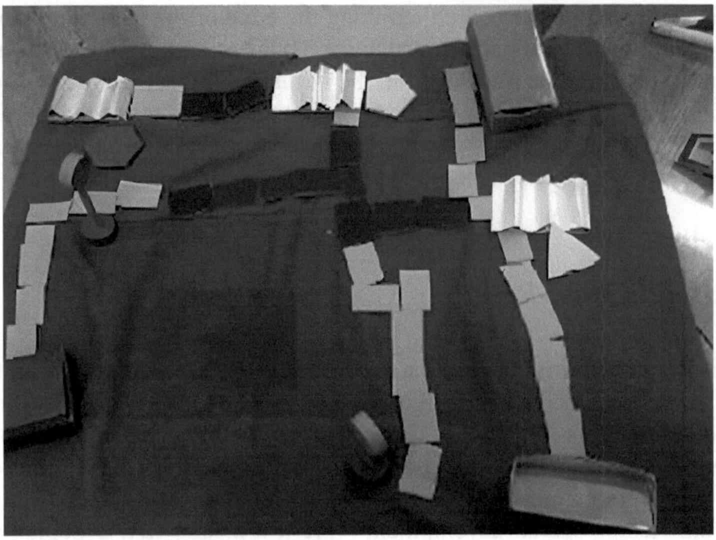

Fig. 11.13 Graphic representation of the mental map of the virtual environment navigated

peripheral exploration while navigating in real life, a tendency that is transferred to their navigation in the virtual environment. This situation is only visible through the representations with representative material, in that virtually the users were able to successfully establish the dimensions that correspond to each area of the maze.

Audio Haptic Maze Results

The interview included two sections. In the first section, five statements were presented related to O&M in which the participants had to respond using the frequency scale.

The second section included eight open-ended questions, of which five were related to O&M difficulties in daily life and three related to the users' perception of the contribution of the videogame to their skills. In general, the users claimed experiencing difficulties in the use of cane techniques. In addition, despite knowing certain techniques, they did not always use them as a problem-solving strategy. Regarding the use of their remaining senses, they preferred to use hearing as a first option to obtain information from their everyday surroundings. In general, to perform tasks involving independent movement through unfamiliar spaces, they required the support of third parties, which was also the case in familiar spaces when they decided to change their habitual route. In this way, the users in the sample represented homogenous characteristics in accordance to the results of the interviews.

For the O&M test, the entire set of participants was analyzed according to the videogame interface group. The following dimensions and subdimensions of the O&M test were analyzed. Each dimension was evaluated through the sum of indicators that contained sensory development (SD, min-value = 0, max-value = 70), which included the subdimensions audio sensory development (ASD, min-value = 0, max-value = 24) and haptic sensory development (HSD, min-value = 0, max-value = 46), and also the tempo-spatial development dimension (TSD, min-value = 0, max-value = 48), the O&M techniques dimension (O&MT, min-value = 0, max-value = 24), and the global indicator (min-value = 0, max-value =142). The global indicator is the sum of SD plus TSD and O&MT. The SD dimension is the sum of ASD plus HSD.

In obtaining the results for the 12 users in the sample, a t-test was performed to compare the means of the indicators obtained for the pre-test and the post-test of the entire group. All the dimensions presented increased in their post-test means compared to the pre-test means. However, these differences in the averages were statistically significant only in the ASD dimension (pre-test mean = 21.420; post-test mean = 23.250; $t = -4.005$; $p < 0.05$), HSD dimension (pre-test mean = 42.830; post-test mean = 44.500; $t = -3.079$; $p < 0.05$), SD dimension (pre-test mean = 64.250; post-test mean = 67.750; $t = -5.326$; $p < 0.05$), O&MT dimension (pre-test mean = 16.170; post-test mean = 19.080; $t = -2.907$; $p < 0.05$), and the global indicator (pre-test mean = 120.170; post-test mean = 132.000; $t = -4.366$; $p < 0.05$).

Complementary to this, a MANOVA test was applied to the post-test data, considering the three user groups (audio, haptics, and haptic+audio) as factors. According to the MANOVA analysis, the mean vectors for the different groups did not present statistical differences between them. That is, the results for the different dimensions do not differ in function of the interface that defined the groups. It is possible that our study sample size was underpowered to detect such differences.

On this basis, we can infer that in general, the use of the videogame allowed for improving the associated cognitive skills to the dimensions ASD, HSD, SD, O&MT, and the global indicator. This happens in all the interfaces studied.

Discussion

MovaWii Discussion

The results obtained regarding O&M skills in users who are blind demonstrated the positive impact of the videogame on such skills. The most significant increases were presented in the development of techniques without mobility aides dimension and in the development of spatial concepts subdimension. At the beginning of the intervention, these dimensions presented high degrees of difficulty, as they included indicators that required the learning of new content provided by the videogame. The increase in the spatial concepts subdimension was a result of the hardware support that the videogame provided to the users regarding the ability to establish their positions in space using their own corporality and understanding that their movements generate changes in space. These changes are manageable and modifiable according to their own spatial needs, directly influencing the orientation that the learners chose when navigating the virtual environment to develop each of the requested activities and to eventually achieve the objective of finding the elements that had been placed within the environment.

Regarding the tactile kinesthetic sensory-perceptual development subdimension, it is possible to affirm that although the incorporation of hardware elements allowed learners to work on behavior related to this dimension, it is necessary to utilize more training time for such skills based on the establishment and integration of the icons proposed to represent a variety of textures, sensations, and shapes of the elements present in the virtual environment.

In relation to the development of psychomotor skills in the learners, the limits of the system (based on its abstract components) made it partially more difficult for the user to be able to integrate the necessary behavior into the experience. Most of the users were more focused on achieving the actions than the way in which they used their bodies and related psychomotor behaviors, and especially those regarding laterality, which were necessary to understand the process that they were participating in.

Finally, regarding the interaction and level of acceptance of the proposed software and hardware that the learners displayed, most of the students did not express any discomfort or discontent with the system. In fact, the use of the Wiimote device ended up being a motivating element, in relating it with the use of the cane and in understanding that through this device, it was feasible to generate an interaction with the videogame through actions geared towards achieving the proposed objectives of the game. Such actions include generating navigation routes that made it possible to find the hidden jewel in the virtual environment. In the same way, it is necessary to mention that a more prolonged work process with the device would make it possible to use a cane prototype, given that it was used more as a joystick than as a cane during the observed intervention experiences.

Audio Haptic Maze Discussion

Regarding the cognitive impact, the results of this study show that all the audio and haptic icons are useful for establishing navigational paths in the virtual environment. The icons that allow the users to measure the spaces that they navigate are especially helpful for this process, not only to establish a mental map of the virtual environment but to apply this information to real navigational contexts as well. This was corroborated by the results regarding the effect that the intervention had on the users in the "O&M skills" dimension.

The results allow for the confirmation that all the users within the 10–12-year-old age group presented significant development of their O&M skills as a result of their interaction with the AHM videogame. The results also indicate that the "O&M skills" dimension was that which experienced the most significant quantitative development, which is directly related to the efficiency of the user's movements when navigating within the videogame's virtual environment.

As far as the results for the 13–15-year-old age group are concerned, all of the users presented a development in their O&M skills after having completed the cognitive tasks. There was an important increase in their scores because of their interaction with the videogame, although this increase was not statistically significant in the "O&M skills" dimension. Case studies were observed in which some users were seen to develop the skills involved in entire indicators that had not been present in the pre-test. One example of this is the development of techniques for the search and location of objects in the environment, which became visible in the videogame when the users had to locate the treasure chests that contained the keys needed to open the doors of the maze.

Audiopolis Discussion

Interaction with the Audiopolis videogame led to markedly high-performance levels in the users during the training tasks. This is denoted by a high mastering of the users concerning the concepts and components that the videogame is mainly based.

In relation to the cognitive tasks, it is important to mention that the level of complexity increases from task 1 to task 12. This is mainly due to the ramping up of the map size, producing an increase in difficulty for the activities involved in the tasks.

The virtual environment, as a simulation of a space with urban characteristics, allowed learners to work within a "safe environment." When performing the search tasks, the learners applied their prior knowledge to test and reinforce previously acquired concepts. In this way, their predisposition to learning was favored by using the videogame. The learners were observed to be highly motivated while performing the various activities.

The learners were also able to create new strategies for solving the problems regarding movement through a virtual space with Audiopolis. Such strategies included going backwards to become reoriented while on a route, circling around different objects, and guiding movements by sound or touch to get to know the boundaries of a space. In general, the group of learners displayed an increase in navigational skills by using the videogame, which can be observed through the speed with which they surpassed the various stages, moving through the game with increasing efficiency.

The use of different interfaces in the videogame helped to generate a positive effect on the learning of O&M skills. The statistical results regarding the difference in the means obtained between the pre-test and the post-test of the entire group resulted in an increase that was statistically significant for some dimensions. These dimensions included the sensory development dimension (in addition to the audio sensory development and haptic sensory development subdimensions), the O&M

techniques dimension, and the global indicator of O&M dimension. A second statistical analysis determined that the results did not differ by segmenting each interface group.

The level obtained in pre-test indicators can be considered high if we consider the maximum possible values. This left a small margin for improvement in post-test indicators consistent with a possible ceiling effect for performance.

Consequently, an increase in the sample of users employed eventually would be needed to validate these findings.

Conclusions

The results demonstrated the creation of a videogame that allows for the development of O&M skills in school-age learners who are blind, in serving as a supportive tool for the construction of a mental map of a virtually navigated space through the integration of its audio and haptic components. The results showed that playing and training with the videogames improved the development of O&M skills in learners who are blind.

The contribution of these works is to show how, through the integration of multimodal interfaces into a videogame, the development of O&M skills can be promoted in blind learners. The playful aspects of the game and its associated technology positively influenced the motivation of end users.

The audio, haptic, and combined audio-haptic stimuli aided in generating an increased understanding of the participants' senses. It was observed that in order to orient themselves, the users preferred the use of hearing rather than touch.

In addition, (in the case of MovaWii) the learners were able to transfer the information obtained for use in the real-world environment, where they were able to navigate autonomously and efficiently.

The game presented limitations in the development of abstract representation that end users could achieve working with the proposed interfaces. We attempted to overcome these limitations by proposing the use of low and bounded complexity spaces in the game (number of items, size of the maze, and choices of paths to follow). As future work plans, we intend to expand the complexity of the virtual environment.

It is proposed as future work to explore how learners construct their mental models. In this research, the evaluation criteria of the graphic representation of the navigated virtual environment were based on the accuracy of representation achieved by learners. However, it will be pertinent and appropriate to study how users represent mental maps, focusing the analysis on the utility for themselves related to the functional elements of the environment.

Finally, it is proposed to increase the sample base to investigate potential differences between the distinct interface groups utilized and to analyze the learning of spatial layout of unknown environments.

Acknowledgments This report was funded by the Chilean National Fund for Science and Technological Development (FONDECYT) (FONDECYT 1150898) and by the Chilean National Research and Development Agency's (ANID) Basal Funding for Scientific and Technology Centers of Excellence, project number FB0003.

References

Agrawal, V., & Singh, V. (2020, October). Haptic structuring assistive innovation for individuals who are visually impaired. *International Journal of Engineering and Advanced Technology, 10*(1), 98–102.

Anirudha, A. R., Swati, R. S. G., Biswarup, G., & Neogi, N. B. (2015). An overview on tactile display, haptic investigation towards beneficial for blind person. *International Journal of Scientific and Engineering Research, 6*(5), 88–95.

Aubert, D., Lenay, C., Ollive, T., & Roccamatisi, R. (2022). A first approach to tactile maps and web contents for visually impaired and blind people with a sensory supplementation system (Tactos). In *Cahiers COSTECH – Cahiers Connaissance, organisation et systèmes techniques.* UTC – Laboratoire Costech. ⟨hal-03667521⟩.

Ballesteros, S. (1993). Percepción Háptica de Objetos y Patrones Realzados: Una Revisión. Departamento de Psicología Básica. Universidad Nacional de Educación a Distancia. *Psicothema, 5*(2), 311–321.

Carvalho, J., Guerreiro, T., Duarte, L., & Carriç, L. (2012, September). Audio-based Mobile puzzle gaming for blind people. In: *MOBACC 2012: Mobile accessibility workshop at MobileHCI 2012*, San Francisco, USA.

Crandall, R., & Karado, E. (2021). Designing pedagogically effective haptic Systems for Learning: A review. *Applied Sciences, 11*(14), 6245. 1-29. https://doi.org/10.3390/app11146245

Crossan, A., & Brewster, S. (2006). Two-handed navigation in a haptic virtual environment. In *Proceedings of international conference on human factors in computing systems* (pp. 676–681). Montréal, Québec, (Canada).

da Silveira Nunes, S., & Lomonaco, J. F. B. (2008). Desarrollo de conceptos en ciegos congénitos: caminos de adquisición del conocimiento. *Psicologia Escolar e Educacional, 12*(1), 119–138. ISSN 1413-8557.

De Felice, F., Renna, F., Attolico, & Distante, A. (2005). Haptic fruition of 3D virtual scene by blind people. In M. Ali & F. Esposito (Eds.), *Proceedings of the 18th international conference on Innovations in Applied Artificial Intelligence (IEA/AIE'2005)* (pp. 269–278). Springer-Verlag.

Espinosa, M. A., Ungar, S., Ochaita, E., Blades, M., & Spencer, C. (1998). Comparing methods for introducing blind and visually impaired people to unfamiliar urban environment. *Journal of Environmental Psychology, 18*, 277–287.

Evett, L., Battersby, S., Ridley, A., & Brown, D. (2009). An interface to virtual environments for people who are blind using Wii technology - mental models and navigation. *Journal of Assistive Technologies, 3*(2), 26–34.

Façanha, A., Darin, T., Viana, W., & Sánchez, J. (2020). *ACM Transactions on Accessible Computing (TACCESS), 13*(2), 1–42.

Frauenberger, C., & Noisternig, M. (2003). 3D audio interfaces for the blind. In: *Proceedings of the 2003 international conference on auditory display*, Boston, MA, USA, July 6–9 (pp. 1–4).

GauBert, N., Bülthoff, H. H., & Wallraven, C. (2011, September). Similarity and categorization: From vision to touch. *Acta Psychologica, 138*(1), 219–230. https://doi.org/10.1016/j.actpsy.2011.06.007

GauBert, N., Waterkamp, S., Fleming, R. W., & Bülthoff, I. (2012). Haptic categorical perception of shape. *PLoS One, 7*(8), e43062. Published online 2012 August 10. https://doi.org/10.1371/journal.pone.0043062

Giudice, N., Benjamin, A. G., Toni Kaplan, S., Anderson, R. K., & Cioffi, J. F. (2020). Use of an indoor navigation system by sighted and blind travelers: Performance similarities across visual status and age. *ACM Transactions on Accessible Computing, 13*(3), 1–27. https://doi.org/10.1145/3407191

Goldman, R. (1969, May). Another approach to evaluating speech sound discrimination. *Exceptional Children, 35*(9), 745–747.

Guerreiro, J., Ahmetovic, D., Sato, D., Kitani, K., & Asakawa, C. (2019, May). Airport accessibility and navigation assistance for people with visual impairments. In *CHI '19: Proceedings of the 2019 CHI conference on human factors in computing systems* (Paper No.: 16) (pp. 1–14). https://doi.org/10.1145/3290605.3300246

Guerreiro, J., Daisuke Sato, D., Ahmetovic, E. O.-B., Kitani, K. M., & Asakawa, C. (2020, March). Virtual navigation for blind people: Transferring route knowledge to the real-World. *International Journal of Human Computer Studies, 135*, 102369. https://doi.org/10.1016/j.ijhcs.2019.102369

Heller, M. A., Brackett, D. D., Scroggs, E., Allen, A. C., & Green, S. (2001). Haptic perception of the horizontal by blind and low-vision individuals. *Perception, 30*(5), 601–610.

Homa, D., Kahol, K., Tripathi, P., Bratton, L., & Panchanathan, S. (2009, May). Haptic concepts in the blind. *Attention, Percept & Psychophys, 71*(4), 690–698. https://doi.org/10.3758/APP.71.4.690

Hu, W., Lin, T., Sakai, K., Imamiya, A., & Omata, M. (2006). Setup consistent visual textures for haptic surfaces in a virtual reality world. In C. Stephanidis & M. Pieper (Eds.), *Proceedings of the 9th conference on user interfaces for all (ERCIM'06)* (pp. 78–87). Springer.

Huang, Y. (2009). Exploration of interface usability in a haptic 3D virtual labyrinth for visually impaired users. In: *Proceedings of IADIS interfaces and human computer interaction (IHCI)*. ALGALVE, Portugal, June 17–23, 2009.

Jain, S. (2012). *Assessment of audio interfaces for use in smartphone based spatial learning systems for the blind.* Master of Science Thesis in Spatial Information Science and Engineering. University of Maine.

Jütte, R. (2008). Haptic perception: An historical approach. In M. Grunwald (Ed.), *Human haptic perception: Basics and applications* (pp. 3–13). ISBN 978-3-7643-7611-6.

Kim, H. N. (2010). *Usable accessibility and haptic user interface design approach.* Doctoral Thesis in Industrial and Systems Engineering. Virginia Polytechnic Institute and State University.

Konstantinosa, P., Panagiotisa, K., Elenia, K., Marinaa, M., Asimisa, V., & Valarib, E. (2015). Audio-haptic map: An orientation and mobility aid for individuals with blindness. *Procedia Computer Science, 67*(2015), 223–230.

Lahav, O., & Mioduser, D. (2002). Multisensory virtual environment for supporting blind Person's acquisition of spatial cognitive mapping, orientation, and mobility skills. In *Proceedings of the international conference on disability, virtual reality and associated technologies, ICDVRAT 2002*, Veszprém, Hungary (pp. 213–220).

Lahav, O., & Mioduser, D. (2004). Blind persons' acquisition of spatial cognitive mapping and orientation skills supported by virtual environments, In *Proceeding of the 5th, ICDVRAT 2004*, Oxford, UK (pp. 131–138).

Lahav, O., & Mioduser, D. (2008a). Construction of cognitive maps of unknown spaces using a multi-sensory virtual environment for people who are blind. *Computers in Human Behavior, 24*(3), 1139–1155.

Lahav, O., & Mioduser, D. (2008b). Haptic-feedback support for cognitive mapping of unknown spaces by people who are blind. *International Journal on Human-Computer Studies, 66*, 23–35.

Lange, B, Flynn, S., Chang, C., Ahmed, A., Geng, Y., Utsav, K., Xu, M., Seok, D., Cheng, S., & Rizzo, A. (2010, 31 August–2 September). Development of an interactive rehabilitation game using the Nintendo WiiFit balance board for people with neurological injury, In *Proceedings 8th international conference on disability, virtual reality and associated technologies*, ICDVRAT 2010 (pp. 249–254). Viña del Mar/Valparaíso.

Loomis, J., Marston, J., Golledge, R., & Klatzky, R. (2005). Personal guidance system for visually impaired people: Comparison of spatial displays for route guidance. *Journal of Visual Impairment Blindness, 99*(4), 219–232.
Lumbreras, M., & Sánchez, J. (1999). Interactive 3D sound hyperstories for blind children. In *Proceedings of the SIGCHI conference on human factors in computing systems: The CHI Is the Limit, CHI '99*, Pittsburgh, Pennsylvania, United States, May 15–20 1999, (pp. 318–325).
Lutz, R. (2006, September). Prototyping and evaluation of landcons: Auditory objects that support wayfinding for blind travelers. *SIGACCESS Accessibility and Computing, 86*, 8–11. Available from: http://doi.acm.org/10.1145/1196148.1196150
Murphy, E., Kuber, R., Strain, P., McAllister, G., & Yu, W. (2007). Developing sounds for a multimodal Interface: Conveying spatial information to visually impaired web users. In *Proceedings of the 13th international conference on auditory display (ICAD 2007)*, Montréal, Canada, June 26–29, 2007.
Norman, J. F., Norman, H. F., Clayton, A. M., Lianekhammy, J., & Zielke, G. (2004, February). The visual and haptic perception of natural object shape. *Perception & Psychophysics, 66*(2), 342–351.
Oakley, I., McGee, M. R., Brewster, S., & Gray, P. (2000). Putting the feel in 'look and feel'. In *Proceedings of the SIGCHI conference on human factors in computing systems. CHI '00* (pp. 415–422). ACM.
Pawluk, D. T. V., Adams, R. J., & Kitada, R. (2015, July–September 1). Designing haptic assistive Technology for Individuals who are Blind or visually impaired. *IEEE Transactions on Haptics, 8*(3), 258–278.
Reuters. (2009). *Novint awarded subcontract to develop physical rehabilitation game for military*, Edition U.S., Tuesday September 1, 2009, 8:02am EDT. Available from: http://www.reuters.com/article/2009/09/01/idUS132915+01-Sep-2009+MW20090901
Rosa, A., & Ochaita, E. (1993). *Psicología de la ceguera*. Alianza editorial. ISBN 84-206-6539-8.
Sánchez, J. (2008, November). User-centered technologies for blind children. *Human Technology Journal, 45*(2), 96–122.
Sánchez, J., & Elías, M. (2007). Guidelines for designing mobility and orientation software for blind children. In C. Baranauskas et al. (Eds.), *INTERACT 2007, lectures notes of computer science* (LNCS 4662, Part 1) (pp. 375–388).
Sánchez, J., & Espinoza, M. (2011). Audio haptic videogaming for navigation skills in learners who are blind. In *The proceedings of the 13th international ACM SIGACCESS conference on computers and accessibility (ASSETS '11)* (pp. 227–228). ACM.
Sánchez, J., & Mascaró, J. (2011). Audiopolis, navigation through a virtual city using audio and haptic interfaces for people who are blind. In Constantine Stephanidis (Ed.), *Proceedings of the 6th international conference on universal access in human-computer interaction: Users' diversity – volume part II (UAHCI'11)* (Vol. Part II, pp. 362–371). Springer-Verlag.
Sánchez, J., & Tadres, A. (2010). Augmented reality application for the navigation of people who are blind. In *Proceedings of the 8th international conference series on disability, virtual reality and associated technologies, ICDVRAT 2010*, Viña del Mar, Chile, August 31–September 2, 2010 (pp. 51–60).
Sánchez, J., Tadres, A., Pascual-Leone, A., & Merabet, L. (2009). Blind children navigation through gaming and associated brain plasticity. In *Proceedings of the IEEE virtual rehabilitation 2009 international conference*, June 29–July 2, 2009, Haifa, Israel (pp. 29–36).
Sánchez, J., Sáenz, M., & Garrido, J. (2010a, November). Usability of a multimodal video game to improve navigation skills for blind children. *ACM Transactions on Accessible Computing, 3*(2), Article 7, 29 pages.
Sánchez, J., Sáenz, M., Pascual-Leone, A., & Merabet, L. (2010b). Enhancing navigation skills through audio gaming. In *Proceedings of the 28th of the international conference extended abstracts on human factors in computing systems (CHI EA '10)* (pp. 3991–3996). ACM.

Sarmiento, L. C. (2003). *Ayudas aumentativas en discapacitados visuales para la representación espacial utilizando las tecnologías de la información y las comunicaciones*. Tesis de Maestría en TIAE.

Siu, A. F., Sinclair, M., Ofek, E., Holz, C., Kovacs, R., & Cutrell, E. (2020, April). Virtual reality without vision: a haptic and auditory white cane to navigate complex virtual worlds. In *CHI '20: Proceedings of the 2020 CHI conference on human factors in computing systems* (pp. 1–13). https://doi.org/10.1145/3313831.3376353

Squire, K. (2003). Video games in education. *International Journal of Intelligent Simulations and Gaming, 2*(1), 49–62.

Steinkuehler, C. (2004). Learning in massively multiplayer online games. In Y. B. Kafai, W. A. Sandoval, N. Enyedy, A. S. Nixon, & F. Herrera (Eds.), *In proceedings of the 6th international conference of the learning sciences* (pp. 521–528). Erlbaum.

Travieso, D. (2007, June). Haptic and proprioceptive experience. Fundación Infancia y Aprendizaje. *Estudios de Psicología, 28*(2), 141–153(13).

Warren, D. H. (1994). *Blindness and children: An individual differences approach*. Cambridge University Press. Mentioned in Ungar, S.: Cognitive mapping without visual experience: In Kitchin, R. & Freundschuh, S. (Eds.). *Cognitive mapping: Past present and future*. London: Routledge (2000).

Williams, R. (2010). Finger tracking and gesture interfacing using the Nintendo\® Wiimote. In *Proceedings of the 48th annual southeast regional conference (ACM SE '10)*. ACM, Article 11, 4 pages.

Williams, M. A., Galbraith, C., Kane, S. K., & Hurst, A. (2014, October). "Just let the cane hit it": how the blind and sighted see navigation differently. In *ASSETS '14: Proceedings of the 16th international ACM SIGACCESS conference on Computers & accessibility* (pp. 217–224). https://doi.org/10.1145/2661334.2661380

Yu, W., & Brewster, S. (2002). Comparing two haptic interfaces for multimodal graph rendering. In *Proceedings of the 10th symposium on haptic interfaces for virtual environment and Teleoperator systems (Haptics 2002)* (pp. 3–9). IEEE.

Yu, W., Ramloll, R., & Brewster, S. (2000). Haptic graphs for blind computer users. In S. Brewster & R. Murray-Smith (Eds.), *Proceedings of the first international workshop on haptic human-computer interaction* (pp. 41–51). Springer.

Yu, W., Kangas, K., & Brewster, S. (2003). Web-based haptic applications for blind people to create virtual graphs. In *Proceedings of the 11th symposium on haptic interfaces for virtual environment and teleoperator systems, HAPTICS'03* (pp. 318–325). IEEE Computer Society.

Yuan, B. (2009). *Towards generalized accessibility of video games for the visually impaired*, PhD dissertation, University of Nevada, Reno, Reno, NV, USA. Advisors S Frederick, C Harris, and E Folmer. AAI3355610.

Yuan, B., & Folmer, E. (2008). Blind hero: Enabling guitar hero for the visually impaired. In *Proceedings of the 10th international ACM SIGACCESS conference on computers and accessibility* (pp. 69–176).

Zhao, Y., Bennett, C. L., Benko, H., Cutrell, E., Holz, C., Morris, M. R., & Sinclair, M. (2018, April). Enabling people with visual impairments to navigate virtual reality with a haptic and auditory cane simulation. In *CHI '18: Proceedings of the 2018 CHI conference on human factors in computing systems* (Paper No.: 116) (pp. 1–14). https://doi.org/10.1145/3173574.3173690

Index

E. Brooks, D. J. Brown (eds.), *Virtual Reality Games for Rehabilitation*, Virtual Reality Technologies for Health and Clinical Applications,
https://doi.org/10.1007/978-1-0716-3371-7

MIX
Papier aus verantwortungsvollen Quellen
Paper from responsible sources
FSC® C105338

If you have any concerns about our products,
you can contact us on
ProductSafety@springernature.com

In case Publisher is established outside the EU,
the EU authorized representative is:
Springer Nature Customer Service Center GmbH
Europaplatz 3, 69115 Heidelberg, Germany

Printed by Libri Plureos GmbH
in Hamburg, Germany